IMAGING FOR
STUDENTS

IMAGING FOR STUDENTS

Fourth edition

David A Lisle
Consultant Radiologist at the
Royal Children's and Brisbane Private
Hospitals; and Associate Professor of
Medical Imaging, University of
Queensland Medical School,
Brisbane, Australia

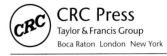

CRC Press
Taylor & Francis Group
Boca Raton London New York

CRC Press is an imprint of the
Taylor & Francis Group, an **informa** business

CRC Press
Taylor & Francis Group
6000 Broken Sound Parkway NW, Suite 300
Boca Raton, FL 33487-2742

10 0769717 15

© 2012 by David A. Lisle
CRC Press is an imprint of Taylor & Francis Group, an informa business

Printed and bound in India by Replika Press Pvt. Ltd.

No claim to original U.S. Government works
Printed on acid-free paper
International Standard Book Number: 978-1-4441-2182-7   (Softcover)

**Library of Congress Cataloging-in-Publication Data and
The British Library Cataloging in Publication Data are available**

**Visit the Taylor & Francis Web site at
http://www.taylorandfrancis.com**

**and the CRC Press Web site at
http://www.crcpress.com**

To my wife Lyn and our daughters Victoria, Charlotte and Margot

Contents

Preface

This fourth edition of *Imaging for Students* builds on the content of the previous three editions to present an introduction to medical imaging. In the years since the previous edition, imaging technologies have continued to evolve. The efforts of researchers have contributed to the evidence base, such that a clearer picture is emerging as to the appropriate use of imaging for a range of clinical indications.

The aims of this edition remain the same as for the previous three editions:

1. To provide an introduction to the various imaging modalities, including an outline of relevant risks and hazards.
2. To outline a logical approach to plain film interpretation and to illustrate the more common pathologies encountered.
3. To provide an approach to the appropriate requesting of imaging investigations in a range of clinical scenarios.

With these aims in mind, the book is structured in a logical, clinically orientated fashion. Chapter 1 gives a brief outline of each of the imaging modalities, including advantages and disadvantages. Chapter 1 finishes with a summary of commonly encountered risks and hazards. This is essential information for referring doctors, weighing up the possible benefits of an investigation against its potential risks.

The chapters covering the spine, the respiratory, cardiovascular, gastrointestinal and musculoskeletal systems include sections on 'how to read' the relevant plain films. Summary boxes that list investigations of choice are provided at the end of most chapters. This edition also includes a new chapter entitled 'Imaging in oncology', designed to summarize the increasingly common and diverse uses of medical imaging in the treatment and follow-up of patients with cancer.

Those of us working in the field of medical imaging continue to be challenged by the often conflicting forces of clinical demand, continued advances in technology and the need to contain medical costs. My ongoing hope with this new edition of *Imaging for Students* is that medical students and junior doctors may see medical imaging for what it is: a vital part of modern medicine that when used appropriately, can contribute enormously to patient care.

David Lisle
Brisbane, June 2011

Acknowledgements

As with previous editions, many people have assisted me in the preparation of this book. I have been inspired by the enquiring minds and enthusiasm of the radiology trainees with whom it has been my privilege to work at Christchurch Hospital, Redcliffe District Hospital and the Royal Children's Hospital in Brisbane. My thanks go to the following for providing images: Professor Alan Coulthard, Dr Susan King, Jenny McKenzie, Sarah Pao and Dr Tanya Wood. Sincere thanks also to Dr Joanna Koster and Stephen Clausard at Hodder Arnold publishers for their continued trust and encouragement. Finally, and most importantly, my unfailing gratitude goes to my family for their continued support and forbearance.

We will not cease from exploration and
the end of all our exploring will be to
arrive where we started and know the
place for the first time.

TS Eliot

1 Introduction to medical imaging

1.1 RADIOGRAPHY (X-RAY IMAGING)

1.1.1 Conventional radiography (X-rays, plain films)

X-rays are produced in an X-ray tube by focusing a beam of high-energy electrons onto a tungsten target. X-rays are a form of electromagnetic radiation, able to pass through the human body and produce an image of internal structures. The resulting image is called a radiograph, more commonly known as an 'X-ray' or 'plain film'. The common terms 'chest X-ray' and 'abdomen X-ray' are widely accepted and abbreviated to CXR and AXR.

As a beam of X-rays passes through the human body, some of the X-rays are absorbed or scattered producing reduction or attenuation of the beam. Tissues of high density and/or high atomic number cause more X-ray beam attenuation and are shown as lighter grey or white on a radiograph. Less dense tissues and structures cause less attenuation of the X-ray beam, and appear darker on radiographs than tissues of higher density. Five principal densities are recognized on plain radiographs (Fig. 1.1), listed here in order of increasing density:

1. Air/gas: black, e.g. lungs, bowel and stomach
2. Fat: dark grey, e.g. subcutaneous tissue layer, retroperitoneal fat
3. Soft tissues/water: light grey, e.g. solid organs, heart, blood vessels, muscle and fluid-filled organs such as bladder
4. Bone: off-white
5. Contrast material/metal: bright white.

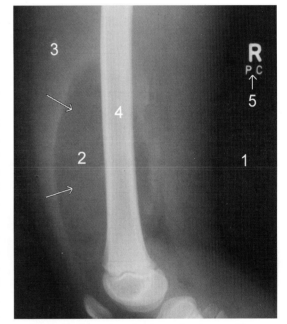

Figure 1.1 The five principal radiographic densities. This radiograph of a benign lipoma (arrows) in a child's thigh demonstrates the five basic radiographic densities: (1) air; (2) fat; (3) soft tissue; (4) bone; (5) metal.

1.1.2 Computed radiography, digital radiography and picture archiving and communication systems

In the past, X-ray films were processed in a darkroom or in freestanding daylight processors. In modern practice, radiographic images are produced digitally using one of two processes, computed radiography (CR) and digital radiography (DR). CR employs cassettes that are inserted into a laser reader following X-ray exposure. An analogue-digital converter (ADC) produces a digital image. DR uses a detector screen containing silicon detectors that produce an electrical signal when exposed to X-rays. This signal is analysed to produce a digital image. Digital images obtained by CR and DR are sent to viewing workstations for interpretation. Images may also be recorded on X-ray film for portability and remote viewing. Digital radiography has many advantages over conventional radiography, including the ability to perform various manipulations on the images including:

- Magnification of areas of interest (Fig. 1.2)
- Alteration of density
- Measurements of distances and angles.

Many medical imaging departments now employ large computer storage facilities and networks known as picture archiving and communication systems (PACS). Images obtained by CR and DR are stored digitally, as are images from other modalities including computed tomography (CT), magnetic resonance imaging (MRI), ultrasound (US) and scintigraphy. PACS systems allow instant recall and display of a patient's imaging studies. Images can be displayed on monitors throughout the hospital in wards, meeting rooms and operating theatres as required.

1.1.3 Fluoroscopy

Radiographic examination of the anatomy and motion of internal structures by a constant stream of X-rays is known as fluoroscopy. Uses of fluoroscopy include:

- Angiography and interventional radiology
- Contrast studies of the gastrointestinal tract (Fig. 1.3)
- Guidance of therapeutic joint injections and arthrograms
- Screening in theatre
  - General surgery, e.g. operative cholangiography
  - Urology, e.g. retrograde pyelography
  - Orthopaedic surgery, e.g. reduction and fixation of fractures, joint replacements.

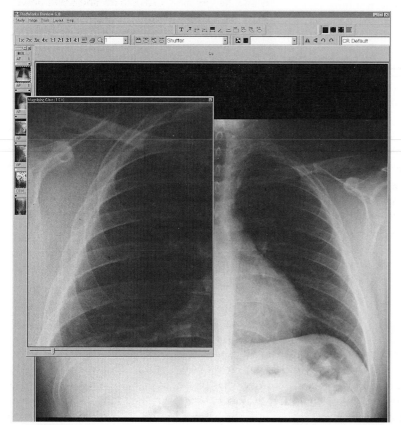

Figure 1.2 Computed radiography. With computed radiography images may be reviewed and reported on a computer workstation. This allows various manipulations of images as well as application of functions such as measurements of length and angle measurements. This example shows a 'magnifying glass' function, which provides a magnified view of a selected part of the image.

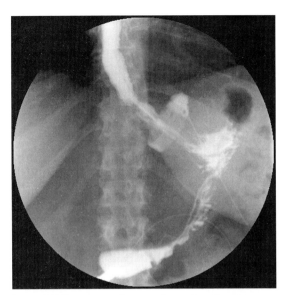

Figure 1.3 Fluoroscopy: Gastrografin swallow. Gastric band applied laparoscopically for weight loss. Gastrografin swallow shows normal appearances: normal orientation of the gastric band, gastrografin flows through the centre of the band and no obstruction or leakage.

Fluoroscopy units fall into two categories: image intensifier and flat panel detector (FPD). Image intensifier units have been in use since the 1950s. An image intensifier is a large vacuum tube that converts X-rays into light images that are viewed in real time via a closed circuit television chain and recorded as required. FDP fluoroscopy units are becoming increasingly common in angiography suites and cardiac catheterization laboratories ('cath labs'). The FDP consists of an array of millions of tiny detector elements (DELs). Most FDP units work by converting X-ray energy into light and then to an electric signal. FDP units have several technical advantages over image intensifier systems including smaller size, less imaging artefacts and reduced radiation exposure.

1.1.4 Digital subtraction angiography

The utility of fluoroscopy may be extended with digital subtraction techniques. Digital subtraction is a process whereby a computer removes unwanted information from a radiographic image. Digital subtraction is particularly useful for angiography, referred to as DSA. The principles of digital subtraction are illustrated in Fig. 1.4.

A relatively recent innovation is rotational 3D fluoroscopic imaging. For this technique, the fluoroscopy unit rotates through 180° while acquiring images, producing a cine display that resembles a 3D CT image. This image may be rotated and reorientated to produce a greater understanding of anatomy during complex diagnostic and interventional procedures.

1.2 CONTRAST MATERIALS

The ability of conventional radiography and fluoroscopy to display a range of organs and structures may be enhanced by the use of various contrast materials, also known as contrast media. The most common contrast materials are based on barium or iodine. Barium and iodine are high atomic number materials that strongly absorb X-rays and are therefore seen as dense white on radiography.

For demonstration of the gastrointestinal tract with fluoroscopy, contrast materials may be swallowed or injected via a nasogastric tube to outline the oesophagus, stomach and small bowel, or may be introduced via an enema tube to delineate the large bowel. Gastrointestinal contrast materials are usually based on barium, which is non-water soluble. Occasionally, a water-soluble contrast material based on iodine is used for imaging of the gastrointestinal tract, particularly where aspiration or perforation may be encountered (Fig. 1.3).

Iodinated (iodine containing) water-soluble contrast media may be injected into veins, arteries, and various body cavities and systems. Iodinated contrast materials are used in CT (see below), angiography (DSA) (Fig. 1.4) and arthrography (injection into joints).

1.3 CT

1.3.1 CT physics and terminology

CT is an imaging technique whereby cross-sectional images are obtained with the use of X-rays. In CT scanning, the patient is passed through a rotating gantry that has an X-ray tube on one side and a set of detectors on the other. Information from the detectors is analysed by computer and displayed as a grey-scale image. Owing to the use of computer analysis, a much greater array of densities can be

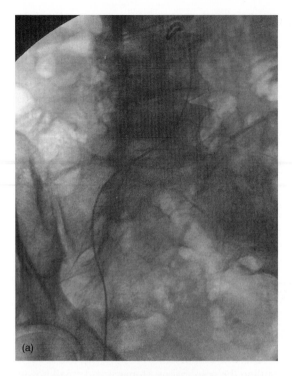
(a)

displayed than on conventional X-ray films. This allows accurate display of cross-sectional anatomy, differentiation of organs and pathology, and sensitivity to the presence of specific materials such as fat or calcium. As with plain radiography, high-density objects cause more attenuation of the X-ray beam and are therefore displayed as lighter grey than objects of lower density. White and light grey objects are therefore said to be of 'high attenuation'; dark grey and black objects are said to be of 'low attenuation'.

By altering the grey-scale settings, the image information can be manipulated to display the various tissues of the body. For example, in chest CT where a wide range of tissue densities is present, a good image of the mediastinal structures shows no lung details. By setting a 'lung window' the lung parenchyma is seen in detail (Fig. 1.5).

The relative density of an area of interest may be measured electronically. This density measurement is given as an attenuation value, expressed in Hounsfield units (HU) (named for Godfrey

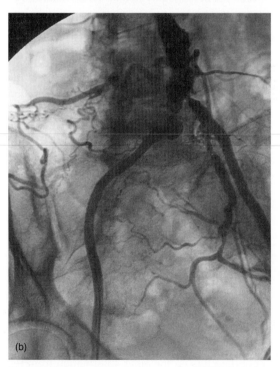
(b)

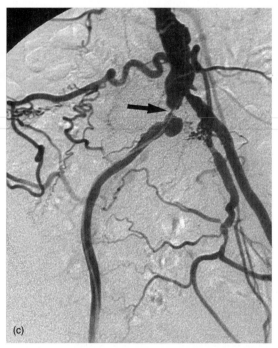
(c)

Figure 1.4 Digital subtraction angiography (DSA). (a) Mask image performed prior to injection of contrast material. (b) Contrast material injected producing opacification of the arteries. (c) Subtracted image. The computer subtracts the mask from the contrast image leaving an image of contrast-filled arteries unobscured by overlying structures. Note a stenosis of the right common iliac artery (arrow).

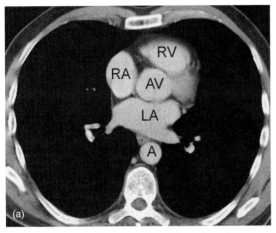
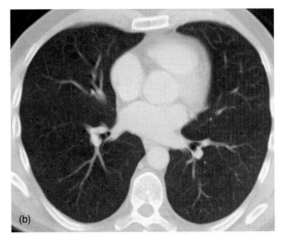

Figure 1.5 CT windows. (a) Mediastinal windows showing mediastinal anatomy: right atrium (RA), right ventricle (RV), aortic valve (AV), aorta (A), left atrium (LA). (b) Lung windows showing lung anatomy.

Hounsfield, the inventor of CT). In CT, water is assigned an attenuation value of 0 HU. Substances that are less dense than water, including fat and air, have negative values (Fig. 1.6); substances of greater density have positive values. Approximate attenuation values for common substances are as follows:

- Water: 0
- Muscle: 40
- Contrast-enhanced artery: 130
- Cortical bone: 500
- Fat: −120
- Air: −1000

1.3.2 Contrast materials in CT

Intravenous iodinated contrast material is used in CT for a number of reasons, as follows:
- Differentiation of normal blood vessels from abnormal masses, e.g. hilar vessels versus lymph nodes (Fig. 1.7)
- To make an abnormality more apparent, e.g. liver metastases
- To demonstrate the vascular nature of a mass and thus aid in characterization
- CT angiography (see below).

Oral contrast material is also used for abdomen CT:
- Differentiation of normal enhancing bowel loops from abnormal masses or fluid collections (Fig. 1.8)
- Diagnosis of perforation of the gastrointestinal tract
- Diagnosis of leaking surgical anastomoses
- CT enterography.

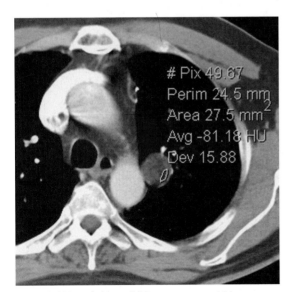

Figure 1.6 Hounsfield unit (HU) measurements. HU measurements in a lung nodule reveal negative values (−81) indicating fat. This is consistent with a benign pulmonary hamartoma, for which no further follow-up or treatment is required.

For detailed examination of the pelvis and distal large bowel, administration of rectal contrast material is occasionally used.

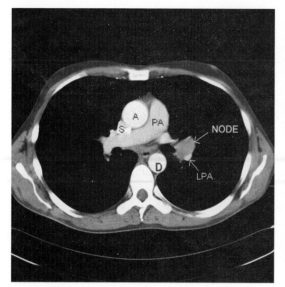

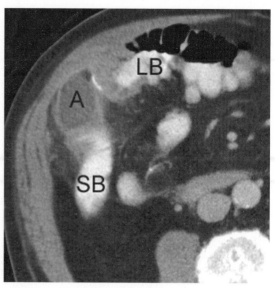

Figure 1.7 Intravenous contrast. An enlarged left hilar lymph node is differentiated from enhancing vascular structures: left pulmonary artery (LPA), main pulmonary artery (PA), ascending aorta (A), superior vena cava (S), descending aorta (D).

Figure 1.8 Oral contrast. An abscess (A) is differentiated from contrast-filled small bowel (SB) and large bowel (LB).

1.3.3 Multidetector row CT

Helical (spiral) CT scanners became available in the early 1990s. Helical scanners differ from conventional scanners in that the tube and detectors rotate as the patient passes through on the scanning table. Helical CT is so named because the continuous set of data that is obtained has a helical configuration.

Multidetector row CT (MDCT), also known as multislice CT (MSCT), was developed in the mid to late 1990s. MDCT builds on the concepts of helical CT in that a circular gantry holding the X-ray tube on one side and detectors on the other rotates continuously as the patient passes through. The difference with MDCT is that instead of a single row of detectors multiple detector rows are used. The original MDCT scanners used two or four rows of detectors, followed by 16 and 64 detector row scanners. At the time of writing, 256 and 320 row scanners are becoming widely available.

Multidetector row CT allows the acquisition of overlapping fine sections of data, which in turn allows the reconstruction of highly accurate and detailed 3D images as well as sections in any desired plane. The major advantages of MDCT over conventional CT scanning are:

- Increased speed of examination
- Rapid examination at optimal levels of intravenous contrast concentration
- Continuous volumetric nature of data allows accurate high-quality 3D and multiplanar reconstruction.

MDCT therefore provides many varied applications including:
- CT angiography: coronary, cerebral, carotid, pulmonary, renal, visceral, peripheral
- Cardiac CT, including CT coronary angiography and coronary artery calcium scoring
- CT colography (virtual colonoscopy)
- CT cholangiography
- CT enterography
- Brain perfusion scanning
- Planning of fracture repair in complex areas: acetabulum, foot and ankle, distal radius and carpus
- Display of complex anatomy for planning of cranial and facial reconstruction surgery (Fig. 1.9).

1.3.4 Limitations and disadvantages of CT

- Ionizing radiation (see below)
- Hazards of intravenous contrast material (see below)

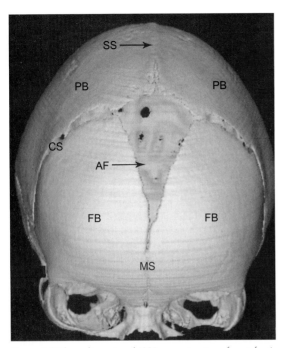

Figure 1.9 Three-dimensional (3D) reconstruction of an infant's skull showing a fused sagittal suture. Structures labelled as follows: frontal bones (FB), parietal bones (PB), coronal sutures (CS), metopic suture (MS), anterior fontanelle (AF) and fused sagittal suture (SS). Normal sutures are seen on 3D CT as lucent lines between skull bones. Note the lack of a normal lucent line at the position of the sagittal suture indicating fusion of the suture.

Solid organs, fluid-filled structures and tissue interfaces produce varying degrees of sound wave reflection and are said to be of different echogenicity. Tissues that are hyperechoic reflect more sound than tissues that are hypoechoic. In an US image, hyperechoic tissues are shown as white or light grey and hypoechoic tissues are seen as dark grey (Fig. 1.10). Pure fluid is anechoic (reflects virtually no sound) and is black on US images. Furthermore, because virtually all sound is transmitted through a fluid-containing area, tissues distally receive more sound waves and hence appear lighter. This effect is known as 'acoustic enhancement' and is seen in tissues distal to the gallbladder, the urinary bladder and simple cysts. The reverse effect, known as 'acoustic shadowing', occurs with gas-containing bowel, gallstones, renal stones and breast malignancy.

US scanning is applicable to:
- Solid organs, including liver, kidneys, spleen and pancreas
- Urinary tract
- Obstetrics and gynaecology
- Small organs including thyroid and testes
- Breast
- Musculoskeletal system.

- Lack of portability of equipment
- Relatively high cost.

1.4 US

1.4.1 US physics and terminology

US imaging uses ultra-high-frequency sound waves to produce cross-sectional images of the body. The basic component of the US probe is the piezoelectric crystal. Excitation of this crystal by electrical signals causes it to emit ultra-high-frequency sound waves; this is the piezoelectric effect. Sound waves are reflected back to the crystal by the various tissues of the body. These reflected sound waves (echoes) act on the piezoelectric crystal in the US probe to produce an electric signal, again by the piezoelectric effect. Analysis of this electric signal by a computer produces a cross-sectional image.

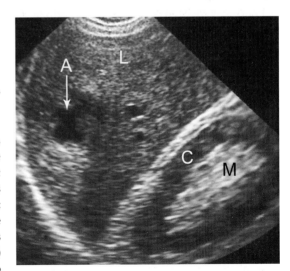

Figure 1.10 An abscess in the liver demonstrates tissues of varying echogenicity. Note the anechoic fluid in the abscess (A), moderately echogenic liver (L), hypoechoic renal cortex (C) and hyperechoic renal medulla (M).

An assortment of probes is available for imaging and biopsy guidance of various body cavities and organs including:

- Transvaginal US (TVUS): accurate assessment of gynaecological problems and of early pregnancy up to about 12 weeks' gestation
- Transrectal US (TRUS): guidance of prostate biopsy; staging of rectal cancer
- Endoscopic US (EUS): assessment of tumours of the upper gastrointestinal tract and pancreas
- Transoesophageal echocardiography (TOE): TOE removes the problem of overlying ribs and lung, which can obscure the heart and aorta when performing conventional echocardiography.

Advantages of US over other imaging modalities include:

- Lack of ionizing radiation, a particular advantage in pregnancy and paediatrics
- Relatively low cost
- Portability of equipment.

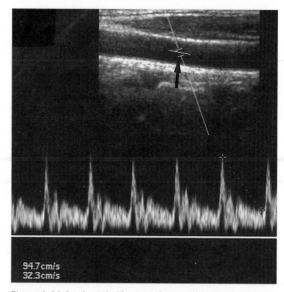

Figure 1.11 Duplex US. The Doppler sample gate is positioned in the artery (arrow) and the frequency shifts displayed as a graph. Peak systolic and end diastolic velocities are calculated and also displayed on the image in centimetres per second.

1.4.2 Doppler US

Anyone who has heard a police or ambulance siren speed past will be familiar with the influence of a moving object on sound waves, known as the Doppler effect. An object travelling towards the listener causes sound waves to be compressed giving a higher frequency; an object travelling away from the listener gives a lower frequency. The Doppler effect has been applied to US imaging. Flowing blood causes an alteration to the frequency of sound waves returning to the US probe. This frequency change or shift is calculated allowing quantitation of blood flow. The combination of conventional two-dimensional US imaging with Doppler US is known as Duplex US (Fig. 1.11).

Colour Doppler is an extension of these principles, with blood flowing towards the transducer coloured red, and blood flowing away from the transducer coloured blue. The colours are superimposed on the cross-sectional image allowing instant assessment of presence and direction of flow. Colour Doppler is used in many areas of US including echocardiography and vascular US. Colour Doppler is also used to confirm blood flow within organs (e.g. testis to exclude torsion) and to assess the vascularity of tumours.

1.4.3 Contrast-enhanced US

The accuracy of US in certain applications may be enhanced by the use of intravenously injected microbubble contrast agents. Microbubbles measure 3–5 μm diameter and consist of spheres of gas (e.g. perfluorocarbon) stabilized by a thin biocompatible shell. Microbubbles are caused to rapidly oscillate by the US beam and, in this way, microbubble contrast agents increase the echogenicity of blood for up to 5 minutes following intravenous injection. Beyond this time, the biocompatible shell is metabolized and the gas diffused into the blood. Microbubble contrast agents are very safe, with a reported incidence of anaphylactoid reaction of around 0.014 per cent. Contrast-enhanced US (CEUS) is increasingly accepted in clinical practice in the following applications:

- Echocardiography
  - Better visualization of blood may increase the accuracy of cardiac chamber measurement and calculation of ventricular function
  - Improved visualization of intracardiac shunts such as patent foramen ovale

- Assessment of liver masses
  - Dynamic blood flow characteristics of liver masses visualized with CEUS may assist in diagnosis, similar to dynamic contrast-enhanced CT and MRI.
  - CEUS may also be used for follow-up of hepatic neoplasms treated with percutaneous ablation or other non-surgical techniques.

1.4.4 Disadvantages and limitations of US

- US is highly operator dependent: unlike CT and MRI, which produce cross-sectional images in a reasonably programmed fashion, US relies on the operator to produce and interpret images at the time of examination.
- US cannot penetrate gas or bone.
- Bowel gas may obscure structures deep in the abdomen, such as the pancreas or renal arteries.

1.5 SCINTIGRAPHY (NUCLEAR MEDICINE)

1.5.1 Physics of scintigraphy and terminology

Scintigraphy refers to the use of gamma radiation to form images following the injection of various radiopharmaceuticals. The key word to understanding scintigraphy is 'radiopharmaceutical'. 'Radio' refers to the radionuclide, i.e. the emitter of gamma rays.

The most commonly used radionuclide in clinical practice is technetium, written in this text as ^{99m}Tc, where 99 is the atomic mass, and the 'm' stands for metastable. Metastable means that the technetium atom has two basic energy states: high and low. As the technetium transforms from the high-energy state to the low-energy state, it emits a quantum of energy in the form of a gamma ray, which has energy of 140 keV (Fig. 1.12).

Other commonly used radionuclides include gallium citrate (^{67}Ga), thallium (^{201}Tl), indium (^{111}In) and iodine (^{131}I).

The 'pharmaceutical' part of radiopharmaceutical refers to the compound to which the radionuclide is bound. This compound varies depending on the tissue to be examined.

For some applications, such as thyroid scanning, free technetium (referred to as pertechnetate) without a binding pharmaceutical is used.

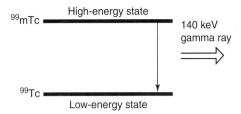

Figure 1.12 Gamma ray production. The metastable atom ^{99m}Tc passes from a high-energy to a low-energy state and releases gamma radiation with a peak energy of 140 keV.

The gamma rays emitted by the radionuclides are detected by a gamma camera that converts the absorbed energy of the radiation to an electric signal. This signal is analysed by a computer and displayed as an image (Fig. 1.13). The main advantages of scintigraphy are:
- High sensitivity
- Functional information is provided as well as anatomical information.

A summary of the more commonly used radionuclides and radiopharmaceuticals is provided in Table 1.1.

1.5.2 Single photon emission CT and single photon emission CT–CT

Single photon emission CT (SPECT) is a scintigraphic technique whereby the computer is programmed to analyse data coming from a single depth within the patient. SPECT allows greater sensitivity in the detection of subtle lesions overlain by other active structures (Fig. 1.14). The accuracy of SPECT may be further enhanced by fusion with CT. Scanners that combine SPECT with CT are now widely available. SPECT–CT fuses highly sensitive SPECT findings with anatomically accurate CT images, thus improving sensitivity and specificity.

The main applications of SPECT–CT include:
- ^{99m}Tc-MDP bone scanning
- ^{201}Tl cardiac scanning
- ^{99m}Tc-MIBG staging of neuroblastoma
- Cerebral perfusion studies.

1.5.3 Positron emission tomography and positron emission tomography–CT

Positron emission tomography (PET) is an established imaging technique, most commonly

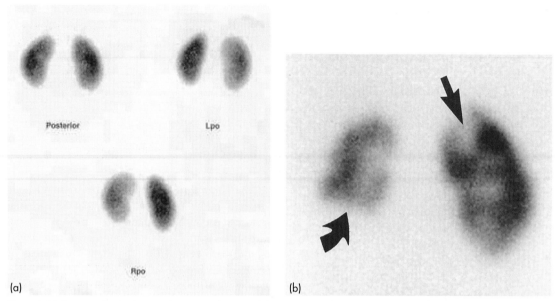

Figure 1.13 Scintigraphy (nuclear medicine): renal scan with ^{99m}Tc-DMSA (dimercaptosuccinic acid). (a) Normal DMSA scan shows normally shaped symmetrical kidneys. (b) DMSA scan in a child with recurrent urinary tract infection shows extensive right renal scarring, especially of the lower pole (curved arrow), with a smaller scar of the left upper pole (straight arrow).

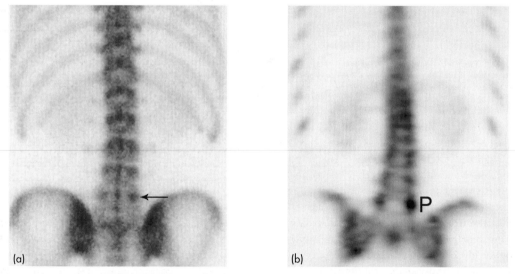

Figure 1.14 Single photon emission CT (SPECT). (a) Scintigraphy in a man with lower back pain shows a subtle area of mildly increased activity (arrow). (b) SPECT scan in the coronal plane shows an obvious focus of increased activity in a pars interarticularis defect (P).

used in oncology. PET ulitizes radionuclides that decay by positron emission. Positron emission occurs when a proton-rich unstable isotope transforms protons from its nucleus into neutrons and positrons. PET is based on similar principles to other fields of scintigraphy whereby an isotope is attached to a biological compound to form a radiopharmaceutical, which is injected into the patient.

The most commonly used radiopharmaceutical

Table 1.1 Radionuclides and radiopharmaceuticals in clinical practice.

Clinical application	Radiopharmaceutical
Bone scintigraphy	^{99m}Tc-methylene diphosphonate (MDP) ^{99m}Tc-hydroxymethylene diphosphonate (HDP)
Thyroid imaging	^{99m}Tc (pertechnetate)
Parathyroid imaging	^{99m}Tc-sestamibi
Renal scintigraphy	^{99m}Tc-mercaptoacetyltriglycerine (MAG3) ^{99m}Tc-diethyltriaminepentaacetic acid (DTPA)
Renal cortical scan	^{99m}Tc-dimercaptosuccinic acid (DMSA)
Staging/localization of neuroblastoma or phaeochromocytoma	^{123}I-metaiodobenzylguanidine (MIBG) ^{131}I-MIBG
Myocardial perfusion imaging	^{201}Thallium (^{201}Tl) ^{99m}Tc-sestamibi (MIBI) ^{99m}Tc-tetrofosmin
Cardiac gated blood pool scan	^{99m}Tc-labelled red blood cells
Ventilation/perfusion lung scan (VQ scan)	Ventilation: ^{99m}Tc-DTPA aerosol or similar Perfusion: ^{99m}Tc-macroaggregated albumen (MAA)
Hepatobiliary imaging	^{99m}Tc-iminodiacetic acid analogue, e.g. DISIDA or HIDA
Gastrointestinal motility study	^{99m}Tc-sulphur colloid in solid food ^{99m}Tc-DTPA in water
Gastrointestinal bleeding study	^{99m}Tc-labelled red blood cells
Meckel diverticulum scan	^{99m}Tc (pertechnetate)
Inflammatory bowel disease	^{99m}Tc-hexamethylpropyleneamineoxime (HMPAO) ^{99m}Tc -labelled sucralfate
Carcinoid/neuroendocrine tumour	^{111}In-pentetreotide (Octreoscan™)
Infection imaging	Gallium citrate (^{67}Ga) ^{99m}Tc-HMPAO-labelled white blood cells
Cerebral blood flow imaging (brain SPECT)	^{99m}Tc-HMPAO (Ceretec™)

in PET scanning is FDG (2-deoxyglucose labelled with the positron-emitter fluorine-18). FDG is an analogue of glucose and therefore accumulates in areas of high glucose metabolism. Positrons emitted from the fluorine-18 in FDG collide with negatively charged electrons. The mass of an electron and positron is converted into two 511 keV photons, i.e. high-energy gamma rays, which are emitted in opposite directions to each other. This event is known as annihilation (Fig. 1.15).

The PET camera consists of a ring of detectors that register the annihilations. An area of high concentration of FDG will have a large number of annihilations and will be shown on the resulting image as a 'hot spot'. Normal physiological uptake of FDG occurs in the brain (high level of glucose metabolism), myocardium, and in the renal collecting systems, ureters and bladder.

The current roles of PET imaging may be summarized as follows:
- Oncology
  - Tumour staging
  - Assessment of tumour response to therapy
  - Differentiate benign and malignant masses, e.g. solitary pulmonary nodule
  - Detect tumour recurrence

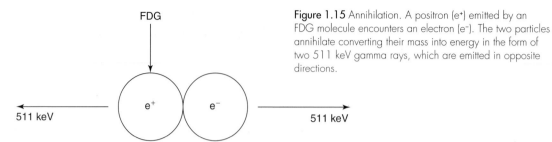

FDG

e⁺   e⁻

511 keV   511 keV

Figure 1.15 Annihilation. A positron (e⁺) emitted by an FDG molecule encounters an electron (e⁻). The two particles annihilate converting their mass into energy in the form of two 511 keV gamma rays, which are emitted in opposite directions.

- Cardiac: Non-invasive assessment of myocardial viability in patients with coronary artery disease
- Central nervous system
  - Characterization of dementia disorders
  - Localization of seizure focus in epilepsy.

As with other types of scintigraphy, a problem with PET is its non-specificity. Put another way, 'hot spots' on PET may have multiple causes, with false positive findings commonly encountered. The specificity of PET may be increased by the use of scanners that fuse PET with CT or MRI. PET–CT fusion imaging combines the functional and metabolic information of PET with the precise cross-sectional anatomy of CT (Fig. 1.16). Advantages of combining PET with CT include:

- Reduced incidence of false positive findings in primary tumour staging
- Increased accuracy of follow-up of malignancy during and following treatment.

PET–CT scanners are now widely available and have largely replaced stand alone PET scanners in modern practice. At the time of writing, PET–MR scanners are also becoming available in research and tertiary institutions.

1.5.4 Limitations and disadvantages of scintigraphy

- Use of ionizing radiation
- Cost of equipment
- Extra care required in handling radioactive materials
- The main disadvantage of scintigraphy is its nonspecificity; as described above, this may be reduced by combining scintigraphy with CT or MRI.

1.6 MRI

1.6.1 MRI physics and terminology

MRI uses the magnetic properties of spinning hydrogen atoms to produce images. The first step

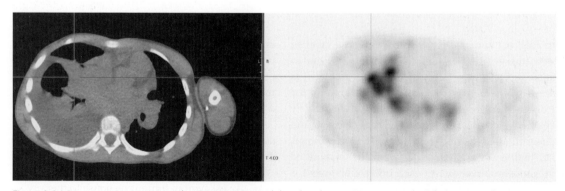

Figure 1.16 Positron emission tomography–CT (PET–CT): Hodgkin's lymphoma. CT image on the left shows neoplastic lymphadenopathy, collapsed lung and pleural effusion. Corresponding FDG-PET image on the right shows areas of increased activity corresponding to neoplastic lymphadenopathy. Collapsed lung and pleural effusion do not show increased activity, thus differentiating neoplastic from non-neoplastic tissue.

in MRI is the application of a strong, external magnetic field. For this purpose, the patient is placed within a large powerful magnet. Most current medical MRI machines have field strengths of 1.5 or 3.0 tesla (1.5T or 3T). The hydrogen atoms within the patient align in a direction either parallel or antiparallel to the strong external field. A greater proportion aligns in the parallel direction so that the net vector of their alignment, and therefore the net magnetic vector, will be in the direction of the external field. This is known as longitudinal magnetization.

A second magnetic field is applied at right angles to the original external field. This second magnetic field is known as the radiofrequency pulse (RF pulse), because it is applied at a frequency in the same part of the electromagnetic spectrum as radio waves. A magnetic coil, known as the RF coil, applies the RF pulse. The RF pulse causes the net magnetization vector of the hydrogen atoms to turn towards the transverse plane, i.e. a plane at right angles to the direction of the original, strong external field. The component of the net magnetization vector in the transverse plane induces an electrical current in the RF coil. This current is known as the MR signal and is the basis for formation of an image. Computer analysis of the complex MR signal from the RF receiver coils is used to produce an MR image.

Note that in viewing MRI images, white or light grey areas are referred to as 'high signal'; dark grey or black areas are referred to as 'low signal'. On certain sequences, flowing blood is seen as a black area referred to as a 'flow void'.

Each medical MRI machine consists of a number of magnetic coils:
- 1.5T or 3T superconducting magnet
- Gradient coils, contained in the bore of the superconducting magnet, used to produce variations to the magnetic field that allow image formation
  - Rapid switching of these gradients causes the loud noises associated with MRI scanning
- RF coils are applied to, or around, the area of interest and are used to transmit the RF pulse and to receive the RF signal
  - RF coils come in varying shapes and sizes depending on the part of the body to be examined

- Larger coils are required for imaging the chest and abdomen, whereas smaller extremity coils are used for small parts such as the wrist or ankle.

1.6.2 Tissue contrast and imaging sequences

Much of the complexity of MRI arises from the fact that the MR signal depends on many varied properties of the tissues and structures being examined, including:
- Number of hydrogen atoms present in tissue (proton density)
- Chemical environment of the hydrogen atoms, e.g. whether in free water or bound by fat
- Flow: blood vessels or CSF
- Magnetic susceptibility
- T1 relaxation time
- T2 relaxation time.

By altering the duration and amplitude of the RF pulse, as well as the timing and repetition of its application, various imaging sequences use these properties to produce image contrast. Terms used to describe the different types of MR imaging sequences include spin echo, inversion recovery and gradient-recalled echo (gradient echo).

1.6.2.1 Spin echo

Spin echo sequences include T1-weighted, T2-weighted and proton density. The following is a brief explanation of the terms 'T1' and 'T2'.

Following the application of a 90° RF pulse, the net magnetization vector lies in the transverse plane. Also, all of the hydrogen protons are 'in phase', i.e. spinning at the same rate. Upon cessation of the RF pulse, two things begin to happen:
- Net magnetization vector rotates back to the longitudinal direction: longitudinal or T1 relaxation
- Hydrogen atoms dephase (spin at slightly varying rates): transverse or T2 relaxation (decay).

The rates at which T1 and T2 relaxation occur are inherent properties of the various tissues. Sequences that primarily use differences in T1 relaxation rates produce T1-weighted images. Tissues with long T1 values are shown as low signal while those with shorter T1 values are displayed as higher signal. Gadolinium produces T1 shortening; tissues or structures that enhance with gadolinium-based contrast materials show increased signal on T1-weighted images.

T2-weighted images reflect differences in T2 relaxation rates. Tissues whose protons dephase slowly have a long T2 and are displayed as high signal on T2-weighted images. Tissues with shorter T2 values are shown as lower signal (Fig. 1.17).

Proton density images are produced by sequences that accentuate neither T1 nor T2 differences. The signal strength of proton density images mostly reflects the density of hydrogen atoms (protons) in the different tissues. Proton density images are particularly useful in musculoskeletal imaging for the demonstration of small structures, as well as articular cartilage (Fig. 1.18).

1.6.2.2 Gradient-recalled echo (gradient echo)

Gradient-recalled echo (GRE) sequences are widely used in a variety of MRI applications. GRE sequences are extremely sensitive to the presence of substances that cause local alterations in magnetic properties. Examples of such substances include iron-containing haemosiderin and ferritin found in chronic blood. GRE sequences are used in neuroimaging to look for chronic blood in patients with suspected vascular tumours, previous trauma or angiopathy. An extension of GRE sequences in the brain known as susceptibility-weighted imaging (SWI) uses subtraction techniques to remove unwanted information and thereby increase sensitivity. GRE sequences also allow extremely rapid imaging and are used for imaging the heart and abdomen.

1.6.2.3 Inversion recovery

Inversion recovery sequences are used to suppress unwanted signals that may obscure pathology. The two most common inversion recovery sequences are used to suppress fat (STIR) and water (FLAIR). Fat suppression sequences such as STIR (short TI-inversion recovery) are used for demonstrating pathology in areas containing a lot of fat, such as

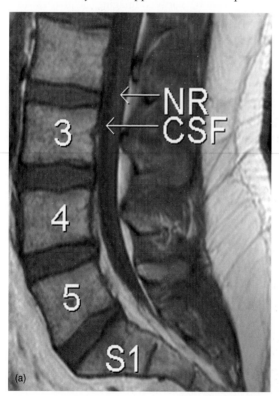
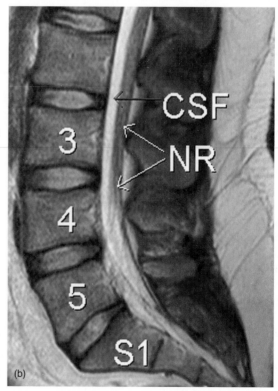

Figure 1.17 MRI of the lower lumbar spine and sacrum. (a) Sagittal T1-weighted image. Note: dark cerebral spinal fluid (CSF). (b) Sagittal T2-weighted image. Note: bright CSF; nerve roots (NR).

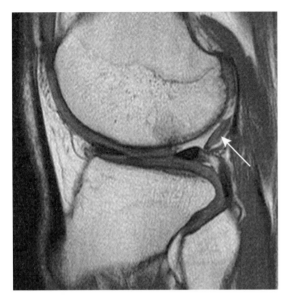

Figure 1.18 Proton density (PD) sequence. Sagittal PD MRI of the knee shows a cartilage fragment detached from the articular surface of the lateral femoral condyle (arrow).

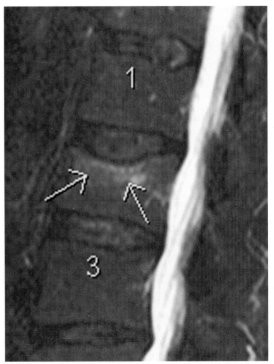

Figure 1.19 Short tau inversion recovery (STIR) sequence. Sagittal STIR MRI of the lumbar spine shows a crush fracture of L2. Increased signal within L2 on STIR (arrows) indicates bone marrow oedema in a recent fracture.

the orbits and bone marrow. STIR sequences allow the delineation of bone marrow disorders such as oedema, bruising and infiltration (Fig. 1.19). FLAIR (fluid-attenuated inversion recovery) sequences suppress signals from CSF and are used to image the brain. FLAIR sequences are particularly useful for diagnosing white matter disorders such as multiple sclerosis.

1.6.3 Functional MRI sequences

1.6.3.1 Diffusion-weighted imaging

Diffusion-weighted imaging (DWI) is sensitive to the random Brownian motion (diffusion) of water molecules within tissue. The greater the amount of diffusion, the greater the signal loss on DWI. Areas of reduced water molecule diffusion show on DWI as relatively high signal.

Diffusion-weighted imaging is the most sensitive imaging test available for the diagnosis of acute cerebral infarction. With the onset of acute ischaemia and cell death there is increased intracellular water (cytotoxic oedema) with restricted diffusion of water molecules. An acute infarct therefore shows on DWI as an area of relatively high signal.

1.6.3.2 Perfusion-weighted imaging

In perfusion-weighted imaging (PWI) the brain is rapidly scanned following injection of a bolus of contrast material (gadolinium). The data obtained may be represented in a number of ways including maps of regional cerebral blood volume, cerebral blood flow, and mean transit time of the contrast bolus. PWI may be used in patients with cerebral infarct to map out areas of brain at risk of ischaemia that may be salvageable with thrombolysis.

1.6.3.3 Magnetic resonance spectroscopy

Magnetic resonance spectroscopy (MRS) uses different frequencies to identify certain molecules in a selected volume of tissue, known as a voxel. Following data analysis, a spectrographic graph of certain metabolites is drawn. Metabolites of interest include lipid, lactate, NAA (N-acetylaspartate), choline, creatinine, citrate and myoinositol. Uses of MRS include characterization of metabolic brain disorders in children, imaging of dementias, differentiation of recurrent cerebral tumour from radiation necrosis, and diagnosis of prostatic carcinoma.

1.6.3.4 Blood oxygen level-dependent imaging

Blood oxygen level-dependent (BOLD) imaging is a non-invasive functional MRI (fMRI) technique used for localizing regional brain signal intensity changes in response to task performance. BOLD imaging depends on regional changes in concentration of deoxyhaemoglobin, and is therefore a tool to investigate regional cerebral physiology in response to a variety of stimuli. BOLD fMRI may be used prior to surgery for brain tumour or arteriovenous malformation (AVM), as a prognostic indicator of the degree of postsurgical deficit.

1.6.4 Magnetic resonance angiography and magnetic resonance venography

Flowing blood can be shown with different sequences as either signal void (black) or increased signal (white). Magnetic resonance angiography (MRA) refers to the use of these sequences to display arterial anatomy and pathology. Computer reconstruction techniques allow the display of blood vessels in 3D as well as rotation and viewing of these blood vessels from multiple angles. MRA is most commonly used to image the arteries of the brain, although is also finding wider application in the imaging of renal and peripheral arteries.

MRI of veins is known as magnetic resonance venography (MRV). MRV is most commonly used in neuroimaging to demonstrate the venous sinuses of the brain. For certain applications, the accuracy of MRA and MRV is increased by contrast enhancement with intravenous injection of Gd-DTPA.

1.6.5 Contrast material in MRI

Gadolinium (Gd) is a paramagnetic substance that causes T1 shortening and therefore increased signal on T1-weighted images. Unbound Gd is highly toxic and binding agents, such as diethylenetriamine pentaacetic acid (DTPA), are required for *in vivo* use. Gd-DTPA is non-toxic and used in a dose of 0.1 mmol per kilogram.

Indications for the use of Gd enhancement in MRI include:
- Brain
    - Inflammation: meningitis, encephalitis
    - Tumours: primary (Fig. 1.20), metastases

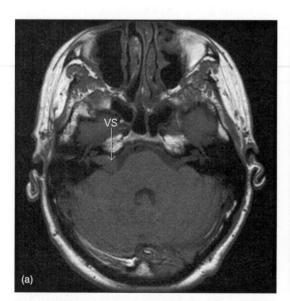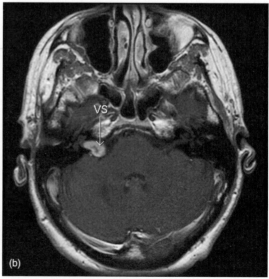

Figure 1.20 Intravenous contrast in MRI: vestibular schwannoma. (a) Transverse T1-weighted image of the posterior fossa shows a right-sided mass. (b) Following injection of gadolinium the mass shows intense enhancement, typical of vestibular schwannoma (VS). (See also Fig. 11.10.)

- Tumour residuum/recurrence following treatment
- Spine
  - Postoperative to differentiate fibrosis from recurrent disc protrusion
  - Infection: discitis, epidural abscess
  - Tumours: primary, metastases
- Musculoskeletal system
  - Soft tissue tumours
  - Intra-articular Gd-DTPA: MR arthrography
- Abdomen
  - Characterization of tumours of liver, kidney and pancreas.

1.6.6 Applications and advantages of MRI

Widely accepted applications of MRI include:
- Imaging modality of choice for most brain and spine disorders
- Musculoskeletal disorders, including internal derangements of joints and staging of musculoskeletal tumours
- Cardiac MR is an established technique in specific applications including assessment of congenital heart disease and aortic disorders
- MR of the abdomen is used in adults for visualization of the biliary system, and for characterization of hepatic, renal, adrenal and pancreatic tumours
- In children, MR of the abdomen is increasingly replacing CT for the diagnosis and staging of abdominal tumours
- MRA is widely used in the imaging of the cerebral circulation and in some centres is the initial angiographic method of choice for other areas including the renal and peripheral circulations.

Particular advantages of MRI in clinical practice include:
- Excellent soft tissue contrast and characterization
- Lack of artefact from adjacent bones, e.g. pituitary fossa
- Multiplanar capabilities
- Lack of ionizing radiation.

1.6.7 Disadvantages and limitations of MRI

- Time taken to complete examination

- Young children and infants usually require general anaesthesia
- Patients experiencing pain may require intravenous pain relief
- For examination of the abdomen, an antispasmodic, such as intravenous hyoscine, may be required to reduce movement of the bowel
- Safety issues related to ferromagnetic materials within the patient, e.g. surgical clips, or electrical devices such as pacemakers (see below)
- High auditory noise levels: earplugs should be provided to all patients undergoing MRI examinations
- Claustrophobia
  - Modern scanners have a wider bore and claustrophobia is less of a problem than in the past; intravenous conscious sedation may occasionally be required
- Problems with gadolinium: allergy (extremely rare) and nephrogenic systemic fibrosis (see below).

1.7 HAZARDS ASSOCIATED WITH MEDICAL IMAGING

Hazards associated with modern medical imaging are outlined below, and include:
- Exposure to ionizing radiation
- Anaphylactoid reactions to iodinated contrast media
- Contrast-induced nephropathy (CIN)
- MRI safety issues
- Nephrogenic systemic sclerosis (NSF) due to Gd-containing contrast media.

1.7.1 Exposure to ionizing radiation

1.7.1.1 Radiation effects and effective dose

Radiography, scintigraphy and CT use ionizing radiation. Numerous studies, including those on survivors of the atomic bomb attacks in Japan in 1945, have shown that ionizing radiation in large doses is harmful. The risks of harm from medical radiation are low, and are usually expressed as the increased risk of developing cancer as a result of exposure. Public awareness of the possible hazards of medical radiation is growing and it is important for doctors who refer patients for X-rays, nuclear medicine scans or CT scans to have at least a basic understanding of radiation effects and the principles of radiation protection.

Radiation effects occur as a result of damage to cells, including cell death and genetic damage. Actively dividing cells, such as are found in the bone marrow, lymph glands and gonads are particularly sensitive to radiation effects. In general, two types of effects may result from radiation damage: stochastic and deterministic. Deterministic effects are due to cell death and include radiation burns, cataracts and decreased fertility. Severity of deterministic effects varies with dose and a dose threshold usually exists below which the effect will not occur. For stochastic effects, the probability of the effect, not its severity is regarded as a function of dose. Theoretically, there is no dose threshold below which a stochastic effect will not occur. The most commonly discussed stochastic effect is increased cancer risk due to radiation exposure.

Radiation dose from medical imaging techniques is usually expressed as effective dose. The concept of effective dose takes into account the susceptibilities of the various tissues and organs, as well as the type of radiation received. The SI unit of effective dose is joules per kilogram and is referred to as the sievert (Sv): $1\,Sv = 1.0\,J\,kg^{-1}$. The effective dose provides a means of calculating the overall risk of radiation effects, especially the risk of cancer.

At the time of writing, there is a debate in the medical literature and the public domain about the risks of radiation exposure due to medical imaging. Those who subscribe to the 'no threshold' theory maintain that there is an increased risk of fatal cancer from any medical imaging examination that uses ionizing radiation. Figures such as a 1 in 2000 lifetime attributable risk of fatal cancer from a single CT of the abdomen may be quoted. Opponents of this theory point to a lack of evidence. In any case, most providers and consumers of medical imaging would agree that it is desirable for referring doctors to have some knowledge of the levels of possible radiation exposure associated with common imaging tests. Furthermore, there is widespread acceptance within the medical imaging community that radiation exposure should be minimized.

To try to make sense of quoted effective doses, there is a tendency to list figures against the number of frontal CXRs that might produce the same dose. Another common factor used for comparison is the amount of background radiation that is received as a normal process. This varies depending on location, but is generally 2–3 mSv per year. Another comparison used is the amount of radiation exposure as a result of flying in an airliner, usually quoted as hours of flying at 12 000 metres. A 20-hour flight from Australia to London would result in an exposure of about 0.1 mSv, the equivalent of about five CXRs. Some typical effective doses (mSv) and relevant comparisons are listed in Table 1.2.

1.7.1.2 The ALARA principle

The basic rule of radiation protection is that all justifiable radiation exposure is kept as low as is reasonably achievable (ALARA principle). This can be achieved by keeping in mind the following points:

- Each radiation exposure is justified on a case-by-case basis.
- The minimum number of radiographs is taken and minimum fluoroscopic screening time used.
- Mobile equipment is only used when the patient is unable to come to the radiology department.
- US or MRI should be used where possible.
- Children are more sensitive to radiation than adults and are at greater risk of developing radiation-induced cancers many decades after the initial exposure.
- In paediatric radiology, extra measures may be taken to minimize radiation dose including gonad shields and adjustment of CT scanning parameters.

1.7.1.3 Pregnancy

Extra measures should also be taken for the care of women of reproductive age:

- Radiation exposure of abdomen and pelvis should be minimized.
- All females of reproductive age asked if they could be pregnant prior to radiation exposure.
- Multilingual signs posted in the medical imaging department asking patients to notify the radiographer of possible pregnancy.

As organogenesis is unlikely to be occurring in an embryo in the first 4 weeks following the last menstrual period, this is not considered a critical

Table 1.2 Effective doses of some common examinations.

Imaging test	Effective dose (mSv)	Equivalent number of CXRs	Equivalent time of background exposure	Equivalent hours of flying at 12 000 metres
CXR frontal	0.02	1	3 days	4
CXR lateral	0.04	2	6 days	8
Limb X-ray	0.02	1	3 days	4
Lumbar spine X-ray	1.5	75	6 months	300
AXR	0.7	35	3 months	150
CT head	2	100	8 months	400
CTPA	8	400	2 years	1200
CT abdomen	2–10	100–500	8 months–3 years	400–1800
DEXA bone densitometry	0.001	0.05	<1 day	<1
Mammogram	0.7	35	3 months	150

period for radiation exposure. Organogenesis commences soon after the time of the first missed period and continues for the next three to four months. During this time, the fetus is considered to be maximally radiosensitive. Radiographic or CT examination of the abdomen or pelvis should be delayed if possible to a time when fetal sensitivity is reduced, i.e. post-24 weeks' gestation or ideally until the baby is born. Where possible, MRI or US should be used. Radiographic exposure to remote areas such as chest, skull and limbs may be undertaken with minimal fetal exposure at any time during pregnancy. For nuclear medicine studies in the post-partum period, it is advised that breastfeeding be ceased and breast milk discarded for 2 days following the injection of radionuclide.

1.7.2 Anaphylactoid contrast media reactions

Most patients injected intravenously with iodinated contrast media experience normal transient phenomena, including a mild warm feeling plus an odd taste in the mouth. With modern iodinated contrast media, vomiting at the time of injection is uncommon. More significant adverse reactions to contrast media may be classified as mild, intermediate or severe anaphylactoid reactions:

- Mild anaphylactoid reactions: mild urticaria and pruritis
- Intermediate reactions: more severe urticaria, hypotension and mild bronchospasm
- Severe reactions: more severe bronchospasm, laryngeal oedema, pulmonary oedema, unconsciousness, convulsions, pulmonary collapse and cardiac arrest.

Incidences of mild, intermediate and severe reactions with non-ionic low osmolar contrast media are 3, 0.04 and 0.004 per cent, respectively. Fatal reactions are exceedingly rare (1:170 000). All staff working with iodinated contrast materials should be familiar with CPR, and emergency procedures should be in place to deal with reactions, including resuscitation equipment and relevant drugs, especially adrenaline. Prior to injection of iodinated contrast media, patients should complete a risk assessment questionnaire to identify predisposing factors known to increase the risk of anaphylactoid reactions including:

- History of asthma: increases the risk by a factor of 10
- History of atopy: increases the risk by a factor of 10
- Previous anaphylactoid reaction to iodinated contrast media: 40 per cent risk of further reactions.

A history of allergy to seafood does not appear to be associated with an increased risk of contrast media reactions. There is no convincing evidence that pretreatment with steroids or an antihistamine reduces the risk of contrast media reactions.

1.7.3 Contrast-induced nephropathy

Contrast-induced nephropathy (CIN) refers to a reduction of renal function (defined as greater than 25 per cent increase in serum creatinine) occurring within 3 days of contrast medium injection. Most cases of CIN are self-limiting with resolution in 1–2 weeks. Dialysis may be required in up to 15 per cent. Risk factors for the development of CIN include:

- Pre-existing impaired renal function, particularly diabetic nephropathy
- Dehydration
- Sepsis
- Age >60 years
- Recent organ transplant
- Multiple myeloma.

Estimated glomerular filtration rate (eGFR) is generally seen as a better measure of renal function for risk assessment. eGRF accounts for age and sex and is calculated by formula from serum creatinine. CIN is very rare in patients with eGFR >60 mL/min. eGFR should be measured prior to contrast medium injection if there is a known history of renal disease or if any of the above risk factors is present.

The risk of developing CIN may be reduced by the following measures:

- Risk factors should be identified by risk assessment questionnaire.
- Use of other imaging modalities in patients at risk including US or non-contrast-enhanced CT.
- Use of minimum possible dose where contrast medium injection is required.
- Adequate hydration before and after contrast medium injection.
- Various pretreatments have been described, such as oral acetylcysteine; however, there is currently no convincing evidence that anything other than hydration is beneficial.

1.7.4 MRI safety issues

Potential hazards associated with MRI predominantly relate to the interaction of the magnetic fields with metallic materials and electronic devices. Reports exist of objects such as spanners, oxygen cylinders and drip poles becoming missiles when placed near an MRI scanner; the hazards to personnel are obvious. Ferromagnetic materials within the patient could possibly be moved by the magnetic field causing tissue damage. Common potential problems include metal fragments in the eye and various medical devices such as intracerebral aneurysm clips. Patients with a past history of penetrating eye injury are at risk for having metal fragments in the eye and should be screened prior to entering the MRI room with radiographs of the orbits.

MRI compatible aneurysm clips and other surgical devices have been available for many years. MRI should not be performed until the safety of an individual device has been established. The presence of electrically active implants, such as cardiac pacemakers, cochlear implants and neurostimulators, is generally a contraindication to MRI unless the safety of an individual device is proven. MRI compatible pacemakers are now becoming available.

1.7.5 Nephrogenic systemic sclerosis

Nephrogenic systemic sclerosis (NSF) is a rare complication of some Gd-based contrast media in patients with renal failure. Onset of symptoms may occur from one day to three months following injection. Initial symptoms consist of pain, pruritis and erythema, usually in the legs. As NSF progresses there is thickening of skin and subcutaneous tissues, and fibrosis of internal organs including heart, liver and kidneys. Identifying patients at risk, including patients with known renal disease, diabetes, hypertension and recent organ transplant, may reduce the risk of developing NSF following injection of Gd-based contrast media. eGFR should be measured in those at risk. Decisions can then be made regarding injection, choice of Gd-based medium, and possible use of alternative imaging tests.

1.7.6 Risk reduction in MRI

A standard questionnaire to be completed by the patient prior to MRI should cover relevant factors such as:

- Previous surgical history
- Presence of metal foreign bodies including aneurysm clips, etc.
- Presence of cochlear implants and cardiac pacemakers
- Possible occupational exposure to metal fragments and history of penetrating eye injury
- Previous allergic reaction to Gd-based contrast media
- Known renal disease or other risk factors relevant to NSF as outlined above.

2 Respiratory system and chest

2.1 INTRODUCTION

Although this chapter is primarily concerned with investigation of diseases of the lung, other chest structures including the aorta and skeletal structures will be discussed, particularly in the context of trauma. A more complete discussion of imaging the heart and aorta may be found in Chapter 3.

Common symptoms due to respiratory disease include cough, production of sputum, haemoptysis, dyspnoea and chest pain. These symptoms may be accompanied by systemic manifestations including fever, weight loss and night sweats. Accurate history plus findings on physical examination, in particular auscultation of the chest, are vital in directing further investigation and management. History and examination may be supplemented by relatively simple tests, such as white cell count, erythrocyte sedimentation rate (ESR), and sputum analysis for culture or cytology. A variety of pulmonary function tests may also be performed including spirometry, measurements of gas exchange, such as CO diffusing capacity and arterial blood gas, and exercise testing. In some cases, more sophisticated and invasive tests, such as flexible fibreoptic bronchoscopy, bronchoalveolar lavage and video-assisted thorascopic surgery (VATS), may be required.

CXR is requested for virtually all patients with respiratory symptoms. This chapter begins with a suggested approach to CXR interpretation, followed by notes on common findings. CT is the next most commonly performed investigation for diseases of the respiratory system and chest. An outline of the common uses and techniques of chest CT is provided, followed by notes on investigation of the patient with haemoptysis, diagnosis and staging of bronchogenic carcinoma, and chest trauma.

2.2 HOW TO READ A CXR

This section is an introduction to the principles of CXR interpretation. An overview of the standard CXR projections is followed by a brief outline of normal radiographic anatomy. Some notes on assessment of a few important technical aspects are then provided, as well as an outline of a suggested systematic approach.

2.2.1 Projections performed

In general, two radiographic views, posteroanterior (PA) and lateral, are used in the assessment of most chest conditions. Exceptions where a PA view alone would suffice include:
- Infants and children
- 'Screening' examinations, e.g. for immigration, insurance or diving medicals
- Follow-up of known conditions seen well on the PA, e.g. pneumonia following antibiotics, metastases following chemotherapy, pneumothorax following drainage.

2.2.1.1 PA erect

To obtain a PA erect CXR, the patient is positioned standing with his or her anterior chest wall up against the X-ray film. The X-ray tube lies behind the patient so that X-rays pass through in a posterior to anterior direction.

Reasons for performing the film PA:

- Accurate assessment of cardiac size due to minimal magnification
- Scapulae able to be rotated out of the way.

Reasons for performing the film erect:
- Physiological representation of blood vessels of mediastinum and lung. In the supine position, mediastinal veins and upper lobe vessels may be distended leading to misinterpretation. In particular, a normal mediastinum may look abnormally wide on supine CXR
- Gas passes upwards: pneumothorax is more easily diagnosed, as is free gas beneath the diaphragm
- Fluid passes downwards: pleural effusion is more easily diagnosed.

2.2.1.2 Lateral

Reasons for performing a lateral CXR:
- Further view of lungs, especially those areas obscured on the PA film, e.g. posterior segments of lower lobes, areas behind the hila, left lower lobe, which lies behind the heart on the PA
- Further assessment of cardiac configuration
- Further anatomical localization of lesions
- More sensitive for pleural effusions
- Good view of thoracic spine.

2.2.1.3 Other projections

In certain circumstances, projections other than those outlined above may be required.

Anteroposterior (AP)/supine X-ray:
- Acutely ill or traumatized patients, and patients in intensive care and coronary care units
- Mediastinum and heart appear wider on an AP/supine film due to venous distension and magnification.

Expiratory film:
- Increased sensitivity for small pneumothorax: in expiration the lung is smaller while the pneumothorax does not change in volume
- Suspected bronchial obstruction with air trapping, e.g. inhaled foreign body in a child: in expiration the normal lung reduces in volume while the lung with an obstructed airway remains inflated.

Decubitus film:
- Radiograph performed with the patient lying on their side
- Used occasionally in patients too ill to stand where pleural effusion or pneumothorax are suspected and not definitely diagnosed on an AP film.

Oblique views may be used for suspected rib fracture, or to display other chest wall pathologies.

2.2.2 Radiographic anatomy

2.2.2.1 PA erect

Look at a normal PA chest radiograph (Fig. 2.1) and try to identify the following features:
- The trachea in the midline, plus its division into right and left main bronchi
- Right paratracheal stripe: thin line on the right margin of the trachea
  - May be lost or thickened in the presence of lymphadenopathy
- Azygos vein: small convex opacity, which sits in the concavity formed by the junction of the trachea and right main bronchus
- Superior vena cava (SVC): straight line, continuous inferiorly with the right heart border
- Right heart border: formed by the right atrium, outlined by the aerated right middle lobe
- Right hilum: midway between the diaphragm and lung apex
  - Formed by the right main bronchus and right pulmonary artery, and their lobar divisions
- Aortic arch, sometimes termed the aortic 'knuckle'
- Descending aorta can be traced downwards from aortic arch as a line to the left of the spine
  - Descending aorta may be obscured by a posterior mediastinal mass, or by pathology in the left lower lobe
- Main pulmonary artery: slightly convex line between aortic arch and left heart border
- Left hilum: posterior to main pulmonary artery and extending laterally
  - Formed by left main bronchus and left pulmonary artery and their main lobar divisions

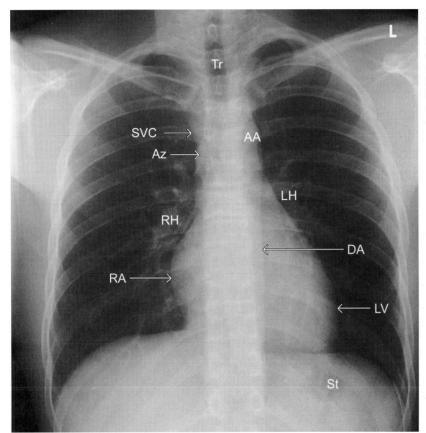

Figure 2.1 Normal PA CXR. Note the following structures: trachea (Tr), superior vena cava (SVC), azygos vein (Az), right hilum (RH), right atrium (RA), aortic arch (AA), left hilum (LH), left ventricle (LV), descending aorta (DA) and stomach (St).

- Left heart border: formed by the left ventricle, except in cases where the right ventricle is enlarged
- Left atrial appendage lies on the upper left cardiac border; it is not seen unless enlarged.

2.2.2.2 Lateral

The lateral view is usually performed with the patient's arms held out horizontally. Look at a normal lateral chest radiograph (Fig. 2.2) and try to identify the following features:

- Humeral heads: round opacities projected over the lung apices
  - Should not be mistaken for abnormal masses
- Trachea: air-filled structure in the upper chest, midway between the anterior and posterior chest walls
- Posterior aspect of the aortic arch: convexity posterior to the trachea

- Trachea can be followed inferiorly to the carina where the right and left main bronchi may be seen end-on as round lucencies
- Left main pulmonary artery forms an opacity posterior and slightly superior to the carina
- Right pulmonary artery forms an opacity anterior and slightly inferior to the carina
- Posterior cardiac border: formed by the left atrium superiorly and the left ventricle inferiorly
- Anterior cardiac border: formed by right ventricle
- Main pulmonary artery forms a convex opacity continuous with the right upper cardiac border.

2.2.3 Technical assessment

Prior to making a diagnostic assessment it is worthwhile to pause briefly to assess the technical quality of the PA film.

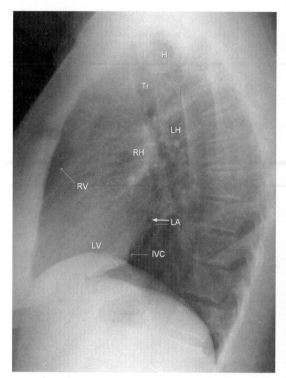

Figure 2.2 Normal lateral CXR. Note the following structures: trachea (Tr), humeral head (H), right hilum (RH), left hilum (LH), right ventricle (RV), left atrium (LA), left ventricle (LV) and inferior vena cava (IVC).

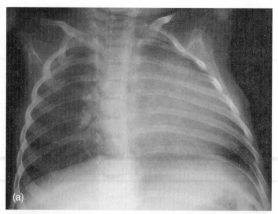

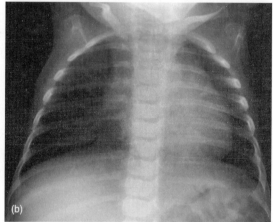

Figure 2.3 Effects of rotation. (a) CXR of an infant with rotation producing significant anatomical distortion. Note the asymmetry of the ribs and apparent cardiac enlargement. (b) A normally centred CXR shows normal anatomy.

Centring of the patient:
- With proper centring of the patient the lung apices and both costophrenic angles should be visualized.

Rotation:
- Rotation may cause anatomical distortion (Fig. 2.3).
- The easiest way to ensure that there is no rotation is to check that the spinous processes of the upper thoracic vertebrae lie midway between the medial ends of the clavicles.

Degree of inspiration:
- Inadequate inspiration may lead to overdiagnosis of pulmonary opacity or collapse.
- With an adequate inspiration the diaphragms should lie at the level of the fifth or sixth ribs anteriorly, and in children trachea should be straight.

2.2.4 Diagnostic assessment

The most important factor in the interpretation of any medical imaging investigation is the clinical context. Accurate interpretation of the CXR may be difficult or impossible in the absence of relevant and accurate clinical information.
- Is the patient febrile or in pain?
- Is there haemoptysis or shortness of breath?
- Are there relevant results from other tests such as spirometry or bronchoscopy?

Another important factor is the time course of any abnormality. Comparison with any previous CXR is often very useful to assess whether visible abnormalities are acute or chronic.

When starting to look at chest radiographs, use of a systemic checklist approach as outlined below will assist in the detection of relevant findings (Tables 2.1 and 2.2).

Table 2.1 Checklist for PA view.

Structure/ anatomical region	Specific features
Heart	Position, size, configuration, calcification
Pulmonary blood vessels	Compare size of upper and lower lobe vessels
Mediastinum	Trachea, aorta, superior vena cava, azygos vein
Right and left hilum	Compare relative size, density and position
Lungs	Check lungs from top to bottom, and from central to peripheral
'Hidden areas'	Behind the heart
	Behind each hilum
	Behind the diaphragms
	Lung apices
Lung contours	Mediastinal margins, cardiac borders, diaphragms
Pleural spaces	Check around periphery of lung for pleural effusion, pneumothorax, pleural plaques and calcification
Bones and chest wall	Ribs, clavicles, scapulae and humeri
Other	Check below the diaphragm for free gas and to ensure that the stomach bubble is in correct position beneath the left diaphragm
	In female patients, check that both breast shadows are present and that there has not been a previous mastectomy
	Check the axillae and lower neck for masses or surgical clips

Table 2.2 Checklist for lateral view.

Structure/ anatomical region	Specific features
Heart	Position, size, configuration, calcification
Mediastinum	Trachea, aorta
Right and left hilum	Compare relative size, density and position
Lungs	Retrosternal airspace, between posterior surface of sternum and anterior surface of heart
	Identify both hemidiaphragms
	Posterior costophrenic angles: very small pleural effusions are seen with greater sensitivity than the PA film
Bones	Sternum and thoracic spine

2.3 COMMON FINDINGS ON CXR

Please see Chapter 3 for notes on assessment of the heart and pulmonary vascular patterns on CXR.

2.3.1 Diffuse pulmonary shadowing

Anatomically, functionally and radiologically the lungs may be divided into two compartments, the alveoli (airspaces) and the interstitium. The interstitium refers to soft tissue structures between the alveoli, and includes branching distal bronchi and bronchioles, accompanying arteries, veins and lymphatics, plus supporting connective tissue. The most distal small bronchioles are called terminal bronchioles. Distal to each terminal bronchiole, the lung acinus consists of multiple generations of tiny respiratory bronchioles and alveolar ducts. The alveoli or airspaces arise from the respiratory bronchioles and alveolar ducts. Disease processes that affect the lung may involve the alveoli or the interstitium, or both. One of the most important factors in narrowing the differential diagnosis of diffuse pulmonary shadowing is the ability to differentiate alveolar from interstitial shadowing.

2.3.1.1 Alveolar opacification

Different causes of alveolar opacification (oedema, inflammatory fluid, blood, protein or tumour cells) have the same soft tissue density on CXR. Because appearances are often non-specific, definite diagnosis is usually only made where the CXR findings are correlated with the clinical signs and symptoms.

CXR signs of alveolar shadowing:
- Opacity tends to appear rapidly after the onset of symptoms
- Fluffy, ill-defined areas of opacification
- Areas of consolidation tend to coalesce
- Air bronchograms (Fig. 2.4): air-filled bronchi can be seen as they are outlined by surrounding consolidated lung; air bronchograms are not seen in pleural or mediastinal processes.

Three patterns of distribution of alveolar shadowing tend to occur:
- Segmental or lobar distribution
- Bilateral opacification spreading from the hilar regions into the lungs with relative sparing of the peripheral lungs, sometimes referred to as a 'bat wing' distribution
- Bilateral opacification involving the peripheral lungs with relative sparing of the central regions, sometimes referred to as 'reversed bat wing' distribution.

Alveolar opacification may be acute or chronic. Differential diagnosis lists based on distribution of changes plus whether changes are acute or chronic may be developed.

2.3.1.2 Causes of alveolar opacification

Segmental/lobar alveolar pattern:
- Pneumonia (see below)
- Segmental/lobar collapse (see below)
- Pulmonary infarct
- Alveolar cell carcinoma
- Contusion (associated with rib fractures, pneumothorax and other signs of trauma).
  Acute bilateral central 'bat wing' pattern:
- Pulmonary oedema (Fig. 2.5)
- Pneumonia: *Pneumocystis jiroveci* pneumonia; TB; viral pneumonias; Mycoplasma
- Pulmonary haemorrhage: Goodpasture's syndrome; anticoagulants; bleeding diathesis: haemophilia, disseminated intravascular coagulation (DIC).

Causes of pulmonary oedema:
- Cardiac failure

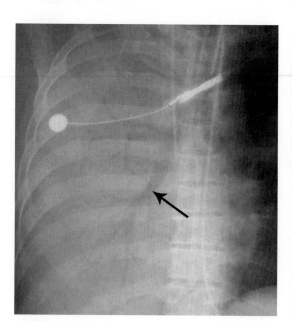

Figure 2.4 Air bronchograms (arrow) indicating extensive alveolar opacification.

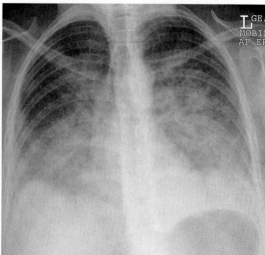

Figure 2.5 'Bat wing' pattern: pulmonary oedema. Extensive bilateral airspace opacification shows parahilar distribution known as the 'bat wing' pattern with relative sparing of the lung periphery.

- Adult respiratory distress syndrome (ARDS)
- Fluid overload
- Drowning and other causes of aspiration
- Head injury or other causes of raised intracranial pressure
- Drugs and poisons (e.g. snake venom, heroin overdose)
- Hypoproteinaemia (e.g. liver disease)
- Blood transfusion reaction.

Chronic bilateral central 'bat wing' pattern:
- Atypical pneumonia: tuberculosis (TB), fungi
- Lymphoma/leukaemia
- Sarcoidosis: interstitial form much more common
- Pulmonary alveolar proteinosis
- Alveolar cell carcinoma: localized form more common.

Reversed 'bat wing' pattern:
- Loeffler's syndrome: transient pulmonary infiltrates associated with blood eosinophilia
- Chronic organizing pneumonia (COP)
- Wegener granulomatosis (Fig. 2.6)
- Fat embolism: occurs 1–2 days after major trauma, particularly with fractures of the large bones of the lower limbs.

2.3.1.3 Interstitial opacification

Three patterns of pulmonary opacification are seen in interstitial processes: linear, nodular and honeycomb pattern. These patterns may occur separately, or together in the same patient with considerable overlap in appearances often encountered.

Linear pattern:
- Network of fine lines running through the lungs
- Lines are due to thickened connective tissue septa
- Kerley A lines: long, thin lines in the upper lobes
- Kerley B lines: short, thin lines predominantly in the lower zones extending 1–2 cm horizontally inwards from the lung surface.

Nodular pattern:
- Nodules due to interstitial disease are small (1–5 mm), well defined and not associated with air bronchograms.
- Nodules tend to be very numerous and are distributed evenly throughout the lungs.

Honeycomb pattern (Fig. 2.7):
- Honeycomb pattern represents the end stage of many of the interstitial processes listed below.
- May also be seen with tuberous sclerosis, amyloidosis, neurofibromatosis and cystic fibrosis.

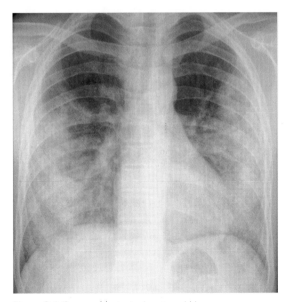

Figure 2.6 'Reversed bat wing' pattern: Wegener granulomatosis. Note the presence of bilateral airspace opacity in a predominantly peripheral distribution with relative sparing of the central parahilar regions.

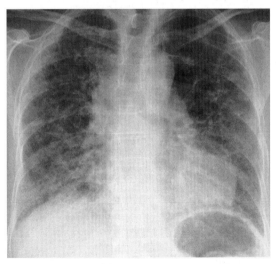

Figure 2.7 Honeycomb lung. Note coarse interstitial opacity throughout both lungs with 'shaggy' appearance of the cardiac borders and hemidiaphragms.

- Honeycomb pattern implies extensive destruction of pulmonary tissue.
- Cysts that range in size from tiny up to 2 cm in diameter replace the lung parenchyma. These cysts have very thin walls.
- Normal pulmonary vasculature cannot be seen.
- Pneumothorax is a frequent complication of honeycomb lung.

The list of interstitial disease processes is extensive. As with alveolar processes, CXR appearances are often non-specific. Short differential diagnosis lists of the more common disorders may be based on whether clinical presentation and CXR findings are acute, subacute or chronic. Chronic diseases may be further subdivided based on their distribution in the lungs, i.e. whether upper or lower zones are predominantly involved.

2.3.1.4 Causes of interstitial opacification

Acute interstitial shadowing:
- Interstitial oedema: Kerley B lines (Fig. 2.8); cardiac enlargement; pleural effusions
- Acute interstitial pneumonia: usually viral.

Subacute interstitial shadowing:
- Lymphangitis carcinomatosis: due to direct malignant infiltration and obstruction of the lymphatic pathways in the pulmonary interstitium
- In patients with a history of carcinoma, lymphangitis carcinomatosis may cause localized or diffuse interstitial shadowing
- Prominent linear and nodular shadowing with Kerley B lines, often associated with mediastinal and/or hilar lymphadenopathy (Fig. 2.9).

Chronic, upper zones:
- TB: upper lobe fibrosis; associated calcification in cavities (Fig. 2.10)
- Sarcoidosis: often associated with hilar lymphadenopathy, although pulmonary involvement alone occurs in 25 per cent of cases
- Silicosis: associated with hilar lymph node calcification and enlargement; may also be associated with large confluent masses, i.e. progressive massive fibrosis (PMF)
- Extrinsic allergic alveolitis
- Bronchopulmonary aspergillosis
- Langerhans cell histiocytosis.

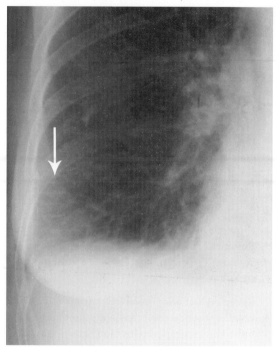

Figure 2.8 Kerley B lines (arrow): interstitial oedema. Note the typical appearance of short linear opacities extending into the lung from the peripheral surface.

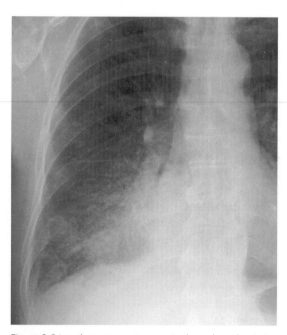

Figure 2.9 Lymphangitis carcinomatosis due to bronchogenic carcinoma. Coarse linear interstitial opacity in the right lower lobe.

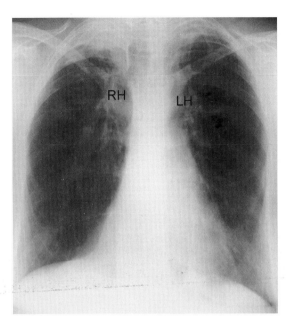

Figure 2.10 Upper lobe fibrosis. Note elevation of right and left hila (RH, LH).

Chronic, lower zones:
- Usual interstitial pneumonia (UIP)
- Asbestosis: may be associated with pleural plaques and calcification, particularly of the diaphragmatic pleura
- Connective tissue disorders: systematic lupus erythematosis (SLE); systemic sclerosis (scleroderma); dermatomyositis/polymyositis.

2.3.2 Lobar pulmonary consolidation and pneumonia

'Pulmonary consolidation' refers to filling of the pulmonary alveoli with fluid (pus, blood and oedema), protein or cells. Radiographic signs of alveolar opacification are described above. Consolidation of a pulmonary lobe or segment is usually due to pneumonia, with other less common causes, such as pulmonary infarct or contusion, usually differentiated on the basis of clinical history. Organisms that commonly cause pneumonia include *Streptococcus pneumoniae, Haemophilus influenzae, Klebsiella pneumoniae* and *Mycoplasma pneumoniae*. Early subtle areas of alveolar shadowing may progress to dense lobar consolidation. Expansion of a lobe with bulging pulmonary fissures may be seen with *Klebsiella*. Necrosis and cavitation may

complicate severe cases of lobar pneumonia. Small pleural effusions commonly accompany pneumonia. More aggressive organisms, such as *Staphylococcus aureus* and *Pseudomonas* may cause more extensive consolidation. This may involve multiple lobes, with cavitation leading to abscess formation. Other complications of pneumonia include empyema and bronchopleural fistula. For further information on pulmonary infections in children, see Chapter 13.

Several radiographic signs may be helpful in localizing areas of pulmonary consolidation. These signs include consolidation adjacent to pulmonary fissures, increased density of the lower thoracic spine on a lateral view and the silhouette sign (Figs 2.11, 2.12, 2.13 and 2.14).

2.3.2.1 Consolidation adjacent to fissures

Straight margins occur in the lungs at the pulmonary fissures. If an area of consolidation or collapse has a straight margin, that margin must abut a fissure and this can help in localization (Fig. 2.11 and Table 2.3).

2.3.2.2 Silhouette sign

The silhouette sign refers to loss of visualization of an anatomical structure or margin due to pathology, and is one of the most important principles in chest radiography. The key to understanding the silhouette

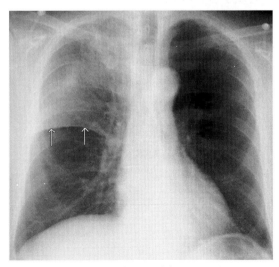

Figure 2.11 Right upper lobe consolidation: pneumonia. Note opacification of the right upper lobe bordered inferiorly by the horizontal fissure (arrows).

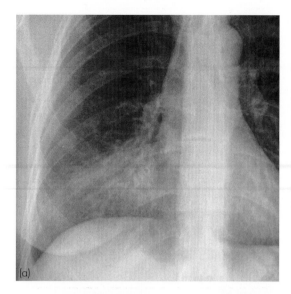

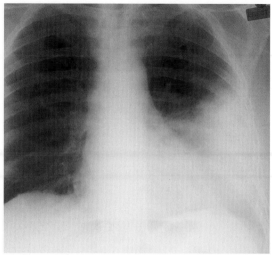

Figure 2.13 Lingula consolidation: pneumonia. Note that consolidation in the lingula obscures the left cardiac border.

object will be seen with conventional radiography if its borders lie beside tissue of different density. This applies especially in the chest where diaphragms, heart and mediastinal structures are well seen due to their lying adjacent to aerated lung. Should a part

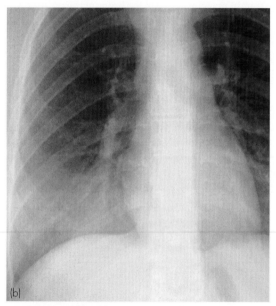

Figure 2.12 Silhouette sign: presence or absence of visible radiographic borders can assist in the diagnosis and localization of pathology as illustrated in these two examples. (a) Consolidation of the right middle lobe obscures the right heart border. (b) Consolidation of the right lower lobe. The right heart border can still be seen.

sign is to remember the five principal densities that are recognized on plain radiographs (see Chapter 1 and Fig. 1.1): air/gas, fat, soft tissue/water, bone and contrast material/metal. The silhouette of an

Table 2.3 Location of pulmonary consolidation or collapse according to fissure abutment.

Lobe of lung	Cause of straight margin
Right upper lobe (Fig. 2.11)	Horizontal fissure inferiorly on PA film. Oblique fissure posteriorly on lateral film
Right middle lobe (Fig. 2.16)	Horizontal fissure superiorly on PA film. Oblique fissure posteriorly on lateral film
Right lower lobe (Fig. 2.17)	Oblique fissure anteriorly on lateral film. Collapse causes rotation and visualization of the oblique fissure on the PA film
Left upper lobe (Fig. 2.18)	Oblique fissure posteriorly on lateral film
Left lower lobe (Fig. 2.19)	Oblique fissure anteriorly on lateral film. Collapse causes rotation and visualization of the oblique fissure on the PA film

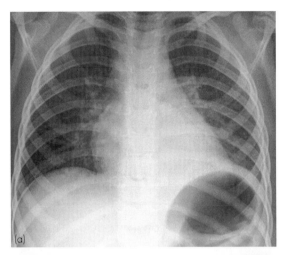

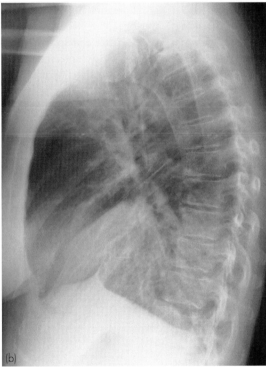

Figure 2.14 Left lower lobe consolidation: pneumonia. (a) On the PA view, consolidation of the left lower lobe produces opacity behind the left heart and loss of definition of the medial aspect of the left diaphragm. (b) On the lateral view, consolidation in either lower lobe may produce apparent increase in density of the lower thoracic vertebral bodies.

Table 2.4 Examples of the silhouette sign in the chest.

Part of lung that is non-aerated	Border that is obscured
Right upper lobe (Fig. 2.11)	Right border of ascending aorta; right mediastinal margin
Right middle lobe (Fig. 2.12)	Right heart border
Right lower lobe (Fig. 2.12)	Right diaphragm
Left upper lobe (Fig. 2.18)	Aortic arch, upper left cardiac border
Left lingula (Fig. 2.13)	Left heart border
Left lower lobe (Fig. 2.14)	Left diaphragm, descending aorta

2.3.2.3 Increased density of lower thoracic spine on the lateral view

On the lateral view, the thoracic vertebral bodies should show a gradual apparent decrease in density as one peruses from top to bottom (see Fig. 2.2). Opacification in the right or left lower lobes may produce an apparent increase in density of the lower thoracic vertebral bodies. This may be the most obvious radiographic sign of lower lobe pneumonia (Fig. 2.14), in particular small areas of consolidation obscured by the heart on the PA view.

2.3.3 Pulmonary collapse

Pulmonary collapse most commonly takes the form of linear or disc-like areas of focal collapse, referred to as linear or discoid atelectasis. Causes of linear atelectasis include:
- Postoperative
- Inflammatory or other painful pathology beneath the diaphragm, e.g. pancreatitis, acute cholecystitis
- Pulmonary embolus
- Following resolution of pneumonia.

More extensive collapse may involve pulmonary segments or lobes. Causes of pulmonary lobar or segmental collapse include:

of lung lying against any of these structures become non-aerated due to collapse, consolidation or a mass, the outline of that structure will no longer be seen (Fig. 2.12 and Table 2.4).

- Bronchial obstruction
  - Tumour
  - Foreign body
  - Mucous plug, e.g. asthma, cystic fibrosis
- Passive collapse due to external pressure on the lung
  - Pneumothorax
  - Pleural effusion or haemothorax
  - Diaphragmatic hernia (neonate)
- Scarring or fibrosis
  - TB (upper lobes)
  - Radiation pneumonitis (post-radiotherapy).

2.3.3.1 General signs of lobar collapse

The most important initial sign for differentiating lobar collapse from consolidation is decreased volume of the affected lung. Other signs of collapse include:

- Displacement of pulmonary fissures
- Local increase in density due to non-aerated lung
- Elevation of ipsilateral hemidiaphragm
- Displacement of hilum
- Displacement of mediastinum towards side of collapse
- Compensatory overinflation of adjacent lobes
- Loss of visualization of anatomical structures: silhouette sign.

2.3.3.2 Specific signs of lobar collapse

Each hilum may be thought of as a hinge, upon which the lung may rotate should there be upper or lower lobe collapse. The upper lobes tend to collapse upwards and anteriorly; the lower lobes collapse inferiorly and posteriorly. This leads to predictable radiographic appearances of the various types of lobar collapse as follows, summarized in Table 2.5 and illustrated with Figs 2.15, 2.16, 2.17, 2.18 and 2.19.

2.3.4 Solitary pulmonary nodule or mass

Solitary pulmonary nodule is a common incidental finding on CXR. The definition of a solitary pulmonary nodule is a spherical lung opacity seen on CXR or CT, measuring less than 3 cm diameter, and not associated with pulmonary collapse or lymphadenopathy. Opacities larger than 3 cm are referred to as masses and are more likely to be malignant.

Differential diagnosis of solitary pulmonary nodule:

- Bronchogenic carcinoma (Fig. 2.20)
- Solitary metastasis
- Granuloma including tuberculoma (Fig. 2.21)
- Carcinoid tumour
- Arteriovenous malformation.

Table 2.5 Specific features of lobar collapse.

Lobe	Direction of collapse	Hilum displacement	Increased density	Silhouette sign
Right upper	Upwards, anterior	Right, upwards	Right upper zone	Right mediastinum
Right middle	Anterior	None	PA: right midzone Lateral: triangular opacity overlying heart	Right heart border
Right lower	Downwards, posterior	Right, downwards	Triangular opacity right base	Right hemidiaphragm
Left upper	Upwards, anterior	Left, upwards	Left upper and midzone	Aortic arch[a] Upper left heart border
Left lower	Downwards, posterior	Left, downwards	Triangular opacity left base, behind heart	Left diaphragm, descending aorta

[a]Note that in complete collapse of the left upper lobe, the aortic arch may be visible. This is because the apical segment of the left lower lobe may be pulled upwards and forwards enough such that aerated lung lies beside the aortic arch.

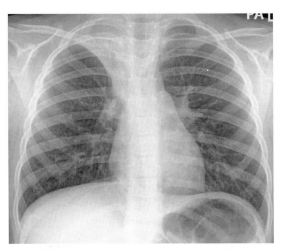

Figure 2.15 Right upper lobe collapse. Note right upper zone opacity with reduced volume of right hemithorax and elevation of the horizontal fissure.

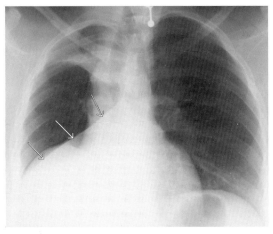

Figure 2.17 Right lower lobe collapse. Triangular opacity behind the right heart (arrows) with loss of definition of the right diaphragm. The right heart border is still seen. Note that in this case the right upper lobe is also collapsed.

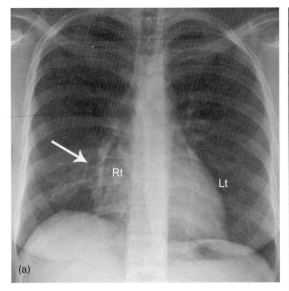

(a)

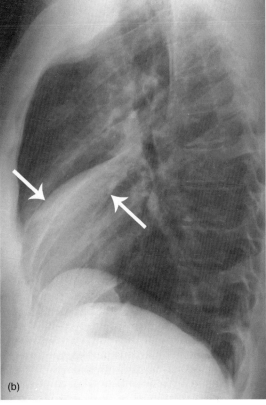

(b)

Figure 2.16 Right middle lobe collapse. (a) PA view shows loss of volume on the right with opacity (arrow) obscuring the right heart border (Rt). Compare this with the left heart border (Lt), which is clearly seen. (b) Lateral view shows the typical triangular-shaped opacity produced by collapsed right middle lobe (arrows).

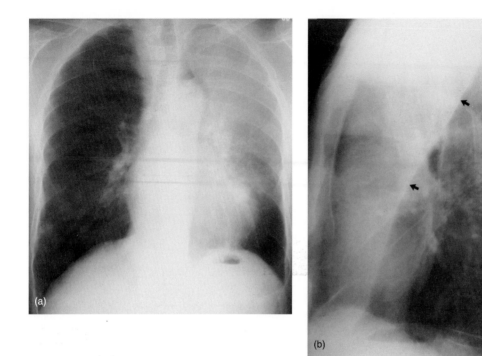

Figure 2.18 Left upper lobe collapse. (a) PA view shows loss of volume on the left and opacity in the left upper zone. The aortic arch is able to be seen due to elevation of the aerated left lower lobe. (b) Lateral view shows the typical pattern of left upper lobe collapse with the oblique fissure pulled upwards and anteriorly (arrows).

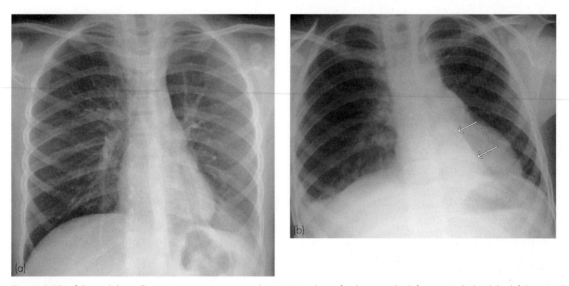

Figure 2.19 Left lower lobe collapse: two separate examples. (a) Note loss of volume on the left, opacity behind the left heart, and blurring of the left diaphragm. (b) A more classical, though less commonly seen pattern of left lower lobe collapse with a sharply defined triangular opacity behind the left heart (arrows).

The aim of investigation and follow-up of pulmonary nodules is to diagnose those that are malignant, and to facilitate early resection.

Features associated with a higher likelihood of malignancy:

- Evidence of rapid growth on serial CXR examinations
- Ill-defined margin
- Size >3 cm
- No calcification.

Features associated with a lower likelihood of malignancy:

- Calcification
- Well-defined margin
- Small size
  - Most granulomas measure 0.3–1.0 cm in diameter
- Unchanged on serial CXR examinations.

Findings on CXR that are sufficiently predictive of a benign aetiology to preclude further investigation are calcification and lack of growth over two years. Comparison with previous CXRs is therefore essential, if these are available. These benign features are present in a minority of solitary pulmonary nodules and most require further imaging investigations, particularly where there are underlying risk factors for lung cancer. Risk factors include cigarette smoking, exposure to asbestos, and a history of lung cancer in a first-degree relative. The two most commonly used imaging investigations for solitary pulmonary nodule are CT and FDG-PET, with CT the first investigation of choice in most instances.

2.3.4.1 CT

CT features suggestive of benign aetiology:

- Small size: risk of malignancy is roughly proportional to nodule size and is about 1 per cent in nodules less than 10 mm diameter
- Calcification
- Fat (see Fig. 1.6)
- Smooth border.

CT features suggestive of malignancy:

- Size >3 cm
- Spiculated (irregular) margin
- Contrast enhancement

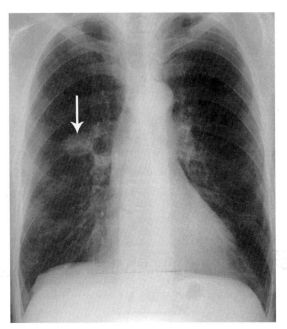

Figure 2.20 Solitary pulmonary nodule (arrow): bronchogenic carcinoma.

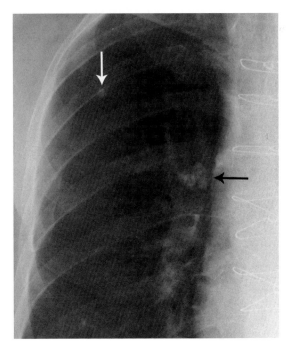

Figure 2.21 Tuberculosis: healed primary. Calcified granuloma in right upper lobe (white arrow) and calcified mediastinal lymph nodes (black arrow).

- Other findings: lymphadenopathy, multiple lung lesions, liver metastases.

The Fleischner Society has developed guidelines for the follow-up of small pulmonary nodules; these guidelines are based on nodule size and patient risk factors (Table 2.6).

Table 2.6 Fleischner Society guidelines for follow-up of pulmonary nodules.

Nodule size	Low-risk patient	High-risk patient
4 mm or less	No follow-up	CT at 12 months; no further if unchanged
4–6 mm	CT at 12 months; no further if unchanged	CT at 6–12 months, then 18–24 months if unchanged
7–8 mm	CT at 6–12 months, then 18–24 months if unchanged	CT at 3–6 months, then at 12 and 24 months if unchanged
>8 mm	CT at 3, 9 and 24 months	CT at 3, 9 and 24 months
	Consider FDG-PET and/or biopsy	Consider FDG-PET and/or biopsy

2.3.4.2 FDG-PET

FDG-PET may be useful to characterize solitary pulmonary nodules where other imaging is unhelpful. FDG-PET is particularly useful for lesions that are not amenable to biopsy. Neoplastic masses show increased uptake of FDG. FDG-PET is unable to accurately characterize lesions less than 1 cm in diameter. False-positive findings may occur in active inflammatory lesions.

2.3.4.3 Biopsy

Lesions that have positive findings for malignancy on CT or FDG-PET usually require biopsy. Biopsy may be performed via bronchoscopy, percutaneously with CT guidance (Fig. 2.22), with VATS, or by open surgical biopsy and resection.

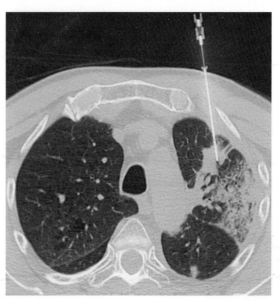

Figure 2.22 Computer tomography-guided lung biopsy.

2.3.5 Multiple pulmonary nodules

Whereas solitary pulmonary nodule is commonly seen as an incidental finding, this is less often the case with multiple pulmonary nodules. More commonly, multiple pulmonary nodules are seen in symptomatic patients, or in patients with underlying pathology, such as immunosuppression or malignancy. The commonest exception to this would be multiple small calcified granulomas, which may indicate previous infection including TB or chicken pox pneumonia (Fig. 2.23).

Differential diagnosis of multiple pulmonary nodules:
- Granulomas
- Metastases (Fig. 2.24)
  - Usually well defined
  - Nodules of varying size
  - More common peripherally and in the lower lobes
  - Cavitation seen in squamous cell carcinomas, sarcomas and metastases from colonic primaries
- Abscesses
  - Cavitation: thick, irregular wall
  - Usually due to *Staphylococcus aureus*

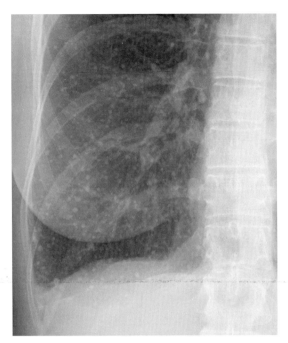

Figure 2.23 Multiple calcified granulomas due to previous chicken pox pneumonia.

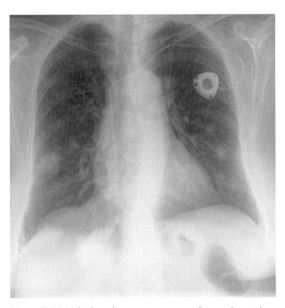

Figure 2.24 Multiple pulmonary metastases from colorectal carcinoma. Note bilateral soft tissue nodules of variable size.

- Fungal infection
  - More common in immunocompromised patients, e.g. bone marrow transplant in children

- Hydatid cysts
  - Often quite large, i.e. 10 cm or more
- Wegener's granulomatosis
  - Cavitation of nodules common
  - Associated paranasal sinus disease
- Multiple arteriovenous malformations.

2.3.6 Mediastinal masses

Signs on CXR that a central opacity or mass lies within the mediastinum rather than the lung include:
- Continuity with the mediastinal outline
- Sharp margin
- Convex margin
- Absence of air bronchograms.

Logical classification and differential diagnosis of mediastinal masses is based on localization to the anterior, middle or posterior mediastinum.

2.3.6.1 Anterior mediastinal mass

Causes of an anterior mediastinal mass:
- Retrosternal goitre
- Thymic tumour
- Thymic cyst
- Lymphadenopathy
  - Hodgkin's disease
  - Metastases
- Aneurysm of ascending aorta.

CXR signs of an anterior mediastinal mass (Fig. 2.25):
- Merge with cardiac border
- Hilar structures can be seen through the mass
- Masses passing upwards into the neck merge radiologically with the soft tissues of the neck and so are not seen above the clavicles
  - This is known as the cervicothoracic sign; a lesion seen above the clavicles must lie adjacent to aerated lung apices, i.e. posterior and within the thorax
- Displaced trachea.

2.3.6.2 Middle mediastinal mass

Differential diagnosis of a middle mediastinal mass includes:
- Lymphadenopathy, mediastinal or hilar
  - Bronchogenic carcinoma, less commonly other tumours (Fig. 2.26)
  - Lymphoma

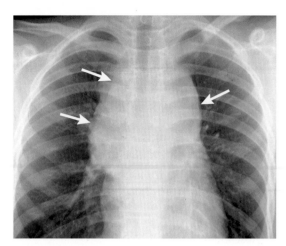

Figure 2.25 Anterior mediastinal mass: Hodgkin's disease. Bilateral anterior mediastinal mass merging with upper cardiac borders (arrows).

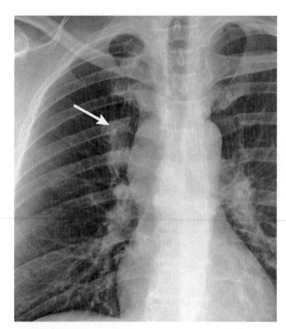

Figure 2.26 Middle mediastinal mass: lymphadenopathy due to bronchogenic carcinoma. Note small mass in right upper lobe (arrow) adjacent to lymphadenopathy.

- Bronchogenic cyst
- Aortic aneurysm.

    CXR signs of a middle mediastinal mass:
- Opacity that merges with the hilar structures and cardiac borders.

2.3.6.3 Posterior mediastinal mass

Differential diagnosis of a posterior mediastinal mass:
- Hiatus hernia
    - Round opacity located behind the heart
    - May contain a fluid level
- Neurogenic tumour
    - Well-defined mass in the paravertebral region (Fig. 2.27)
    - May be associated with erosion or destruction of vertebral bodies or posterior ribs
- Anterior thoracic meningocele
    - Associated with neurofibromatosis
- Neurenteric cyst
    - Associated with vertebral abnormalities
- Aneurysm of descending thoracic aorta
- Paravertebral lymphadenopathy.

    CXR signs of a posterior mediastinal mass:
- Does not obscure heart and middle mediastinal structures
    - Cardiac borders and hila clearly seen
- Posterior descending aorta obscured
- May be underlying vertebral changes.

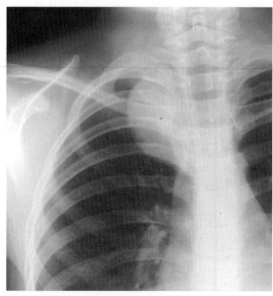

Figure 2.27 Posterior mediastinal mass: neurogenic tumour. Mass can be seen above the clavicle indicating posterior position ('cervicothoracic sign').

2.3.7 Hilar disorders

Each hilar complex as seen on the PA and lateral chest radiographs comprises the proximal pulmonary arteries, bronchus, pulmonary veins and lymph nodes. Hilar lymph nodes are not visualized unless enlarged. In assessing hilar enlargement, be it bilateral or unilateral, one must decide whether it is due to enlargement of the pulmonary arteries, or some other cause like lymphadenopathy or a mass. If the branching pulmonary arteries are seen to converge into an apparent mass, this is a good sign of enlarged main pulmonary artery (hilum convergence sign).

Causes of unilateral hilar enlargement:
- Bronchial carcinoma (Fig. 2.28)
- Infective causes
  - TB
  - Mycoplasma
- Perihilar pneumonia
  - An area of pneumonia lying anterior or posterior to the hilum may cause *apparent* hilar enlargement on the PA film
  - Usually obvious on the lateral film
- Other causes of lymphadenopathy (more commonly bilateral)
  - Lymphoma
  - Sarcoidosis

- Causes of enlargement of a single pulmonary artery
  - Post-stenotic dilatation on the left side due to pulmonary stenosis
  - Massive unilateral pulmonary embolus
  - Pulmonary artery aneurysm (often calcified).

Causes of bilateral hilar enlargement:
- Bilateral pulmonary artery enlargement
  - Pulmonary arterial hypertension
- Lymphoma
  - Often asymmetrical
- Metastatic malignancy
  - Bronchogenic carcinoma
  - Non-pulmonary primary, e.g. testis
- Sarcoidosis (Fig. 2.29)
  - Disease of unknown aetiology characterized by the widespread formation of non-caseating granulomas
  - Chest is the commonest site of involvement
    - Lymphadenopathy alone in 50 per cent
    - Lymphadenopathy plus lung changes in 25 per cent
    - Lung changes alone in 25 per cent

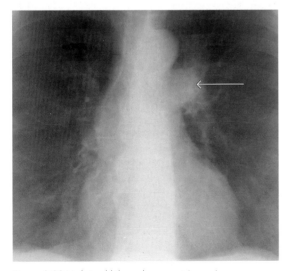

Figure 2.28 Unilateral hilar enlargement (arrow): bronchogenic carcinoma.

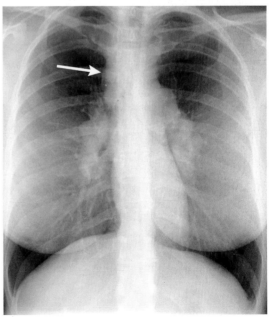

Figure 2.29 Bilateral hilar enlargement: sarcoidosis. PA view showing enlarged right hilum and left hilum due to lymphadenopathy as well as right mediastinal lymphadenopathy (arrow).

- Hilar lymphadenopathy is usually symmetrical and lobulated, and associated with right paratracheal lymphadenopathy
- The lung changes of sarcoidosis consist of small interstitial nodules 2–5 mm diameter spread through both lungs, predominantly in the midzones
- Healing may lead to bilateral upper zone fibrosis
- Extrathoracic sites of involvement with sarcoidosis include liver, spleen, peripheral lymph nodes, CNS, eyes (uveitis), bone, salivary glands and skin (erythema nodosum).

2.3.8 Pleural disorders

Pleural disorders include accumulation of fluid in the pleural spaces (pleural effusion), air leaks (pneumothorax and pneumomediastinum), and pleural soft tissue thickening and plaque formation.

2.3.8.1 Pleural effusion

Pleural effusion refers to accumulation of fluid in the pleural space, between the visceral and parietal pleural layers. The radiographic appearances of pleural effusion are generally the same regardless of the nature of the fluid, which may include transudate, exudate, blood, pus (empyema) or lymph (chylothorax).

Causes of pleural effusion:
- Cardiac failure
  - Bilateral pleural effusions, right usually larger than left
- Malignancy
  - Bronchogenic carcinoma
  - Metastatic
  - Mesothelioma
- Infection
  - Bacterial pneumonia
  - TB
  - Mycoplasma
  - Empyema
  - Subphrenic abscess
- Pulmonary embolus with infarct
- Pancreatitis: effusion is usually left-sided
- Trauma: associated with rib fractures
- Connective tissue disorders

  - Rheumatoid arthritis
  - SLE
- Liver failure
- Renal failure
- Meig's syndrome: associated with ovarian tumour.

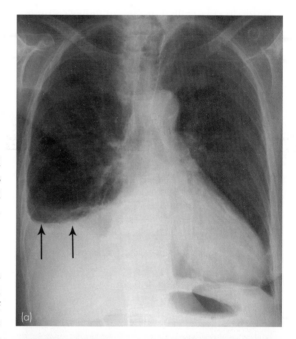

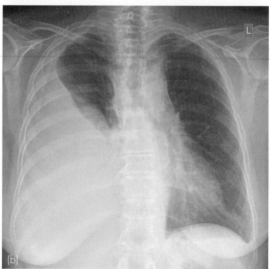

Figure 2.30 Pleural effusion. (a) Pleural effusion producing a fluid level at the right base (arrows). The outer edge of the fluid tracks a small distance up the chest wall producing a typical meniscus shape. (b) Massive right pleural effusion.

Signs of pleural effusion on erect CXR (Fig. 2.30):
- Homogeneous dense opacity at the base of the lung
- Concave upper surface higher laterally than medially, producing a meniscus
- Small pleural effusions produce blunting of the normal sharp angle between the lateral curve of the diaphragm and the inner chest wall, referred to as blunting of the costophrenic angle
- Large pleural effusions displace the mediastinum towards the contralateral side.

The lateral view is more sensitive to the presence of small pleural effusions than the PA view. It is estimated that about 300 mL of fluid is required to show costophrenic angle blunting on the PA, whereas only 100 mL is required to produce this sign (posteriorly) on the lateral view.

Variations to the 'normal' appearance of pleural effusion:
- Loculations, i.e. failure of pleural fluid to layer out in a dependent position
  - Pleural fluid may accumulate laterally or over the lung apices and may resemble pleural masses
- Causes of loculation of pleural fluid include
  - Pleural scarring
  - Distortion of the lung due to collapse, fibrosis or surgery
  - Complex, thick fluid, e.g. empyema
- Fluid accumulating in a pulmonary fissure may mimic a pulmonary mass
- Subpulmonic effusion: fluid trapped beneath the lung produces opacity parallel to the diaphragm with a convex upper margin.

Signs of pleural fluid on supine CXR (Fig. 2.31) include opacity over the lung apex (pleural cap) and increased opacity of the hemithorax, through which lung structures can still be seen. There is often loss of definition of the hemidiaphragm and blunting of the costophrenic angle. The opacity caused by pleural effusion in a supine patient may be differentiated from pulmonary consolidation by the absence of air bronchograms.

2.3.8.2 Pneumothorax

Pneumothorax refers to accumulation of air in the pleural space, between the visceral and parietal pleural layers.

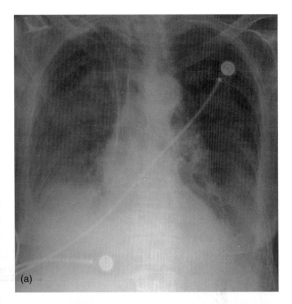
(a)

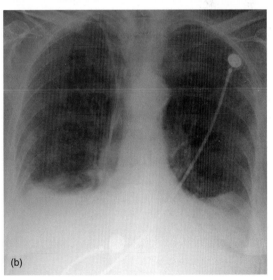
(b)

Figure 2.31 Pleural effusions on supine CXR. (a) Supine CXR: pleural effusions produce vague opacity over both lower zones with poor definition of each hemidiaphragm. Lack of air bronchograms and visualization of pulmonary structures helps differentiate pleural effusions from pulmonary consolidation. (b) Erect CXR confirms the diagnosis of bilateral pleural effusions.

Causes of pneumothorax:
- Spontaneous
  - Tall, thin males
  - Smokers
- Iatrogenic
  - Percutaneous lung biopsy

- • Complication of ventilation
- • Central venous pressure (CVP) line or cardiac pacemaker insertion
- Trauma: associated with rib fractures
- Emphysema
- Malignancy: high incidence with osteogenic sarcoma metastases
- Honeycomb lung
- Lymphangiomyomatosis (LAM): interstitial disease of young women
- Cystic fibrosis.

Pneumothorax is usually well seen on a normal inspiratory PA film. The diagnosis of small pneumothorax may be easier on an expiratory film. This is due to reduced volume of the lung in expiration, which makes the pneumothorax look relatively larger. Whether the film is performed in inspiration or expiration, the sign to look for is the lung edge outlined by air in the pleural space (Fig. 2.32).

Tension pneumothorax occurs with continued air leak from the lung into the pleural space. This results in increased pressure in the pleural space with expansion of the hemithorax and further compression and collapse of the lung.

CXR signs of tension pneumothorax (Fig. 2.33):
- Marked collapse and distortion of the lung
- Increased volume of hemithorax
  - • Displacement of the mediastinum to the contralateral side

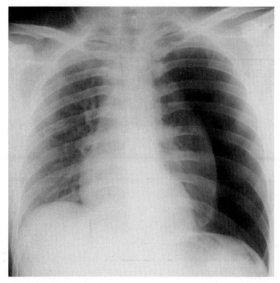

Figure 2.33 Tension pneumothorax. Signs of tension include expansion of the left hemithorax, increased space between the left ribs, shift of the mediastinal structures to the right, and severe collapse of the left lung.

- • Depressed diaphragm
- • Increased space between the ribs.

Supine AP CXR may have to be performed in ICU patients or following severe trauma. Pleural air lays anteromedially and beneath the lung so that the usual appearance of a pneumothorax as described for an erect PA film is not seen.

Signs of pneumothorax on a supine CXR (Fig. 2.34):
- Mediastinal structures including heart border, inferior vena cava (IVC), SVC are sharply outlined by adjacent free pleural air
- Upper abdomen appears lucent due to overlying air
- Deep lateral costophrenic angle.

2.3.8.3 Pneumomediastinum

Pneumomediastinum refers to air leak into the soft tissues of the mediastinum.

Causes of pneumomediastinum:
- Spontaneous: following severe coughing or strenuous exercise
- Asthma
- Foreign body aspiration in neonates
- Chest trauma

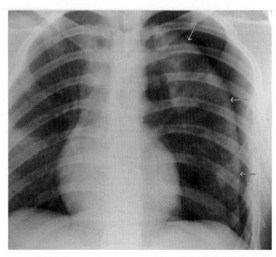

Figure 2.32 Pneumothorax. The edge of the partly collapsed lung (arrows) is outlined by the pneumothorax.

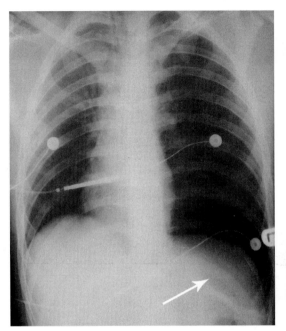

Figure 2.34 Supine pneumothorax. Pneumothorax in a supine patient shows as an area of lucency over the lower left hemithorax and upper left abdomen (arrow). Note also increased volume on the left indicating tension. (See also Fig. 16.3.)

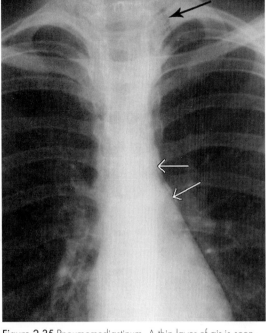

Figure 2.35 Pneumomediastinum. A thin layer of air is seen parallel to the left mediastinal margin (white arrows). Air is also seen tracking into the soft tissues of the neck (black arrow).

- Oesophageal perforation: tumour, severe vomiting and endoscopy.

Radiographic signs of pneumomediastinum are due to air outlining the normal mediastinal structures:
- A strip of air outlining the left side of the mediastinum
- Air around the aorta, pulmonary arteries and pericardium
- Subcutaneous air extending upwards into the soft tissues of the neck (Fig. 2.35).

2.3.8.4 Pleural thickening

Pleural thickening or pleural plaque formation may occur in a variety of circumstances:
- Secondary to trauma
  - Associated with healed rib fractures
  - Dense layer of soft tissue, often calcified
- Following empyema
  - More common over the lung bases
  - Often calcified

- TB
- Asbestos exposure
  - Irregular pleural thickening and pleural plaques (Fig. 2.36)
  - Calcification common, especially of diaphragmatic surface of pleura
  - Note that pleural disease is not asbestosis; the term 'asbestosis' refers to the interstitial lung disease secondary to asbestos exposure
- Mesothelioma
  - Diffuse or localized pleural mass
  - Rib destruction uncommon
  - Large pleural effusions common
  - Pleural plaques elsewhere in 50 per cent
- Pancoast tumour
  - Primary apical lung neoplasm
  - Rib destruction with irregular pleural thickening
- Pleural metastases
  - Often obscured by associated pleural effusion.

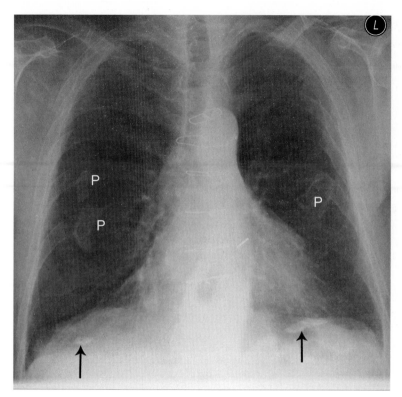

Figure 2.36 Pleural plaques: asbestos exposure. Multiple plaques (P) are seen as well-defined though irregular opacities projected over the lungs. Note also linear regions of pleural calcification (arrows).

Various radiographic appearances related to pleural thickening or plaque formation may be seen:
- Blunting of costophrenic angles, mimicking pleural effusion
- Soft tissue thickening over the lungs, including the lung apices
- Calcification of the pleural surfaces due to previous pleural haemorrhage or infection
- Pleural plaques
  - Convex, pleural-based opacities when seen in profile
  - Less well-defined opacities when not in profile
  - May be calcified, especially with a history of exposure to asbestos.

2.3.9 Emphysema

Emphysema refers to enlarged airspaces secondary to destruction of the alveolar walls. Centrilobular emphysema is the most common form; it occurs in smokers and predominantly affects the upper lobes. Panlobular emphysema is seen in association with alpha-1 antitrypsin deficiency; it tends to predominantly affect the lower lobes.

CXR signs of emphysema (Fig. 2.37):
- Overexpanded lungs
  - Flattening of the diaphragms, best seen on lateral CXR
  - Diaphragms lie below anterior end of sixth rib on frontal view
  - Increased retrosternal airspace on lateral film
  - Beware incorrect diagnosis of pulmonary overexpansion in a young, athletic patient capable of a large inspiration
- Decreased vascular markings in lung fields
- Increased AP diameter of the chest, with in some cases kyphosis and anterior bowing of the sternum
- Bulla formation: bullae are seen as thin-walled air-containing cavities
- Pulmonary arterial hypertension: prominent main pulmonary arteries.

High resolution CT of the lungs (HRCT) may be used to assess accurately the severity and distribution of emphysema, quantitate the percentage of residual healthy lung, and identify associated findings such as bronchogenic carcinoma.

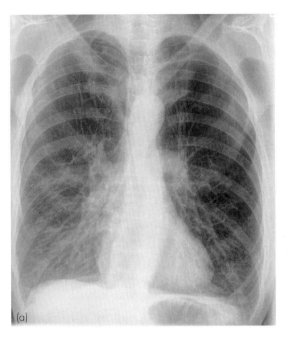

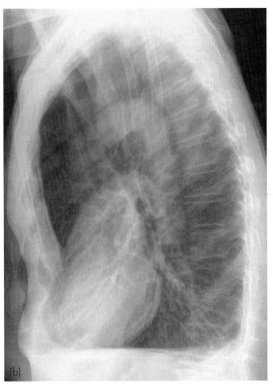

Figure 2.37 Emphysema. (a) PA radiograph showing overexpansion of both lungs. (b) Lateral radiograph showing flattening of the hemidiaphragms and increased size of retrosternal airspace posterior to the sternum.

2.3.10 Tuberculosis

2.3.10.1 Primary TB

Primary TB is usually asymptomatic. The healed pulmonary lesion of primary TB may be seen on CXR as a small, calcified peripheral pulmonary nodule with calcified hilar lymph node (Fig. 2.21).

2.3.10.2 Post-primary pulmonary TB (reactivation TB)

Post-primary TB has a predilection for the apical and posterior segments of the upper lobes, plus the apical segments of the lower lobes. Variable CXR appearances may include ill-defined areas of alveolar consolidation and thick-walled, irregular cavities (Fig. 2.38). Haemoptysis, aspergilloma, tuberculous empyema and bronchopleural fistula may complicate cavitation. Subsequent fibrosis may cause volume loss in the upper lobes. Fibrosis and calcification usually indicate disease inactivity and healing, but one should never diagnose inactive TB on a single CXR; serial films are essential to prove inactivity.

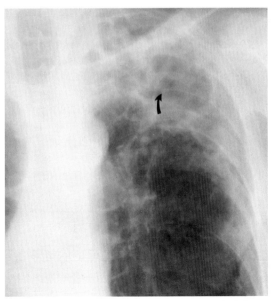

Figure 2.38 Tuberculosis: post-primary. Opacity in the left upper lobe with cavitation (arrow).

2.3.10.3 Miliary TB

Miliary TB occurs due to haematogenous dissemination, which may occur at any time following primary infection. On CXR, miliary TB appears as tiny densities of approximately 2 mm diameter spread evenly through both lungs.

2.3.11 Usual interstitial pneumonia

The term 'idiopathic interstitial pneumonia' refers to a group of diffuse lung diseases that share many features despite being separate disease entities. Diseases classified under this term include usual interstitial pneumonia (UIP), non-specific interstitial pneumonia (NSIP), desquamative interstitial pneumonia (DIP), acute interstitial pneumonia (AIP), lymphoid interstitial pneumonia (LIP) and cryptogenic organizing pneumonia (COP). The commonest form of idiopathic interstitial pneumonia is UIP, also known as idiopathic pulmonary fibrosis.

Usual intersitital pneumonia is a chronic lung disorder characterized by diffuse interstitial inflammation and fibrosis. Peak incidence is 50–60 years of age. Patients present with insidious onset of dyspnoea with exertion. Diagnosis relies on abnormal pulmonary function tests with evidence of restriction and impaired gas exchange, exclusion of other causes of interstitial lung disease, such as connective tissue disorders and drug toxicity, and typical findings on HRCT.

CXR signs of UIP include an interstitial linear pattern, predominantly at the lung bases (Fig. 2.7). This produces an irregular 'shaggy' heart border. As the disease progresses there is loss of lung volume and development of the honeycomb lung pattern. HRCT findings include a peripheral linear pattern involving predominantly the lower lobes. There is often also diffuse density known as a 'ground-glass' pattern. These changes progress over time to a honeycomb pattern, seen on HRCT as coarse irregular linear opacity with cyst-like air spaces (Fig. 2.39).

2.4 CT IN THE INVESTIGATION OF CHEST DISORDERS

CT of the chest may be used in a number of ways including:

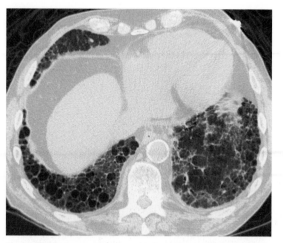

Figure 2.39 Honeycomb lung: high resolution CT (HRCT). HRCT in a patient with end-stage usual interstitial pneumonia shows replacement of normal pulmonary parenchyma with air-filled cysts and coarse linear markings.

- Further characterization of CXR findings
- As a primary investigation of chest disease
- Procedure guidance
- HRCT
- CT pulmonary angiography (CTPA) (see Chapter 3).

2.4.1 CT for further characterization of CXR findings

- Mediastinal mass (Fig. 2.40)
  - Accurate localization
  - Characterization of internal contents of mass: fat, air, fluid and calcification
  - Displacement/invasion of adjacent structures, such as aorta, heart, trachea, oesophagus, vertebral column, chest wall
- Hilar mass
  - Greater sensitivity than plain films for the presence of hilar lymphadenopathy
  - Greater specificity in differentiating lymphadenopathy or hilar mass from enlarged pulmonary arteries
- Characterization of a pulmonary mass seen on CXR
  - More accurate than plain films for the presence of calcification or fat
  - Other factors also well assessed by CT include cavitation and relation of a mass to the chest wall or mediastinum

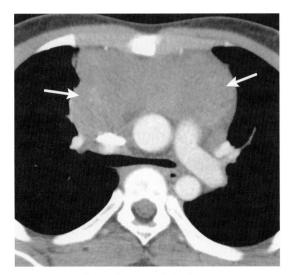

Figure 2.40 Hodgkin's disease: CT. CT shows an anterior mediastinal mass (arrows) due to lymphadenopathy (same patient as Fig. 2.25).

- Intravenous contrast material may help to identify aberrant vessels and arteriovenous malformations
- Suspected vascular anomaly as a cause for abnormality on CXR
  - Azygos continuation of IVC
  - Partial anomalous pulmonary venous drainage
- Characterization of pleural disease
  - CT provides excellent delineation of pleural abnormalities, which may produce confusing appearances on CXR
  - Pleural masses, fluid collections, calcifications and tumours such as mesothelioma are well shown, as are complications such as rib destruction, mediastinal invasion and lymphadenopathy.

2.4.2 Chest CT as primary investigation of choice

- Staging of bronchogenic carcinoma
  - Greater sensitivity than CXR for the presence of mediastinal or hilar lymphadenopathy
  - Greater sensitivity for complications such as chest wall or mediastinal invasion, and cavitation

- Detection of pulmonary metastases
  - CT has greater sensitivity than CXR for the detection of small pulmonary lesions, including metastases
  - This is particularly so in areas of the lung seen poorly on CXR including the apices, posterior segments of the lower lobes, and medial areas that are obscured by the hila
- Chest trauma
  - Exclusion of mediastinal haematoma in a haemodynamically stable patient with a widened mediastinum on CXR following chest trauma
  - CT angiogram to assess aorta (see below)
  - Accurate delineation of chest injuries including pneumothorax, haemothorax, pulmonary contusion
  - Multidetector CT (MDCT) also allows immediate assessment of bony structures including thoracic spine, sternum and ribs
- Diseases of the thoracic aorta
  - Thoracic aortic aneurysm
  - Aortic dissection.

2.4.3 CT for guidance of percutaneous biopsy and drainage procedures

CT-guided biopsy is especially useful for peripheral lesions not amenable to bronchoscopic biopsy.

2.4.4 High resolution CT

High resolution CT is a modified chest CT technique whereby thin 1–2 mm sections provide highly detailed views of the lung parenchyma. There are two methods for performing HRCT:

- Reconstruction of fine sections from MDCT: 1–2 mm sections may be reconstructed from chest CT or CT pulmonary angiography
- 'Traditional' method: 1–2 mm sections obtained at intervals of 10–20 mm through the lungs
  - Lower radiation dose
  - Intravenous contrast material is not used
  - Mediastinal and chest wall structures are less well seen than with MDCT.

Whatever method of acquisition is used, HRCT is used to detect and characterize diffuse lung diseases as follows.

2.4.4.1 Bronchiectasis

High resolution CT is the investigation of choice in the assessment of bronchiectasis (Fig. 2.41). As well as showing dilated bronchi, HRCT accurately shows the anatomical distribution of changes, in addition to complications, such as scarring, collapse, consolidation and mucous plugging.

2.4.4.2 Interstitial lung disease

High resolution CT is more sensitive and specific than plain films in the diagnosis of many interstitial lung diseases. Sarcoidosis, idiopathic interstitial pneumonias, lymphangitis carcinomatosis and Langerhans cell histiocytosis are examples of disorders that have specific appearances on HRCT, often obviating the need for biopsy in these patients. Surgical biopsy is often required for specific diagnosis of interstitial lung disease; HRCT may aid in guiding the operator to the most favourable biopsy site.

2.4.4.3 Atypical infections

High resolution CT provides diagnosis of many atypical infections earlier and with greater specificity than plain CXR. Examples include infections that occur in immunocompromised patients, such as pneumocystis pneumonia, aspergillosis and candidosis. As well as assisting with diagnosis, HRCT may be useful for monitoring disease progress and response to therapy.

2.4.4.4 Chronic lung diseases in children

High resolution CT is used to monitor changes associated with cystic fibrosis, such as mucous plugging and pulmonary collapse, acute infective episodes, and acute bronchopulmonary aspergillosis (ABPA). Other examples of childhood lung disease where HRCT may be helpful include chronic lung disease of infancy and interstitial lung diseases, e.g. neuroendocrine hyperplasia of infancy (NEHI).

2.4.4.5 Normal CXR in symptomatic patients

High resolution CT has a definite role in the assessment of patients with an apparently

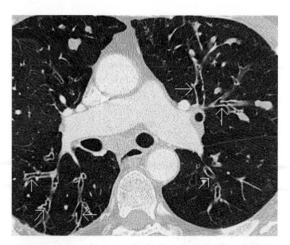

Figure 2.41 Bronchiectasis: high resolution CT. Dilated thick-walled bronchi (arrows). Compare this appearance with the normal lungs in Fig. 1.5b.

normal CXR, despite strong clinical indications of respiratory disease, including dyspnoea, chest pain, haemoptysis and abnormal pulmonary function tests. In such cases, the much greater sensitivity of HRCT may provide a diagnosis or direct further investigations, such as lung biopsy.

2.5 HAEMOPTYSIS

Haemoptysis refers to the expectoration of blood from the tracheobronchial tree or lung. The commonest cause of haemoptysis is erosion of bronchial mucosa in smokers with chronic bronchitis. The next most common cause is bronchogenic carcinoma. Haemoptysis may also be encountered with pulmonary infections, including TB. The initial imaging investigation of haemoptysis is CXR followed by other investigations, such as CT, bronchoscopy or biopsy as required.

Massive haemoptysis is defined as expectoration of more than 300 mL of blood per 24 hours. Causes of massive haemoptysis include arteriovenous malformation and erosion of bronchial arteries in association with bronchiectasis. Investigation of massive haemoptysis consists of urgent CXR followed by angiography. Selective angiography of the bronchial arteries with identification of a bleeding site may be followed by embolization. If this is not curative, surgical removal of the affected segment or lobe may be required.

2.6 DIAGNOSIS AND STAGING OF BRONCHOGENIC CARCINOMA (LUNG CANCER)

For principles of cancer staging please see Chapter 14.

Bronchogenic carcinoma is classified into small cell lung cancer (SCLC) and non-small cell lung cancer (NSCLC). SCLS accounts for about 15 per cent of new cases of bronchogenic carcinoma and is more aggressive than NSCLC. The TNM system is used to stage bronchogenic carcinoma:

- 'T' includes features such as tumour size and evidence of chest wall or mediastinal invasion.
- 'N' refers to regional hilar or mediastinal lymph node involvement.
- 'M' refers to distant metastasis.

Small cell lung cancer is often staged using a two-stage system, where patients are classified as having limited or extensive disease. Limited disease implies tumour confined to one hemithorax and to regional lymph nodes. Limited stage usually implies that the tumour is confined to a region small enough to be treated with radiotherapy. Extensive disease describes SLSC that has spread to the contralateral lung or lymph nodes, or to distant organs.

The majority of bronchogenic carcinomas are initially diagnosed on CXR. CXR may be performed for investigation of a specific symptom, such as haemoptysis or weight loss in a smoker. Alternatively, bronchogenic carcinoma may be an incidental finding on a CXR performed for other reasons, such as pre-anaesthetic or as part of a routine medical check-up. The usual appearance of a bronchogenic carcinoma on CXR is a pulmonary mass (Fig. 2.20). Complications of bronchogenic carcinoma that may produce a more complex appearance on CXR include:

- Segmental/lobar collapse (Fig. 2.42)
- Persistent areas of consolidation
- Hilar lymphadenopathy
- Mediastinal lymphadenopathy
- Pleural effusion
- Invasion of adjacent structures: mediastinum, chest wall
- Metastases: lungs, bones.

CT is the imaging modality of choice for the staging of bronchogenic carcinoma. CT is more

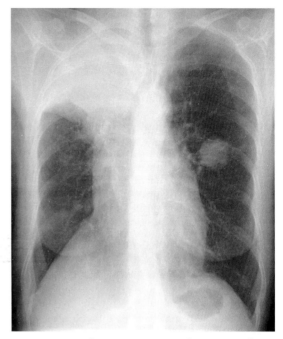

Figure 2.42 Bronchogenic carcinoma. A large mass at the right hilum is associated with collapse of the right upper lobe. Soft tissue mass in the left lung due to a metastasis.

accurate than CXR for the diagnosis of mediastinal lymphadenopathy, hilar lymphadenopathy, mediastinal invasion and chest wall invasion. CT may also be used for primary diagnosis where the CXR is negative and the presence of a tumour is suspected on clinical grounds, e.g. haemoptysis, positive sputum cytology or paraneoplastic syndrome. FDG-PET may complement CT in the staging of bronchogenic carcinoma. PET–CT has a high negative predictive value such that a negative PET scan can obviate the need for other imaging or more invasive studies.

Diagnosis of cell type is important, first to confirm the diagnosis of bronchogenic carcinoma, and second to classify the tumour. Tumour cells may be obtained from sputum cytology or from aspiration of pleural fluid. More commonly, some form of invasive biopsy will be required as follows:

- Centrally located tumours: bronchoscopy and biopsy
- Peripheral tumours: CT-guided biopsy (Fig. 2.22)

- Very small masses, or tumours in difficult locations, such as deep to the scapula: open biopsy or video-assisted thoracoscopic surgery.

2.7 CHEST TRAUMA

CXR is the initial investigation of choice in suspected or known chest trauma. CXR is usually performed in this context as part of a 'trauma series', which also includes a lateral radiograph of the cervical spine and a frontal radiograph of the pelvis. CXR in the setting of acute trauma is often performed with the patient in the supine position, leading to a number of potential problems with interpretation:

- The mediastinum appears widened due to normal distension of venous structures.
- Pleural fluid may be more difficult to diagnose in the absence of a fluid level.
- Pneumothorax may be more difficult to diagnose.

Findings to look for on the CXR of a trauma patient:

- Pneumothorax (Figs 2.32, 2.33 and 2.34)
- Pneumomediastinum
- Subcutaneous emphysema (Fig. 2.43)
  - Streaky gas lucencies in the soft tissues of the chest wall

- Commonly tracks superiorly into soft tissues of the neck
- May extend into muscle in which case gas lucencies are seen outlining bundles of muscle fibres
- Haemothorax (Fig. 2.44)
  - Appearance as described for pleural effusion
- Haemopneumothorax (Fig. 2.45)
  - Combination of fluid and air in the pleural cavity produces a sharply defined fluid level

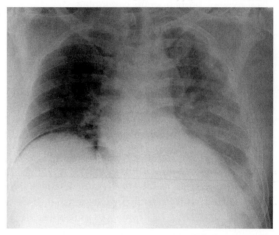

Figure 2.44 Haemothorax producing opacification of the left hemithorax on supine CXR. Note multiple rib fractures.

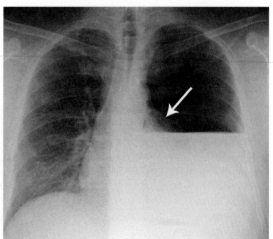

Figure 2.45 Haemopneumothorax. Note that a combination of air and fluid in the pleural space produces a straight line without the typical meniscus of a pleural effusion. Compare this appearance with Fig. 2.30. In this case, there is also evidence of tension with increased volume on the left and marked collapse and distortion of the left lung (arrow).

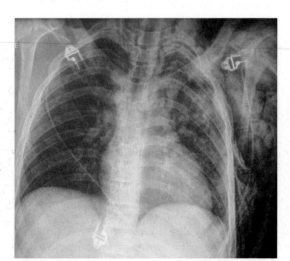

Figure 2.43 Chest trauma due to high speed motor vehicle accident: CXR. Note multiple rib fractures, ill-defined opacity left upper lobe due to contusion, extensive subcutaneous air in the left chest wall tracking upwards into the neck.

- Fluid level extends to the chest wall without forming a meniscus
- Pulmonary contusion
  - Focal area of alveolar shadowing that appears within hours of the trauma and usually clears after 4 days; usually associated with rib fractures
- Mediastinal haematoma (see below)
- Ruptured diaphragm
  - CXR signs of ruptured diaphragm include herniation of abdominal structures into the chest, apparent elevation of the hemidiaphragm and contralateral mediastinal shift
- Rib fractures
  - Oblique views looking for subtle rib fractures are not advised in the acute situation
  - Fractures of the upper three ribs indicate a high level of trauma, though there is no proven increase in the incidence of great vessel damage
  - Fractures of the lower three ribs have an association with upper abdominal injury (liver, spleen and kidney)
- Flail segment refers to segmental fractures of three or more ribs
  - Flail segment produces paradoxical movement of a segment of the chest wall with respiration
  - This is often very difficult to appreciate clinically and as such flail segment is usually a radiological diagnosis
  - Flail segment has a high incidence of associated injuries, such as pneumothorax, subcutaneous emphysema and haemothorax, and adequate pain management is crucial to prevent lobar collapse and pneumonia
- Fractures of the clavicle, scapula, sternum and humerus may also be seen in association with chest trauma.

2.7.1 Aortic injury

Rupture of the thoracic aorta is the most catastrophic injury associated with chest trauma. Full thickness or complete aortic rupture is usually fatal. Approximately 20 per cent of aortic ruptures are not full thickness, i.e. the outer aortic wall (adventitia) is intact. If left untreated, incomplete aortic rupture has a high mortality rate; delayed complete rupture occurs in most cases within four months of trauma. Only around 5 per cent of incomplete ruptures develop a false aneurysm, associated with a normal lifespan.

Note that incomplete aortic rupture implies an intact adventitia. Therefore, the mediastinal haematoma that occurs in association with incomplete aortic rupture arises from other blood vessels, such as the intercostal or internal mammary arteries or veins. Mediastinal haematoma is associated with, not caused by, aortic injury. Twenty per cent of patients with mediastinal haematoma on CXR or CT will have an aortic injury. Absence of mediastinal haematoma is a reasonably reliable predictor of an intact aorta. CXR signs of aortic rupture are due to the associated mediastinal haematoma (Fig. 2.46):

- Widened mediastinum that may be difficult to assess on a supine film
- Obscured aortic knuckle and other mediastinal structures
- Displacement of trachea and nasogastric tube to the right
- Depression of left main bronchus
- Left haemothorax causing pleural opacification, including depression of the apex of the left lung.

Most aortic injuries occur at the aortic isthmus, just distal to the left subclavian artery.

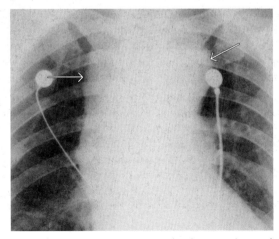

Figure 2.46 Aortic injury: CXR. Note that there is widening of the mediastinum (arrows) with loss of definition of mediastinal structures due to mediastinal haematoma.

Incomplete rupture of the aorta is confirmed by MDCT or transoesophageal echocardiogram (TOE). MDCT is most commonly employed (Fig. 2.47). MDCT has the added advantage of being able to demonstrate accurately most other injuries related to chest trauma. Indications for MDCT in a setting of chest trauma include:

- Definite CXR signs of mediastinal haematoma are present

- CXR is equivocal or normal and aortic injury suspected on clinical grounds.

Transoesophageal echocardiogram may be used as a problem-solving tool in difficult or equivocal cases. Interventional radiology is commonly used to treat aortic rupture, with aortogram and covered stent deployment (Fig. 2.48).

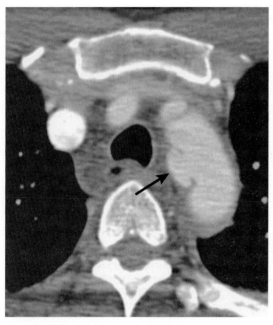

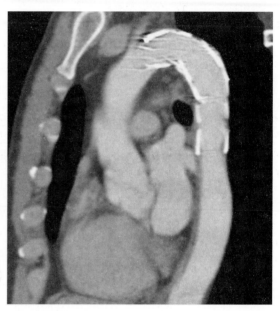

Figure 2.48 Aortic injury post-repair with covered stent: CT.

Figure 2.47 Aortic injury: CT. Contrast-enhanced MDCT shows a localized out-pocketing of the medial wall of the aortic arch indicating a pseudoaneurysm (arrow).

SUMMARY BOX

Clinical presentation	Investigation of choice	Comment
Respiratory symptoms including cough, shortness of breath, pleuritic chest pain, haemoptysis	CXR	CT for further characterization of CXR findings or as specifically indicated, e.g. suspected bronchiectasis
Staging of bronchogenic carcinoma	CT FDG-PET	
Detection of pulmonary metastases	CT	
Solitary pulmonary nodule	CT FDG-PET Biopsy	See Table 2.6 above for guidelines on follow-up of small pulmonary nodules
Massive haemoptysis	CXR Angiography ± embolization	Massive haemoptysis = expectoration >300 mL blood per 24 hours
Chest trauma	CXR CT	

FDG-PET, fluorodeoxyglucose positron emission tomography.

3 Cardiovascular system

3.1 IMAGING OF THE HEART

3.1.1 CXR

The most common use of plain films in cardiac disease is in the assessment of cardiac failure and its treatment.

CXR features relevant to cardiac disease:
- Cardiac position
- Cardiac size
- Specific cardiac chamber enlargement
- Cardiac valve calcification
- Pulmonary vascular pattern
- Pulmonary oedema
- Pleural effusion.

3.1.1.1 Position

The normal cardiac apex is directed towards the left chest wall. About two-thirds of the normally positioned heart lies to the left of midline. Malposition of the heart refers to an abnormally positioned heart, though with normal orientation of chambers and with the apex still pointing to the left. The heart may be malpositioned to one side by collapse of the ipsilateral lung, or by a contralateral space-occupying process, such as tension pneumothorax or large pleural effusion. Dextrocardia refers to reversal of the normal orientation of the heart with the cardiac apex directed to the patient's right. With isolated dextrocardia, other organs, such as liver and stomach, are positioned normally. In situs inversus, all of the organs are reversed and the gastric bubble lies beneath the right diaphragm (Fig. 3.1).

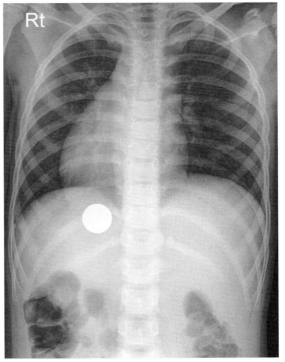

Figure 3.1 Situs inversus: CXR and AXR. Radiographs performed in a six-year-old female for a swallowed coin. Orientation of visible organs is a 'mirror image' of normal with heart and stomach to the right and liver on the left.

3.1.1.2 Cardiac size

Cardiothoracic ratio (CTR) refers to the ratio between the maximum transverse diameter of the heart and the maximum transverse diameter of the chest. CTR is usually expressed as the ratio of these measurements (Fig. 3.2). CTR of greater than 0.5 is said to indicate cardiac enlargement although there are a number of variables, not least of which is the shape of the patient's chest. CTR is unreliable as a one-off measurement; of more significance is an increase in heart size on serial CXRs.

3.1.1.3 Signs of specific chamber enlargement

These signs are shown in Table 3.1.

3.1.1.4 Cardiac valve calcification

Calcification of the mitral valve annulus is common in elderly patients and may be associated with mitral regurgitation (Fig. 3.3). Calcification of the mitral valve leaflets may occur in rheumatic heart disease or mitral valve prolapse. Mitral valve leaflet or annulus calcification is seen on the lateral CXR inferior to a line from the carina to the anterior costophrenic angle, and on the PA CXR inferior to a line from the right cardiophrenic angle to the left hilum.

Aortic valve calcification is associated with aortic stenosis, and is seen on the lateral CXR lying above and anterior to a line from the carina to the anterior costophrenic angle.

3.1.1.5 Pulmonary vascular patterns

The normal pulmonary vascular pattern has the following features:

Table 3.1 Signs of cardiac chamber enlargement.

Cardiac chamber	Radiological signs of enlargement
Right atrium	Bulging right heart border
Left atrium	Prominent left atrial appendage on the left heart border (Fig 3.3)
	Double outline of the right heart border
	Splayed carina with elevation of the left main bronchus
	Bulge of the upper posterior heart border on the lateral view
Right ventricle	Elevated cardiac apex
	Bulging of anterior upper part of the heart border on the lateral view
Left ventricle	Bulging lower left cardiac border with depressed cardiac apex

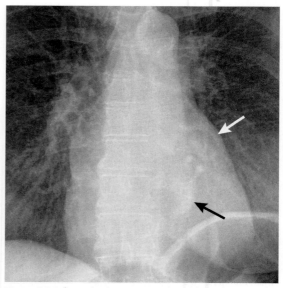

Figure 3.3 Left atrial enlargement and mitral annular calcification. Heart is enlarged with prominence of the left atrial appendage producing a bulge of the upper left cardiac border (white arrow). Curvilinear calcification in the mitral valve annulus (black arrow).

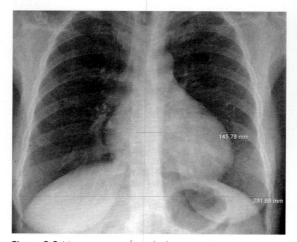

145.78 mm

281.68 mm

Figure 3.2 Measurement of cardiothoracic ratio.

- Arteries branching vertically to upper and lower lobes
- Veins running roughly horizontally towards the lower hila
- Upper lobe vessels smaller than lower lobe vessels on erect CXR
- Vessels difficult to see in the peripheral thirds of the lungs.

Abnormal pulmonary vascular patterns are outlined below:
- Pulmonary venous hypertension
  - Blood vessels in the upper lobes are larger than those in the lower lobes on erect CXR
  - Associated with cardiac failure and mitral valve disease, and often accompanied on CXR by cardiomegaly, pulmonary oedema and pleural effusion
- Pulmonary arterial hypertension (Fig. 3.4)
  - Bilateral hilar enlargement due to enlarged proximal pulmonary arteries with rapid decrease in the calibre of peripheral vessels ('pruning')
  - Associated with long-standing pulmonary disease, including emphysema, multiple recurrent pulmonary emboli, left-to-right shunts (ventricular septal defect (VSD), atrial septal defect (ASD), patent ductus artery (PDA))
- Pulmonary plethora
  - Increased size and number of pulmonary vessels
  - Increased pulmonary blood flow caused by left-to-right cardiac shunts (VSD, ASD, PDA)
- Pulmonary oligaemia
  - General lucency (blackness) of lungs with decreased size and number of pulmonary vessels and small main pulmonary arteries
  - Reduced pulmonary blood flow associated with pulmonary stenosis/atresia, Fallot tetralogy, tricuspid atresia, Ebstein anomaly and severe emphysema.

3.1.2 Echocardiography

Echocardiography combines direct visualization of cardiac anatomy, Doppler analysis of flow rates through valves and septal defects, and colour Doppler. Colour Doppler helps in the identification of septal defects and quantification of gradients across stenotic valves.

Indications for echocardiography include:
- Quantification of cardiac function
  - Systolic function: measurement of ejection fraction
  - Quantification of stroke volume and cardiac output
  - Measurement of chamber volumes and wall thicknesses
  - Diastolic function: measurement of left ventricular 'relaxation'
- Congenital heart disease
- Diagnosis and quantification of valvular dysfunction
- Stress echocardiography: diagnosis of regional wall motion abnormalities induced by exercise as a sign of coronary artery disease
- Miscellaneous: cardiac masses, pericardial effusion, aortic dissection.

The accuracy of echocardiography may be further enhanced by the injection of microbubble contrast agents.

Indications for contrast-enhanced echocardiography include:
- Cardiac chamber visualization and measurement in technically challenging cases

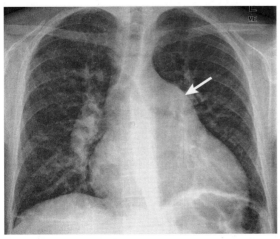

Figure 3.4 Pulmonary arterial hypertension: CXR. Dilated main pulmonary artery produces a bulge of the upper left cardiac border (arrow), higher than the left atrial appendage. Prominent hila due to enlarged right and left pulmonary arteries. Rapid tapering of calibre of pulmonary arteries as they extend through the lungs.

- Diagnosis of intracardiac shunts such as patent foramen ovale.

Transoesophageal echocardiography (TOE) is a specialized echocardiographic technique that uses a transoesophageal probe. TOE overcomes the difficulty of imaging through the anterior chest wall, especially in patients with emphysema in whom the heart may be obscured anteriorly by overexpanded lung. TOE also provides improved imaging of the thoracic aorta and may be used to diagnose aortic diseases such as acute aortic dissection.

3.1.3 CT

Modern multidetector CT (CT) scanners with up to 256 and 320 detectors are able to image the heart and coronary arteries during the diastolic (resting) phase of a single heartbeat (Fig. 3.5).

Current roles of cardiac CT include:
- Quantification of coronary artery calcium expressed as coronary artery calcium score
- CT coronary angiography (CTCA) in patients at risk for coronary artery disease
- CTCA for assessment of coronary artery bypass grafts and stent patency

- Mapping of the anatomy of the left atrium and pulmonary veins prior to radiofrequency catheter ablation for atrial fibrillation.

3.1.4 Scintigraphy: gated myocardial perfusion imaging

Myocardial perfusion scintigraphy is performed with thallium-201 (^{201}Tl), ^{99}mTc-sestamibi or ^{99}mTc-tetrofosmin. Indications for myocardial perfusion imaging include:
- Acute chest pain with normal or inconclusive ECG
- Abnormal stress ECG in patients at low or intermediate risk of coronary artery disease (high-risk patients should have coronary angiography)
- Determine haemodynamic significance of coronary artery disease
- Assess cardiac risk prior to major surgery.

3.1.5 Coronary angiography

Coronary angiography is performed by placement of preshaped catheters into the origins of the coronary arteries and injection of contrast material. Catheters are inserted via femoral artery puncture.

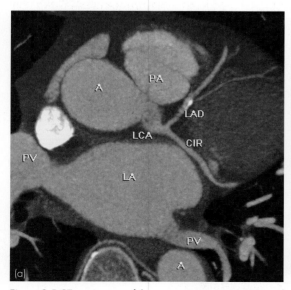
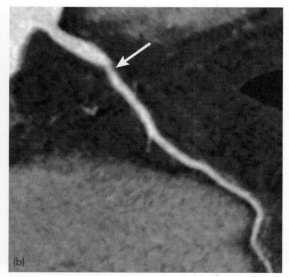

Figure 3.5 CT angiogram of the coronary arteries. (a) Normal anatomy. Note the following structures: aorta (A), pulmonary artery (PA), pulmonary veins (PV), left atrium (LA), left main coronary artery (LCA), left anterior descending artery (LAD) and circumflex artery (CIR). (b) Coronary artery stenosis (arrow).

Coronary angiography is the investigation of choice for quantification of coronary artery stenosis. Coronary angiography may be combined with therapeutic interventions including coronary artery angioplasty and stent deployment. Limitations of coronary angiography are discussed below.

3.1.6 MRI

Cardiac MRI (CMR) is an established modality in the investigation of cardiac disease.

Current applications of CMR include:
- Quantification of cardiac function
  - Calculation of ejection fraction, myocardial thickness and regional wall motion where echocardiography is difficult or equivocal
- Congenital heart disease: complementary to echocardiography
- Cardiac anatomy
  - Cardiomyopathy, left ventricular aneurysm etc. where echocardiography is difficult or equivocal (Fig. 3.6)
- Myocardial viability
- Infarct scan
  - Contrast material accumulates in infarcted myocardium allowing direct visualization on a delayed scan
- Great vessel disease: aortic dissection, coarctation
- Miscellaneous: cardiac masses; pericardial disease.

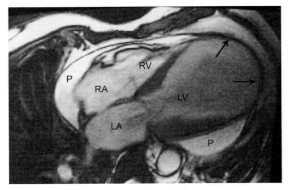

Figure 3.6 Left ventricular aneurysm: MRI. Transverse MR scan showing a four chamber view of the heart. Note the right atrium (RA), right ventricle (RV), left atrium (LA), left ventricle (LV) and pericardial effusion (P). The apex of the left ventricle has a markedly thinned wall and is dilated (arrows).

3.2 CONGESTIVE CARDIAC FAILURE

Dyspnoea may have a variety of causes including cardiac and respiratory diseases, anaemia and anxiety states. Certain features in the clinical history may be helpful in diagnosis, such as whether dyspnoea is acute or chronic, worse at night, or accentuated by lying down (orthopnoea). Initial tests include full blood count, ECG and CXR, followed by pulmonary function tests when a respiratory cause such as emphysema or asthma is suspected. Congestive cardiac failure (CCF) is the most common cardiac cause of dyspnoea. CCF may be caused by systolic or diastolic dysfunction, or a combination of the two. Systolic dysfunction refers to reduction of the amount of blood pumped due to failure of ventricular contraction. Diastolic dysfunction refers to failure of ventricular relaxation between contractions leading to reduced filling of the ventricular chambers.

The most common underlying cause of CCF is ischaemic heart disease. Other causes include valvular heart disease, hypertension, hypertrophic cadiomyopathy, infiltrative disorders like amyloidosis, pericardial effusion or thickening, or congenital heart disease. Imaging is performed to confirm that CCF is the cause of dyspnoea, to quantitate and classify cardiac dysfunction, and to search for underlying causes. CXR and echocardiography are the usual imaging tests employed for the initial assessment of CCF. Coronary artery imaging with CT or angiography is indicated where an ischaemic cause for CCF is suspected.

3.2.1 CXR signs of congestive cardiac failure

- Cardiac enlargement
  - Cardiothoracic ratio is unreliable as a one-off measurement
  - Of more significance is an increase in heart size on serial CXRs
- Pulmonary vascular redistribution
  - Upper lobe blood vessels larger than those in the lower lobes
- Interstitial oedema
  - Reticular (linear) pattern with Kerley B lines (see Fig. 2.8)

- Alveolar oedema
  - Fluffy, ill-defined areas of alveolar opacity in a bilateral central or 'bat wing' distribution (see Fig. 2.5)
- Pleural effusions
  - Pleural effusions associated with CCF tend to be larger on the right.

3.2.2 Echocardiography

Echocardiography may be used to calculate cardiac chamber size and wall thickness, and to diagnose the presence of valvular dysfunction and pericardial effusion. Systolic dysfunction may be diagnosed and quantitated by calculation of left ventricular ejection fraction. Ejection fraction is a measurement of the amount of blood ejected from the left ventricle with systolic contraction. To calculate ejection fraction, the volume of the left ventricle is calculated at the end of diastole (D) and then at the end of systole (S). Left ventricular volume may be calculated by various methods. Figure 3.7 illustrates the modified Simpson's biplane method. Ejection fraction, expressed as a percentage is calculated by the following formula: $D - S/D \times 100$. Normal values for ejection fraction are 70 per cent ± 7 per cent for males and 65 per cent ± 10 per cent for females.

Other measurements, such as stroke volume and cardiac output, may be calculated with echocardiography. Measurements of left ventricular relaxation may also be done to assess diastolic dysfunction.

3.3 ISCHAEMIC HEART DISEASE

3.3.1 Overview of coronary artery disease

Coronary artery disease (CAD) is the leading cause of death worldwide. Mortality and disability rates due to CAD are increasing in industrialized and developing countries.

Coronary artery disease is a diffuse disease of the coronary arteries characterized by atheromatous plaques. Plaques may cause stenosis of coronary arteries producing limitation of blood flow to the myocardium. During the development of atheromatous plaque, the external membranes of coronary arteries may expand outwards. As a result of this arterial remodelling phenomenon, significant coronary atherosclerosis may be present without narrowing of the vessel lumen (non-stenosing plaque). Rupture of atherosclerotic plaques with subsequent arterial thrombosis leads to acute cardiac events (acute cardiac syndrome), such as unstable angina, myocardial infarction and sudden death. Instability and rupture of atherosclerotic plaque is mediated by inflammatory factors, and may occur with stenosing or non-stenosing plaque.

Coronary artery disease with multiple arterial stenoses may present clinically with chronic cardiac disease, most commonly cardiac failure. CCF in this context is caused by pump failure due to ischaemic myocardium. CCF due to CAD is commonly associated with chronic stable angina.

The roles of imaging in CAD include:
- Screening for CAD
- Diagnosis and quantification of CAD in acute cardiac syndrome
- Planning of revascularization procedures including coronary artery bypass graft, and interventional procedures such as angioplasty and coronary artery stent placement
- Assessment of myocardial viability
- Assessment of cardiac function.

3.3.2 Screening for CAD

The traditional approach to prevention of CAD has been identification and reduction of risk factors such as hypertension, tobacco smoking, lack of physical activity, obesity, diabetes and dyslipidaemias. This approach has limited accuracy in predicting the presence of CAD and the occurrence of acute cardiac syndrome. Acute cardiac syndrome may occur in the absence of known risk factors. Furthermore, a large percentage of patients with high risk factors do not suffer a cardiac event.

3.3.2.1 Catheter coronary angiography

In the past, catheter coronary angiography has been the standard method for the diagnosis of CAD. Coronary angiography remains the investigation of choice in acute cardiac syndrome and in patients at high risk for the presence of CAD. The major limitation of coronary angiography is that it only provides an image of the vessel lumen. Only atherosclerotic plaques that cause significant

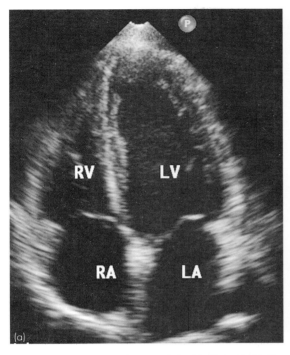

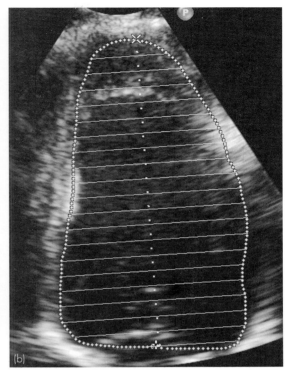

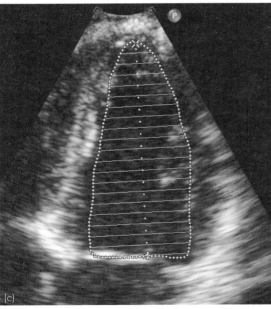

Figure 3.7 Calculation of ejection fraction: echocardiography. (a) Apical four chamber view of the heart: right ventricle (RV), left ventricle (LV), right atrium (RA), left atrium (LA). (b) Measurement of left ventricular volume at end diastole. (c) Measurement of left ventricular volume in systole.

narrowing of the lumen of the coronary artery are diagnosed with coronary angiography. Non-stenosing plaque, which may be at risk of rupture, is not diagnosed with coronary angiography.

3.3.2.2 CT coronary angiography

CT coronary angiography is now an established technique in the diagnosis of CAD. Modern CT scanners with up to 320 rows of detectors are able to scan up to 16 cm in as little as 175 milliseconds. This means that the entire heart may be imaged during the diastolic (resting) segment of a single heartbeat, allowing accurate depiction of the coronary arteries.

CT coronary angiography involves intravenous contrast material injection. CTCA requires a relatively low heart rate; patients with a high heart rate are usually given beta-blocker medication prior to scanning.

Advantages of CTCA over catheter coronary angiography include:
- Relative non-invasiveness
- Ability to image non-stenotic plaque in the vessel wall
- Very high negative predictive value, i.e. a normal CTCA examination is an excellent indicator of the absence of clinically significant CAD.
  Indications for CTCA include:
- Investigation of choice for the diagnosis of CAD in low to intermediate risk patients
- Diagnosis of indeterminate chest pain, specifically exclusion of a cardiac cause.

3.3.2.3 CT calcium scoring

Multidetector CT is highly sensitive to the presence of coronary artery calcification (Fig. 3.8).

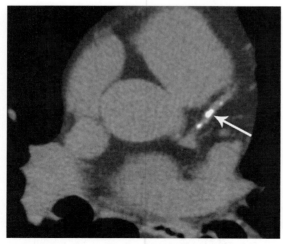

Figure 3.8 CT coronary calcium scoring. Note calcification in the left anterior descending artery (arrow) in a middle-aged male with atherosclerosis of the coronary arteries.

The amount of coronary artery calcification increases with the overall burden of coronary atherosclerotic disease. Computer software programs are able to quantitate coronary artery calcium detected by CT, and provide a coronary calcium score. Calcium scores adjusted for age and gender, in combination with other known risk factors, can help to predict the risk of future cardiac events. A calcium score of zero is a strong indicator of a very low risk of subsequent cardiac events, although it does not exclude non-calcified plaque. Calcium scoring may also be useful for monitoring CAD in patients undergoing medical treatments for risk factor reduction.

3.3.2.4 Exercise stress testing

Screening tests may be performed to identify clinically silent CAD, to calculate the risk of future acute cardiac events, and to identify those patients that may benefit from revascularization procedures. These screening tests are designed to detect abnormalities such as ECG changes or regional ventricular wall motion abnormalities in response to exercise or pharmacologically induced myocardial stress. An abnormal exercise test has a high predictive value for the presence of obstructive CAD.

Methods of exercise stress testing include:
- Stress ECG: ST segment depression induced by exercise
- Stress echocardiogram: segmental wall motion abnormalities induced by exercise
- Myocardial perfusion scintigraphy with thallium-201 (201Tl), ^{99m}Tc-sestamibi or ^{99m}Tc-tetrofosmin.

3.3.3 Acute chest pain

As outlined above, sudden rupture of an atherosclerotic plaque with subsequent arterial thrombosis and occlusion may lead to acute cardiac events, such as sudden death, myocardial infarction and acute unstable angina. The classic symptoms of acute angina are chest pain and tightness radiating to the left arm. Other causes of acute chest pain include aortic dissection, pulmonary embolism, gastro-oesophageal reflux, muscle spasm, and a variety of respiratory causes. Initial workup for a cardiac cause includes ECG and serum markers such as CK-MB and cardiac treponins. Initial imaging assessment in the acute situation consists of a CXR to look for evidence of cardiac failure and to diagnose a non-cardiac cause of chest pain, such as pneumonia or pneumothorax. Coronary angiography is indicated in patients with ECG changes or elevated serum markers. Interventional procedures aimed at restoring coronary blood flow, including coronary artery angioplasty and stent deployment, may also be performed acutely.

3.3.4 Myocardial viability and cardiac function

Further imaging in the setting of CAD and ischaemic heart disease consists of tests of myocardial viability including thallium scintigraphy to assess the amount of viable versus non-viable myocardium, and echocardiography to quantitate cardiac function. Cardiac MRI may also be used to assess myocardial viability and cardiac function in patients with CAD. CMR is able to provide a quantitative assessment of ventricular wall motion and assess myocardial perfusion, at rest and with pharmacologically induced stress. CMR is generally less widely available than myocardial perfusion scintigraphy and echocardiography.

3.3.4.1 Myocardial perfusion scintigraphy

Myocardial perfusion scintigraphy is used to differentiate viable from non-viable myocardium and hence identify those patients who would benefit from coronary revascularization procedures such as angioplasty or bypass graft. Myocardial perfusion scintigraphy is performed with thallium-201 (^{201}Tl), ^{99}mTc-sestamibi or ^{99}mTc-tetrofosmin. FDG-PET is also used in some centres to assess myocardial viability. Following injection of radiopharmaceutical, the heart is put under stress through exercise, or with various pharmacological agents such as dobutamine or dipyridamole. Images are acquired with the heart under stress and then repeated after a period of rest. Reversible ischaemia is seen as a region of reduced tracer activity ('cold' spot) on exercise that returns to normal after 4 hours of rest (Fig. 3.9). An infarct is seen as a 'cold' spot on exercise unchanged after 4 hours of rest.

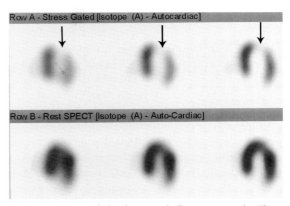

Figure 3.9 Myocardial ischaemia: thallium scintigraphy. The top three images are of the left ventricle after exercise; below these are corresponding images after a rest period. Note the presence of a region of reduced myocardial uptake of thallium with exercise (arrows). There is normal distribution of activity at rest indicating reversible ischaemia rather than established infarction.

3.3.4.2 Echocardiography

Echocardiography is a highly accurate non-invasive method for the quantification of left ventricular ejection fraction. Echocardiography is also able to diagnose complications of myocardial infarction, such as papillary muscle rupture, ventricular septal defect, left ventricular aneurysm and pericardial effusion.

3.3.5 Summary of imaging in CAD

The Framingham risk score is a well-recognized tool used to provide a global risk assessment for future 'hard' cardiac events, including myocardial infarction and sudden death. Based on gender and age, cholesterol and HDL levels, systolic blood pressure and tobacco use, individuals are categorized as low, intermediate or high risk.

Low-risk individuals have no risk factors and comprise about 35 per cent of those tested. Low-risk asymptomatic patients require no imaging. Exceptions to this include insurance medicals and certain occupations, e.g. airline pilots. For such individuals, CTCA is a highly accurate, relatively non-invasive method for excluding CAD.

High-risk individuals have established atheromatous disease and/or multiple risk factors and comprise about 25 per cent of those tested. High-risk or symptomatic patients should be assessed with coronary catheter angiography and tests of myocardial viability. Choice of test will hinge on a number of factors including local expertise and availability, as well as the individual circumstances of the patient.

Intermediate-risk individuals comprise about 40 per cent of those tested and include those with one or more risk factor outside the normal range or a positive family history of CAD. Intermediate-risk individuals are best assessed by non-invasive means including exercise stress tests and CTCA. CTCA is less invasive than coronary catheterization and is highly accurate in the detection of coronary artery plaque. CTCA has a very high negative predictive value and, therefore, is able to reduce the number of normal or negative catheter studies.

3.4 AORTIC DISSECTION

Aortic dissection occurs when a tear in the surface of the intima allows flow of blood into the aortic wall. This creates a false lumen, with re-entry of blood into the true lumen occurring more distally. Dissection may involve the aorta alone or may cause occlusion of major arterial branches.

Aortic dissection usually presents with acute chest pain, often described as a 'tearing' sensation. Chest pain may be anterior, or posterior between the scapulae, and may radiate more distally as the dissection progresses. Aortic dissections are classified by the Stanford system into types A and B:

- Type A: all dissections involving the ascending aorta, with the re-entry site anywhere distally down to and sometimes beyond the aortic bifurcation
- Type B: does not involve ascending aorta; confined to the descending aorta distal to the origin of the left subclavian artery.

Type A dissection has a worse prognosis that type B due to increased risk of coronary artery occlusion, rupture into the pericardium, and aortic valve regurgitation.

CXR is performed in the initial assessment of the patient with chest pain. In the context of suspected aortic dissection, CXR is mainly to exclude other causes of chest pain prior to more definitive investigation. Most of the CXR signs that may be seen with aortic dissection, such as pleural effusion, are non-specific and may be seen in a range of other conditions. Alterations to the contour of the aortic arch and displacement of intimal calcification may be more specific but are only occasionally seen, and then with some difficulty (Fig. 3.10).

Contrast-enhanced CT of the chest is the investigation of choice for suspected aortic dissection (Fig. 3.11). The roles of CT in the evaluation of suspected aortic dissection are:

- Confirm the diagnosis by demonstration of the dissection flap, as well as the true and false lumens; classify the dissection as type A or B
- Identify occlusion of arterial branches, including the coronary arteries
- Demonstration of bleeding: mediastinal haematoma, pleural or pericardial effusion.

Depending on local availability and expertise, TOE or MRI may be used to confirm the diagnosis in difficult or equivocal cases. TOE may also be performed at the bedside in critically ill patients.

3.5 ABDOMINAL AORTIC ANEURYSM

Abdominal aortic aneurysm (AAA) is generally defined as an abdominal aortic diameter of greater than 3 cm. AAA is usually caused by weakening of the aortic wall due to atherosclerosis. This weakening leads to dilatation of the aorta, which is usually progressive. AAA may present clinically as a pulsatile abdominal mass or occasionally with acute abdominal pain due to leakage. More commonly, AAA is an incidental finding on imaging performed for other reasons including US or CT of the abdomen, or X-ray of the lumbar spine. Plain-film signs of AAA may include a soft tissue mass with curvilinear calcification.

3.5.1 US

Most small aneurysms less than 5 cm in diameter may be managed conservatively with regular clinical and imaging surveillance.

Indications for surgical or endoluminal repair include:

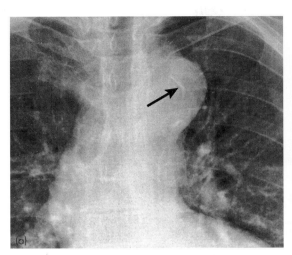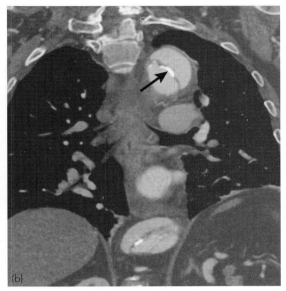

Figure 3.10 Aortic dissection: CXR and CT. (a) CXR shows intimal calcification (arrow) displaced centrally by blood in the false lumen. (b) Coronal contrast-enhanced CT in the same patient shows true lumen and false lumen separated by intimal flap. The intimal flap contains calcification (arrow), which is displaced on CXR.

- Diameter >5.4 cm
- Diameter expansion >1 cm in one year
- Symptoms attributable to AAA.

US is the investigation of choice for initial measurement and definition of AAA.

Based on diameter measurement, further surveillance or management may be recommended as follows:

- 3.0–3.9 cm: repeat US in five years
- 4.0–4.9 cm: repeat US in six months
- >4.9 cm: refer to vascular surgeon.

3.5.2 CT

Except for emergency situations, imaging is usually required for preoperative planning prior to surgical or endoluminal repair of AAA. Multidetector CT is the investigation of choice for measurement, definition of anatomy and diagnosis of complications, such as leakage. Leakage of AAA may be seen on CT as soft tissue surrounding the aneurysm (Fig. 3.12). Treatment planning prior to percutaneous stent placement (see below) requires precise CT measurements of aneurysm diameter and length, distance from renal arteries, diameter

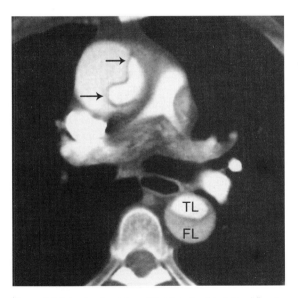

Figure 3.11 Aortic dissection: CT. Note the thin intimal flap in the ascending aorta (arrows). In the descending aorta the flap is seen separating the true lumen (TL) from the false lumen (FL).

and length of common iliac arteries (Fig. 3.13). CT may also be performed after stent deployment or surgical repair for diagnosis of problems such as infection, blockage and endoleak, or less common

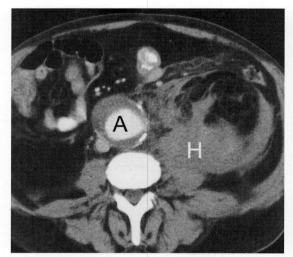

Figure 3.12 Leaking abdominal aortic aneurysm: CT. CT obtained in a patient with acute onset of abdominal pain shows an aortic aneurysm (A) and a large left retroperitoneal haematoma (H).

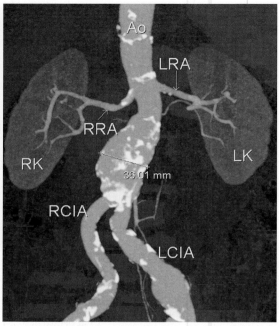

Figure 3.13 Abdominal aortic aneurysm: CT. A reconstructed image from a CT angiogram shows the following structures: aorta (Ao), left and right renal arteries (LRA, RRA), left and right kidneys (LK, RK), left and right common iliac arteries (LCIA, RCIA).

complications such as aortoduodenal fistula and retroperitoneal fibrosis.

3.6 PERIPHERAL VASCULAR DISEASE

The most common clinical presentation of the patient with peripheral vascular disease (PVD) is claudication. Claudication is characterized by muscle pain and weakness, reproducibly produced by a set amount of exercise and relieved by rest. Patients with severe arterial disease may have pain at rest, or tissue changes like ischaemic ulcers and gangrene. Non-arterial causes of claudication, such as spinal stenosis and chronic venous occlusion, may be seen in 25 per cent of cases.

3.6.1 Physiological testing and Doppler US

The diagnosis of PVD in patients with claudication may be confirmed with non-invasive physiological tests:

- Ankle–brachial index (ABI)
- Pulse volume recordings
- Segmental pressures including measurements performed at rest and following exercise.

A normal ABI at rest and following exercise usually excludes significant peripheral arterial

disease, and in such cases no further arterial imaging is required. The non-invasive vascular laboratory combines physiological tests with Doppler US imaging to define those patients requiring angiography and possible further treatment, either surgery or interventional radiology. Signs of arterial stenosis on Doppler US include visible narrowing of the artery seen on 2D and colour images associated with a focal zone of increased flow velocity and an altered arterial wave pattern distally. Doppler US is particularly useful for differentiating focal stenosis from diffuse disease and occlusion. Other arterial abnormalities, such as aneurysm, pseudoaneurysm and arteriovenous malformation (AVM) are well seen, and Doppler US is also useful for postoperative graft surveillance.

Therapy is required if physiological testing with or without Doppler US reveals the presence of significant peripheral arterial disease in a patient with claudication. In these cases, a complete accurate assessment of the arterial system from the aorta to the foot arteries is required. This may consist of CT angiography (CTA), MR angiography (MRA) or catheter angiography. Choice of modality often depends on local expertise and availability.

3.6.2 CTA AND MRA

CT angiography and MRA are used increasingly for planning of therapy for PVD. CTA and MRA are able to obtain highly accurate images of the peripheral vascular system without arterial puncture. MRA generally uses sequences that show flowing blood as high signal (bright white) and stationary tissues as low signal (dark). Intravenous contrast material (gadolinium) is used to enhance blood vessels and reduce scanning times. Problems with MRA include long examination times, inability to image patients with cardiac pacemakers, and artefacts from surgical clips and metallic stents. CTA with multidetector CT has very short examination times, uses less radiation than catheter angiography, and is usually not significantly degraded by stents and surgical clips. CTA has fewer technical problems

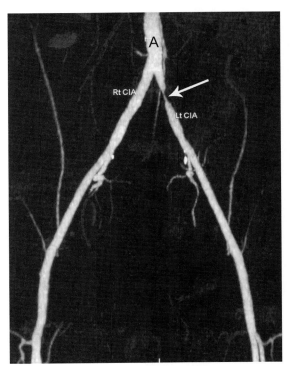

Figure 3.14 Stenosis of left common iliac artery (arrow): CT angiogram.

than MRA and is more widely used for assessment of PVD (Fig. 3.14).

3.6.3 Catheter angiography

Catheter angiography refers to the placement of selective arterial catheters and injection of contrast material to outline arterial anatomy. Most catheters are placed via femoral artery puncture and less commonly via the brachial or axillary artery. Catheter insertion is performed by the Seldinger technique as follows:

- Artery punctured with needle
- Wire threaded through the needle into the artery
- Needle removed leaving the wire in the artery
- Catheter inserted over the wire into the artery.

A wide array of preshaped catheters is available allowing selective catheterization of most major arteries in the body. Postprocedure care following catheter angiography consists of bed rest for a few hours with observation of the puncture site for bleeding and swelling. The complication rate of modern angiography is very low; most complications relate to the arterial puncture:

- Haematoma at the puncture site
- False aneurysm formation
- Arterial dissection
- Embolism due to dislodgement of atheromatous plaques.

Other possible complications of catheter angiography relate to the use of iodinated contrast material (allergy and contrast-induced nephropathy: see Chapter 1).

With the increasing use of less invasive diagnostic methods, such as Doppler US, CT angiography and MR angiography, catheter angiography is less commonly performed for purely diagnostic purposes. Catheter angiography is now more usually performed in association with interventional techniques, such as angioplasty, arterial stent placement and thrombolysis (see below).

3.7 PULMONARY EMBOLISM

Pulmonary embolism (PE) is one of the commonest preventable causes of death in hospital inpatients.

PE is a common cause of morbidity and mortality in postoperative patients, as well as in patients with other risk factors such as prolonged bed rest, malignancy and cardiac failure. Symptoms of PE may include pleuritic chest pain, shortness of breath, cough and haemoptysis; a large number of PEs are clinically silent. Clinical signs. such as hypotension, tachycardia, reduced oxygen saturation and ECG changes (S1 Q3 T3) are non-specific and often absent. As such, the clinical diagnosis of PE is problematical and usually requires confirmation with imaging studies including CXR, CT pulmonary angiography (CTPA), and ventilation/perfusion nuclear lung scan (V/Q scan).

The rate of negative imaging studies can be reduced by assignment of pretest probability of PE in a patient presenting with suggestive history and clinical findings by the use of a logical clinical assessment system and a D-dimer assay. The most widely used clinical model is the Simplified Wells Scoring System in which points are assigned:

- Leg pain, swelling and tenderness suggestive of DVT: 3.0
- Heart rate >100 beats/minute: 1.5
- Immobilization for ≥3 consecutive days: 1.5
- Surgery in the previous 4 weeks: 1.5
- Previous confirmed DVT or PE: 1.5
- Haemoptysis: 1.0
- Malignancy: 1.0
- PE more likely as or more likely than alternate diagnosis: 3.0

Pretest probability is assigned depending on the points score:

- <2.0: low
- 2.0–6.0: moderate
- >6.0: high.

D-dimer is a plasma constituent present when fibrin is released from active thrombus. Various assays for D-dimer are available. Of these, the quantitative enzyme-linked immunosorbent assay (ELISA) has a sensitivity of over 95 per cent, though is highly non-specific. It therefore has a very high negative predictive value. The diagnosis of PE is reliably excluded if the clinical pretest probability is low and the D-dimer assay is negative. In such patients, imaging with CTPA or scintigraphy is not indicated. Imaging is indicated where the clinical pretest probability is moderate or high or where the D-dimer assay is positive.

3.7.1 CXR

The initial imaging investigation in all patients with suspected PE is CXR. Signs of PE on CXR include pleural effusion, localized area of consolidation contacting a pleural surface or a localized area of collapse. These signs are non-specific and often absent. The main role of CXR in this context is to diagnose other causes for the patient's symptoms, such as pneumonia. CXR may also assist in the interpretation of a V/Q scan.

3.7.2 CT pulmonary angiography

In most circumstances, CTPA with multidetector CT is the investigation of choice for confirming the diagnosis of PE. Pulmonary emboli are seen on CTPA as filling defects within contrast-filled blood vessels (Fig. 3.15).

Advantages of CTPA in the investigation of suspected PE:

- Very low percentage of intermediate or equivocal results
- May establish alternate diagnoses, such as pneumonia, aortic dissection, etc.

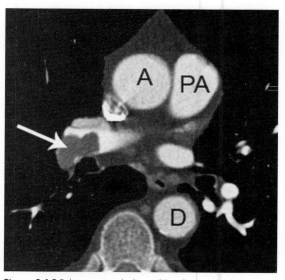

Figure 3.15 Pulmonary embolism: CT pulmonary angiogram. Pulmonary embolus seen as a low density filling defect in the right pulmonary artery (arrow). Note also ascending aorta (A), descending aorta (D), main pulmonary artery (PA).

Disadvantages of CTPA:

- Intravenous injection of iodinated contrast material
- Radiation dose: this is a particular issue in young women as the absorbed radiation dose to the breasts from CTPA is quite high; if scintigraphy is not available or is non-diagnostic, CTPA may be performed using breast shields to reduce the breast radiation dose.

3.7.3 Scintigraphy: V/Q scan

Scintigraphy is indicated if the patient has a history of previous allergic reaction to intravenous contrast material. Scintigraphy may also be indicated in young women as the absorbed radiation dose to the breasts is much lower than with CTPA.

V/Q scan consists of the following:

- Ventilation phase is first performed with the patient breathing a radioactive tracer ^{99}mTc-labelled aerosol
- Perfusion phase in which images are obtained after an intravenous injection of ^{99}mTc-labelled macroalbumen aggregates (MAA). These aggregates have a mean diameter of 30–60 μm and are trapped in the pulmonary microvasculature on first pass through the lungs
- Perfusion phase compared with the ventilation phase.

The diagnostic hallmark of PE is one or more regions of ventilation/perfusion mismatch, i.e. a region of lung where perfusion is reduced or absent and ventilation is preserved. After correlation with an accompanying CXR, lung scans are graded as low, intermediate or high probability of PE. High probability scan is an accurate predictor of PE. Low probability scan accurately excludes the diagnosis. Unfortunately, a large proportion of patients (up to 75 per cent in some series) have an intermediate probability scan.

3.8 DEEP VENOUS THROMBOSIS

Deep venous thrombosis (DVT) of the leg presents clinically with local pain and tenderness accompanied by swelling. Risk factors for development of DVT include:

- Hospitalization and immobilization
- Trauma

- Surgery, particularly surgery to the lower limb, or major abdominal surgery
- Malignancy
- Obesity
- History of previous DVT
- Factor V Leiden.

Sequelae of DVT include:

- Pulmonary embolism
- Recurrent DVT
- Post-thrombotic syndrome, in which venous incompetence and stasis cause chronic leg pain, swelling and venous ulcers.

Doppler US is the investigation of choice for suspected DVT. US is highly accurate in the diagnosis of DVT, and may detect conditions that can mimic DVT, such as ruptured Baker's cyst.

Signs of DVT on US examination (Fig. 3.16):

- Visible thrombus within the vein
- Non-compressibility of the vein
- Failure of venous distension with Valsalva's manoeuvre
- Lack of normal venous Doppler signal
- Loss of flow on colour images.

3.8.1 Upper limb DVT

Upper limb DVT usually presents clinically with acute onset of upper limb swelling. Risk factors for upper limb DVT include:

- Central venous catheters including percutaneously inserted central venous catheter (PICC) lines
- Trauma
- In young adult patients, especially bodybuilders, upper limb DVT may occur secondary to compression of the subclavian vein where it crosses the first rib
- Superior vena cava (SVC) compression by mediastinal tumour or lymphadenopathy.

Doppler US is the first investigation of choice for suspected upper limb DVT. If Doppler US is negative, contrast-enhanced CT is indicated to provide further assessment of the large central veins including the SVC. Venography and thrombolysis may be indicated for acute thrombosis of the axillary or subclavian veins. In cases of SVC compression by tumour or lymph node mass, stent deployment may provide palliation.

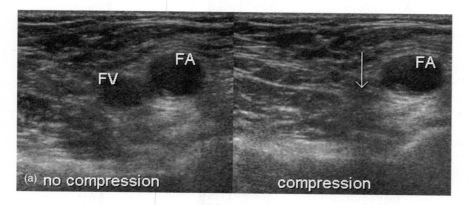

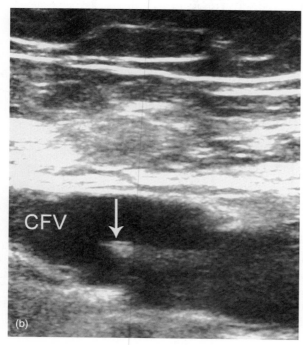

Figure 3.16 Deep venous thrombosis: duplex US. (a) Normal deep veins: duplex US. US images obtained just below the inguinal ligament in the transverse plane showing the common femoral artery (FA) and vein (FV). The common femoral vein is able to be compressed with gentle pressure (arrow), excluding the presence of deep vein thrombosis (DVT). (b) DVT: thrombus is seen as echogenic material (arrow) projecting into the common femoral vein (CFV).

3.9 VENOUS INSUFFICIENCY

For the patient with varicose veins for whom surgery is contemplated, US with Doppler is the imaging investigation of choice for assessment. The competence of a leg vein, deep or superficial, is determined with Doppler US using calf compression and release. A competent vein will show no or minor reflux (reversal of flow) on release of calf compression. Incompetence is defined as reflux of greater than 0.5 seconds in duration.

The following information may be obtained with Doppler US:

- Patency and competence of the deep venous system from the common femoral vein to the lower calf
- Competence and diameter of saphenofemoral junction
- Competence and diameter of long saphenous vein
- Duplications, tributaries, varices arising from the long saphenous vein
- Competence and diameter of the saphenopopliteal junction
- Document location of saphenopopliteal junction

- Anatomical variants of the saphenopopliteal junction
- Course and connections of superficial varicose veins
- Incompetent perforator veins connecting deep system with superficial system and their position in relation to anatomical landmarks such as groin crease, knee crease and medial malleolus.

To assist with surgical planning marks may be placed on the skin over incompetent perforating veins preoperatively. For clarity, a diagram of the venous system based on the US examination is usually provided.

3.10 HYPERTENSION

The vast majority of hypertensive patients have essential hypertension. The clinical challenge is to identify the small percentage of patients with secondary hypertension and to delineate any treatable cause. All hypertensive patients should have a CXR for the diagnosis of cardiovascular complications (cardiac enlargement, aortic valve calcification, cardiac failure) and to establish a baseline for monitoring of future changes or complications such as aortic dissection. Further imaging investigation of hypertension is indicated in the following:

- Children and young adults less than 40 years old
- Hypertension that is severe or malignant in nature
- Failure of antihypertensive medication
- Renal dysfunction
- Certain clinical signs, such as a bruit heard over the renal arteries
- Clinical evidence of endocrine disorders.

The more common causes of secondary hypertension include:
- Renal artery stenosis
- Chronic renal failure
- Endocrine disorders, such as phaeochromocytoma, primary hyperaldosteronism and Cushing syndrome; for notes on imaging of endocrine disorders, please see Chapter 12.

3.10.1 Renal artery stenosis

Initial screening for renal artery stenosis may be performed with Doppler US or scintigraphy.

Doppler US is non-invasive with no radiation required and should be the initial investigation of choice where local expertise is available. A major limitation of US is obscuration of renal arteries by overlying bowel gas and obesity. Scintigraphy with ^{99}mTc-DTPA (diethylenetriamine pentaacetic acid) may be used where US is technically inadequate. The use of an angiotensin-converting enzyme inhibitor such as intravenous captopril increases the accuracy of the study. CT or MR angiography may be used for further relatively non-invasive imaging where the above screening tests are equivocal.

Where the screening tests are positive, renal angiography and interventional radiology are indicated. Most patients with renal artery stenosis are treated with interventional radiology, i.e. percutaneous transluminal angioplasty (PTA) and stent insertion. The goals of treatment with interventional radiology are normal blood pressure, or hypertension that can be controlled medically plus improved renal function.

In some specialist centres, renal vein renin assays may be performed prior to treatment of renal artery stenosis. For renal vein renin assays, catheters are inserted through the femoral vein and positioned in the renal veins. Blood samples are taken from each renal vein to assess renin levels. A relatively high renin level from the side with renal artery stenosis indicates a positive study. A positive renal vein renin assay indicates a favourable outcome from surgery or interventional radiology.

3.11 INTERVENTIONAL RADIOLOGY OF THE PERIPHERAL VASCULAR SYSTEM

3.11.1 Central venous access

Interventional radiologists use a combination of US and fluoroscopic guidance in acquiring long-term access to the central venous system. US is used to obtain initial venous access. US is able to localize the vein, confirm its patency, and diagnose relevant anatomical variants. Fluoroscopic guidance is used to confirm the final position of the catheter. In general, a central venous catheter should be positioned with its tip at the junction of the SVC and right atrium.

Indications for central venous access include:
- Chemotherapy
- Antibiotic therapy
- Hyperalimentation
- Haemodialysis.

Type of device depends largely on the period of time that venous access is required. Most commonly used devices are:
- PICC lines
  - Short- to intermediate-term central venous access
  - Inserted via a peripheral arm vein
  - With US guidance PICC lines may be inserted above the elbow into the basilic or brachial vein; patients generally prefer this over cubital fossa placement as they are able to use their arm
- Tunnelled catheters (Fig. 3.17)
  - Intermediate-term access
  - Internal jugular vein is usually the preferred route for insertion
  - A subcutaneous tunnel is made with blunt dissection from a skin incision in the upper chest wall to the venous access site
  - The venous catheter is pulled through this subcutaneous tunnel with a tunnelling device and inserted into the internal jugular vein
  - The catheter is held at the skin insertion site with a purse-string suture
- Implanted ports
  - Longer-term (three months or more) intermittent access
  - Particularly suitable for cyclical chemotherapy
  - Access ports are made of steel, titanium or plastic
  - A subcutaneous pocket is fashioned in the chest wall for the port
  - Venous access is via the internal jugular or subclavian vein
  - After placement, the skin is sutured over the port.

PICC line insertion requires only local anaesthetic; the other methods usually require sedation, and in some cases including children, general anaesthetic.

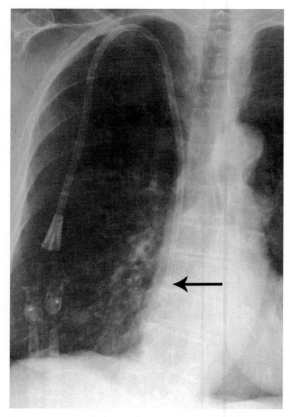

Figure 3.17 Tunnelled central venous port. The tip of the catheter is well positioned at the junction of the superior vena cava and right atrium (arrow).

All venous access techniques are performed under conditions of strict sterility. Complications of venous access may include the following:
- Infection: rate of infection expressed as the number of infections per 10 000 catheter days
  - PICC lines: 4–11
  - Tunnelled catheters: 14
  - Implantation ports: 6
- Catheter blockage due to thrombosis and fibrin sheath formation: 3–10 per cent
- Venous thrombosis (upper limb DVT): 1–2 per cent
- Other complications, such as catheter malposition and kinking, are rare with careful placement.

3.11.2 Endovascular AAA repair

Endoluminal devices combining metallic stents with Dacron® graft material may be used to treat aneurysms of the abdominal aorta. These devices are inserted percutaneously via femoral artery puncture, removing the need for open surgery. Covered stent is the most commonly used endoluminal device for endovascular AAA repair (EVAR). Covered stents consist of a tube of Dacron graft material that is held open by a series of self-expanding stents; usually three components, an inverted 'Y'-shaped graft that sits in the aorta with the lower limbs of the 'Y' projecting into the common iliac arteries, and two shorter grafts for the common iliac arteries.

Aims of endovascular AAA repair:
- Reconstitute a normal lumen in the centre of the aneurysm
- Prevent aneurysm rupture by excluding the aneurysm sac from blood flow and arterial pressure.

Complications of endovascular AAA repair include graft migration, kinking and distortion, and endoleak. Endoleak refers to blood flow in the aneurysm sac outside the graft. Endoleak is an important complication to recognize as it implies that the aneurysm sac is exposed to arterial pressure, increasing the risk of further dilatation and rupture. Postprocedure imaging consists of AXR to confirm graft position and structural integrity plus contrast-enhanced CT to exclude endoleak (Fig. 3.18).

3.11.3 Percutaneous transluminal angioplasty

The usual indication for PTA is a short segment arterial stenosis with associated clinical evidence of limb ischaemia.

PTA consists of the following:
- Arterial puncture
- Wire passed across the arterial stenosis
- Balloon catheter passed over the wire and the balloon dilated to expand the stenosed arterial segment
- Pressure readings proximal and distal to the stenosis pre- and post-dilatation may be performed
- Post-dilatation angiogram performed to assess the result (Fig. 3.19).

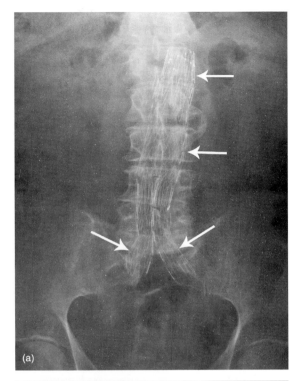

(a)

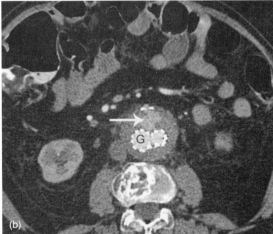

(b)

Figure 3.18 Covered stent (arrows) for aortic aneurysm. (a) AXR shows the position of the stent graft (arrows). (b) CT with intravenous contrast injection shows the stent graft (G) within the aortic aneurysm. Note the presence of contrast enhancement in the aneurysm sac anterior to the graft indicating an endoleak (arrow).

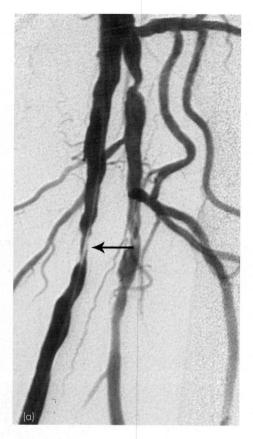
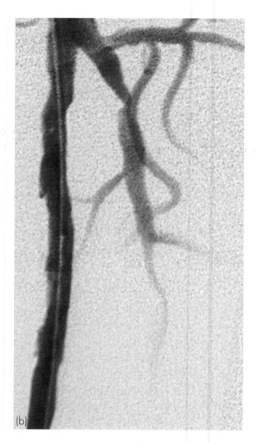

Figure 3.19 Percutaneous transluminal angioplasty (PTA). (a) Catheter angiography shows a stenosis of the superficial femoral artery in the upper thigh (arrow). (b) Following PTA the stenosis is no longer seen.

Postprocedure care following PTA consists of haemostasis and bed rest as for angiography. Patients may be maintained on low-dose aspirin or heparin following a complicated procedure. Complications are uncommon and include arterial occlusion, arterial rupture, haemorrhage and distal embolization.

3.11.4 Arterial stent placement

Arterial stents are commonly used by interventional radiologists in the management of stenotic and occlusive arterial disease. Particular indications for stent deployment include:

- Severe or heavily calcified iliac artery stenosis/ occlusion
- Acute failure of PTA due to recoil of the vessel wall

- PTA complicated by arterial dissection
- Late failure of PTA due to recurrent stenosis.

Arterial stents are of two types: balloon-expandable (Palmaz®) and self-expanding (Wallstent®).

Self-expanding stents consist of stainless steel spring filaments woven into a flexible self-expanding band. Both types of stent are deployed via arterial puncture.

3.11.5 Arterial thrombolysis

Indications for thromboylsis in the peripheral vascular system include:

- Acute, or acute on chronic arterial ischaemia
- Arterial thrombosis complicating PTA
- Surgical graft thrombosis
- Acute upper limb DVT.

Thrombolysis is performed via arterial puncture, or venous puncture for upper limb DVT. A catheter is positioned in or just proximal to the thrombosis followed by infusion of a thrombolytic agent such as urokinase or tissue plasminogen activator (tPA). Regular follow-up angiograms or venograms are performed to ensure dissolution of thrombus with repositioning of the catheter as required. PTA or arterial stent deployment may be performed for any underlying stenosis. The patient is maintained on anticoagulation therapy following successful thrombolysis.

Contraindications to thrombolysis include:
- Bleeding diathesis
- Active or recent bleeding from any source
- Recent surgery, pregnancy or significant trauma.

Complications of thrombolysis may include:
- Haematoma formation at the arterial puncture site
- Distal embolization of partly lysed thrombus
- Systemic bleeding including cerebral haemorrhage, haematuria and epistaxis.

3.11.6 Vascular embolization

Vascular embolization refers to selective delivery of a variety of embolic materials.

Uses of vascular embolization include:
- Control of bleeding
  - Trauma: penetrating injuries; pelvic trauma (Fig. 3.20)
  - Arteriovenous malformations and aneurysms
  - Severe epistaxis

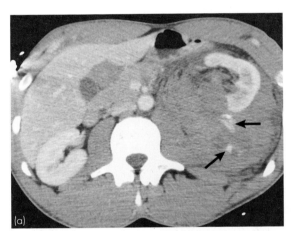

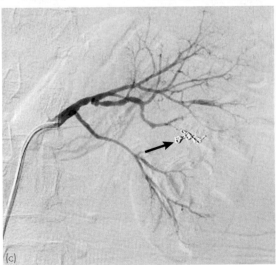

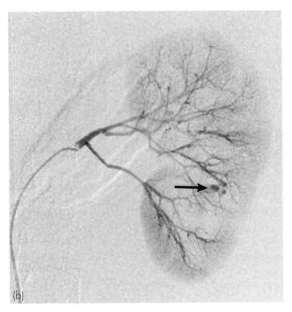

Figure 3.20 Renal trauma and embolization: CT and angiogram. (a) CT post-trauma shows a lacerated left kidney surrounded by a large haematoma. Small pools of extravasated contrast material indicate active bleeding (arrows). (b) Catheter angiogram shows extravasation of contrast material (arrow). (c) Post-embolization angiogram shows embolic material (arrow) with cessation of bleeding.

- Management of tumour
  - Palliative: embolic agents labelled with cytotoxic agents, radioactive isotopes or monoclonal antibodies
  - Definitive treatment for tumours of vascular origin, e.g. aneurysmal bone cyst
  - Preoperative to decrease vascularity or deliver chemotherapy
- Systemic arteriovenous malformation: definitive treatment, preoperative, palliative.

For vascular embolization, the embolic material is delivered through an arterial catheter, either a standard diagnostic angiographic catheter or one of a number of specialized superselective catheters. These include microcatheters, which can be coaxially placed through a larger guiding catheter to gain distal access in small arteries. Embolic materials include:

- Metal coils with or without thrombogenic fibres attached
- Particles such as polyvinyl alcohol particles
- Glue: superglue acrylates
- Detachable balloons: latex or silicon
- Gelfoam pledgets
- Absolute alcohol
- Chemotherapeutic agents
- Resin microspheres loaded ^{90}yttrium.

The type of material used depends on the site, blood flow characteristics, whether a permanent or temporary occlusion is required, type of catheter in use, and personal preference of the operator. Vascular embolization requires high quality imaging facilities, especially digital subtraction angiography, to monitor progress of embolization and to diagnose complications.

Complications of vascular embolization may include:

- Inadvertent embolization of normal structures
- Pain
- Post-embolization syndrome: fever, malaise and leukocytosis 3–5 days after embolization.

3.11.7 Inferior vena cava filtration

In certain situations, self-expanding metal filters may be deployed in the inferior vena cava (IVC) to prevent pulmonary embolus (Fig. 3.21).

Indications for IVC filtration include:

- PE or DVT, where anticoagulation therapy is contraindicated
- Recurrent PE despite anticoagulation
- During surgery in high-risk patients.

Technique of IVC filter insertion:

- Venous puncture, either common femoral or internal jugular vein
- Inferior cavogram is performed to check IVC patency, exclude anatomical anomalies, measure IVC diameter and document the position of the renal veins
- IVC filter deployed via a catheter.

Permanent or removable filters may be used. Complications of IVC filtration are rare and may include femoral vein or IVC thrombosis, perforation of the IVC, and filter migration.

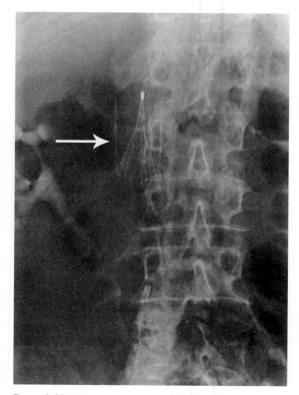

Figure 3.21 Intravenous vena cava filter (arrow).

SUMMARY BOX

Clinical presentation	Investigation of choice	Comment
Congestive cardiac failure	CXR	
	Echocardiography	
Screening for coronary artery disease	Exercise stress testing: ECG, echocardiography, perfusion scintigraphy CT coronary angiography Catheter coronary angiography CT calcium score	Choice of modality depends on multiple factors including: Clinical presentation Cardiac risk factors Local expertise and availability
Myocardial viability	Myocardial perfusion scintigraphy	
	Echocardiography	
Aortic dissection	CT	
Abdominal aortic aneurysm	US for surveillance	
	CT for preoperative planning	
	CT for suspected leak	
Claudication: PVD	Physiological testing and Doppler US CTA/MRA	Catheter angiography largely replaced by CTA and MRA for diagnosis of PVD
Pulmonary embolism	CT pulmonary angiogram	V/Q scintigraphy in selected cases, e.g. allergy to iodinated contrast material
Deep venous thrombosis	Duplex US	
Venous incompetence	Duplex US	
Hypertension: suspected renal artery stenosis	Duplex US	

CTA, CT angiography; ECG, electrocardiogram, MRA, magnetic resonance angiography; PVD, peripheral vascular disease.

4 Gastrointestinal system

4.1 HOW TO READ AN AXR

With the widespread use of US and CT in the imaging of abdominal disorders, the AXR is less commonly performed in modern practice.

Indications for AXR include:
- Suspected intestinal obstruction
- Perforation of the gastrointestinal tract
- Follow-up of urinary tract calculi
- Foreign bodies due to penetrating injuries or ingestion (see Fig. 3.1).

The standard plain film abdominal series consists of three films as follows:
- Supine AP abdomen: standard projection used in all cases
- Erect CXR can be included as part of a routine abdominal series to look for the following
  - Free gas beneath the diaphragm
  - Chest complications of abdominal conditions, e.g. pleural effusion in pancreatitis
  - Chest conditions presenting with abdominal pain, e.g. lower lobe pneumonia
- Erect AP abdomen: used to look for fluid levels and free gas in cases of suspected intestinal obstruction or perforation.

Owing to a number of variable factors including body habitus, distribution of bowel gas and the size of individual organs, such as the liver, the 'normal' AXR may show a wide range of appearances. For this reason, a methodical approach is important and the following check-list of 'things to look for' should be used (Fig. 4.1):
- Hollow organs
  - Stomach
  - Small bowel: generally contains no visible gas, although a few non-dilated gas-filled loops may be seen in elderly patients as a normal finding
  - Large bowel
  - Bladder: seen as a round, soft tissue 'mass' arising from the pelvic floor
- Solid organs: liver, spleen, kidneys, uterus
- Margins: diaphragm, psoas muscle outline, flank stripe, otherwise known as the properitoneal fat line
- Bones: lower ribs, spine, pelvis, hips and sacroiliac joints
- Calcifications
  - Aorta
  - Other arteries: the splenic artery is often calcified in the elderly and is seen as tortuous calcification in the left upper abdomen
  - Phleboliths: small, round calcifications within pelvic veins; very common even in young patients and should not be confused with ureteric calculi
  - Lymph nodes: lymph node calcification may be due to previous infection and is common in the right iliac fossa and the pelvis
  - Costal cartilages commonly calcify in older patients.

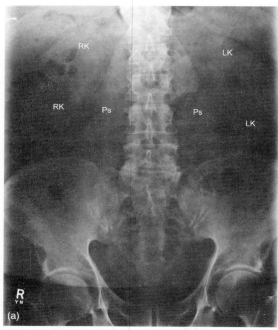
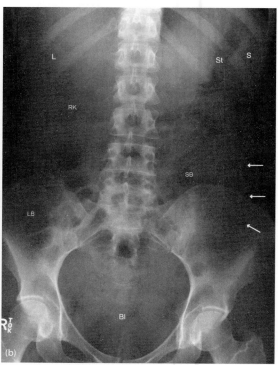

Figure 4.1 Normal AXR. (a) Note the following: right kidney (RK), left kidney (LK), psoas muscles (Ps). According to the principles explained in Chapter 1, the margins of the kidneys and psoas muscles are outlined by retroperitoneal fat. (b) Note the following: liver (L), right kidney (RK), stomach (St), spleen (S), small bowel (SB), large bowel (LB), bladder (Bl) and properitoneal fat stripe (arrows).

4.2 CONTRAST STUDIES OF THE GASTROINTESTINAL TRACT

4.2.1 Barium swallow

Barium swallow is a relatively simple and non-invasive investigation in which the patient is asked to swallow liquid barium and images are obtained as it passes through the oesophagus. Indications for barium swallow include:

- Dysphagia
- Swallowing disorders in the elderly following stroke or central nervous system (CNS) trauma
- Suspected gastro-oesophageal reflux
- Post-oesophageal surgery.

Barium is usually used, although for checking integrity of surgical anastomoses a water-soluble material such as Gastrografin is preferable. Gastrografin should not be used if pulmonary aspiration is suspected as it is highly osmolar and may induce pulmonary oedema if it enters the lungs.

4.2.2 Barium meal: examination of the stomach and duodenum

Barium meal has generally been replaced by endoscopy for the investigation of upper gastrointestinal tract (GIT) symptoms such as dyspepsia, suspected upper GIT bleeding, weight loss or anaemia of unknown cause. Water-soluble contrast material (Gastrografin) is used for assessment of anastomoses post-gastric surgery, including various surgical procedures used for control of obesity, such as gastric banding, sleeve gastrectomy and Roux-en-Y gastric bypass.

4.2.3 Barium follow-through: examination of the small bowel

Barium follow-through or small bowel series is a simple procedure used to demonstrate gross small bowel pathology, such as mechanical obstruction or malrotation. The patient drinks a quantity of barium or Gastrografin and images are acquired until the contrast material either reaches an obstruction or enters the large bowel.

4.2.4 Small bowel enema (enteroclysis)

For enteroclysis, a nasogastric tube is passed into the stomach and with the aid of a steering wire is then guided through the duodenum to the duodenojejunal flexure. A mixture of barium with either water or methyl cellulose is injected rapidly through the tube into the small bowel giving a double-contrast effect. Enteroclysis has largely been replaced in modern practice by CT or magnetic resonance (MR) enterography (see Section 4.5.1 below), as well as a variety of endoscopic techniques including wireless capsule enteroscopy, push enteroscopy, and double- and single-balloon enteroscopy.

4.2.5 Barium enema: examination of the large bowel

For most indications including altered bowel habit, weight loss or anaemia of unknown cause, lower GIT bleeding, and to screen for the presence of colorectal carcinoma or polyps in patients at risk, barium enema has been replaced with colonoscopy. Where colonoscopy is contraindicated or incomplete, imaging assessment of the large bowel is best performed with CT colonography, also known as virtual colonoscopy (see below). Contrast enema studies may be performed for investigation of suspected large bowel pathology in specific circumstances as outlined below, or where colonoscopy and CT colonography are unavailable. Single contrast enema studies with Gastrografin may be useful to outline and define a suspected large bowel obstruction, to define a suspected perforation or to check surgical anastomoses (Fig. 4.2). Single contrast barium enema with dilute barium may be used in children for the diagnosis of large bowel pathology, such as Hirschsprung disease. Barium enema is contraindicated in the presence of acute colitis and toxic megacolon. Complications are very rare and consist of bowel perforation and transient bacteraemia; patients with artificial heart valves should receive antibiotic cover when having a barium enema.

4.3 DYSPHAGIA

Dysphagia refers to the subjective feeling of swallowing difficulty caused by a variety of structural or functional disorders of the oral cavity, pharynx, oesophagus or stomach. Endoscopy is the first investigation of choice when oesophageal malignancy is suspected on clinical grounds. Advantages of endoscopy include direct visualization of the mucosal surface of the oesophagus, performance of biopsies, as well as other interventions, such as dilatation and stent placement. In most other instances, or where endoscopy has limited availability, barium swallow is the simplest and cheapest screening test for the investigation of dysphagia. For many conditions, barium swallow is sufficient for diagnosis; for others it will guide further investigations. Some of the more common findings in patients with dysphagia are outlined below:

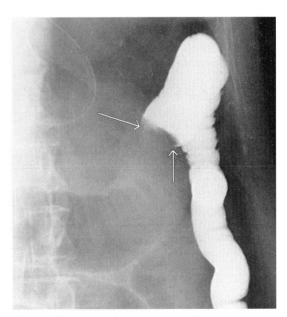

Figure 4.2 Single contrast barium enema showing an obstructing tumour (arrows) in the distal transverse colon.

- Stricture of the oesophagus, i.e. a localized region of constant narrowing
  - Intrinsic stricture due to a disease process of the wall of the oesophagus can usually be differentiated from extrinsic compression on barium swallow
  - Intrinsic stricture of the oesophagus may be due to oesophageal carcinoma, peptic stricture secondary to gastro-oesophageal reflux, corrosive ingestion or systemic sclerosis
  - All strictures seen on barium swallow should undergo endoscopic assessment and biopsy, as should areas of ulceration and mucosal irregularity
  - Stricture due to external compression (extrinsic stricture) may be caused by aberrant blood vessels, mediastinal tumours or lymphadenopathy
  - Extrinsic stricture seen on barium swallow should be investigated further with CT
- Carcinoma of the oesophagus
  - Appearances of oesophageal carcinoma depend on the pattern of tumour growth
  - Early lesions: mucosal irregularity and ulceration
  - More advanced lesions: irregular strictures with elevated margins
  - Further staging: CT to assess local invasion and mediastinal lymphadenopathy, as well as to exclude liver and pulmonary metastases
- Sliding hiatus hernia
  - Range in size from a small clinically insignificant hernia to the entire stomach lying in the thorax (i.e. thoracic stomach), which is at risk of volvulus
  - Hiatus hernia may be seen on CXR as an apparent mass containing a fluid level lying behind the heart
- Pharyngeal pouch (Zenker's diverticulum)
  - Weakness of the posterior wall of the lower pharynx may lead to formation of a pharyngeal pouch
  - Contrast-filled pouch projects posteriorly and to the left above the cricopharyngeus muscle (Fig. 4.3)
  - Pharyngeal pouches may become quite large with a fluid level seen on CXR

- Achalasia
  - Dilated oesophagus that may also be elongated and tortuous with a smoothly tapered lower end
  - CXR signs: fluid level in the mediastinum, absent gastric bubble and evidence of aspiration pneumonia
- Motility disorders of the oesophagus
  - Dysphagia due to abnormal oesophageal motility is common in elderly patients, and may also be seen in association with reflux oesophagitis, early achalasia and various causes of neuropathy including diabetes
- Patients with swallowing disorders due to CNS problems, such as stroke or Parkinson's disease, or following laryngectomy may be assessed with modified barium swallow

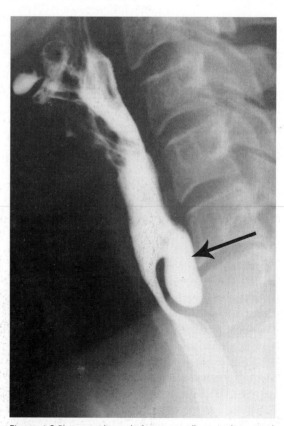

Figure 4.3 Pharyngeal pouch: barium swallow. A pharyngeal pouch (arrow) is seen on a lateral view projecting posteriorly from the lower pharynx.

- Ingestion of liquids and solids of varying consistency under the supervision of a speech therapist and radiologist with video recording of swallowing
- Dysphagia in immunocompromised patients is usually due to infectious oesophagitis
  - Commonest causative organism in HIV-positive patients is *Candida albicans* and dysphagia in these patients is often treated empirically with antifungal therapy
  - Other causes include herpes simplex and cytomegalovirus
  - Endoscopy is indicated to obtain specimens for laboratory analysis if dysphagia in an immunocompromised patient fails to settle on antifungal therapy.

4.4 ACUTE ABDOMEN

Acute abdominal pain is a common clinical problem that encompasses a wide range of pathologies. Key diagnostic points may be obtained from initial history and examination including:

- Location of the pain
- Associated fever
- History of previous or recent surgery
- Prior history of similar pain

- Signs that may indicate intestinal obstruction, such as abdominal distension, vomiting and altered bowel habit.

Clinical history and examination may be accompanied by laboratory investigations, such as white cell count and pancreatic enzymes. Imaging may be used to complement, not replace clinical assessment. Where the diagnosis is obvious on clinical grounds and/or AXR, more sophisticated imaging is not required. Particular indications for AXR in a setting of acute abdomen are suspected bowel obstruction or perforation of the GIT. AXR may be negative or actually misleading in many of the other common causes of acute abdomen. Other imaging modalities, such as CT, US and contrast studies, may be used where appropriate (Fig. 4.4). US is useful for assessment of the solid organs and for the diagnosis of gallstones.

CT has found an increasing role in the assessment of acute abdominal pain. One of the most important reasons for this is the ability of CT to display inflammation or oedema in fat. Inflammatory change is very well shown on CT as streaky soft tissue density or infiltration within the darker fat. This is an extremely useful sign on CT that often helps to localize pathology that may otherwise be overlooked. CT is less sensitive in the assessment of

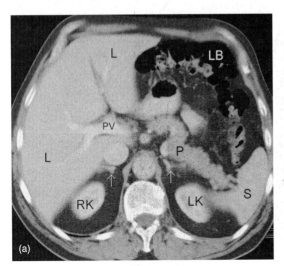
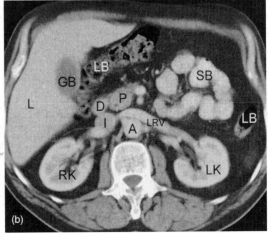

Figure 4.4 Normal abdomen: CT. (a and b) Two separate transverse CT images of the upper abdomen showing the following structures: liver (L), portal vein (PV), right kidney (RK), left kidney (LK), spleen (S), pancreas (P), gallbladder (GB), large bowel (LB), duodenum (D), inferior vena cava (I), aorta (A), left renal vein (LRV), small bowel (SB), adrenal glands (arrows).

very thin or cachectic patients in whom abdominal fat planes may be absent.

4.4.1 Perforation of the gastrointestinal tract

Perforation of the GIT may be due to peptic ulceration, inflammation including acute diverticulitis and appendicitis, and blunt or penetrating injury including iatrogenic trauma. Perforation of the stomach, small intestine and most of the colon produces free gas in the peritoneal cavity. Perforation of the duodenum and posterior rectum results in free retroperitoneal gas.

Radiographic signs of free gas:
- Erect CXR: gas beneath diaphragm (Fig. 4.5)
- Supine abdomen: gas outlines anatomical structures, such as the liver, falciform ligament and spleen; bowel walls are seen as white lines outlined by gas on both sides, i.e. inside and outside the bowel lumen (Fig. 4.6)
- Free gas is also identified on erect abdomen film
- If the patient is too ill to stand then either decubitus or shoot-through lateral films can be performed.

4.4.2 Suspected small bowel obstruction

The clinical presentation of small bowel obstruction (SBO) may include abdominal pain and vomiting, progressing to acute abdomen with abdominal distension and tenderness. Causes of SBO in adults include:
- Adhesions due to previous surgery, trauma or infection
- Strangulated hernia
- Small bowel neoplasm
- Gallstone ileus.

In children, causes of SBO include strangulated hernia, congenital malformation, intussusception and malrotation (see Chapter 13).

4.4.2.1 AXR

AXR is the primary investigation of choice in suspected small bowel obstruction. Situations where AXR may be less accurate include partial or early obstruction, and closed-loop obstruction. The majority of small bowel obstructions are diagnosed with clinical assessment and AXR.

Signs of small bowel obstruction on AXR (Fig. 4.7):
- Dilated small bowel loops, which have the following features
  - Central location

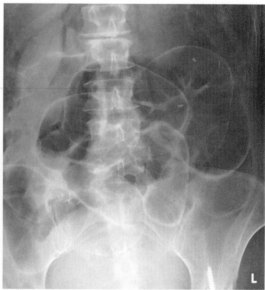

Figure 4.6 Free gas: AXR. Free gas in the peritoneal cavity caused clear delineation of both sides of the bowel wall. Compare the appearances of these bowel lops with those visualized in other images in this chapter. Multiple small surgical clips are also present.

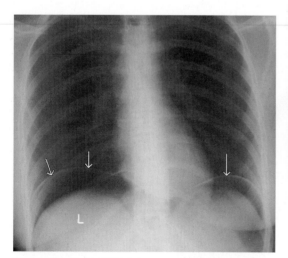

Figure 4.5 Free gas: CXR. Free gas is seen beneath the diaphragm (arrows). Free gas separates the liver (L) from the right diaphragm.

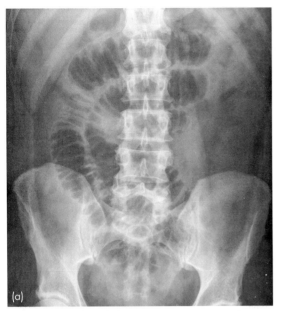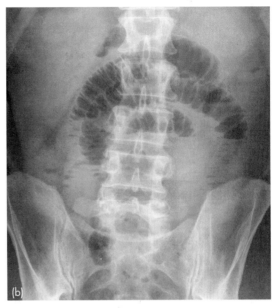

Figure 4.7 Small bowel obstruction. (a) Supine view showing multiple loops of small bowel. Note the features of small bowel loops as described in the text. (b) Erect view showing multiple relatively short fluid levels.

- Numerous
- 2.5–5.0 cm diameter
- Small radius of curvature
- Valvulae conniventes, seen as white lines that are thin, numerous, close together and extend right across the bowel
- Do not contain solid faeces
- Multiple fluid levels on the erect AXR
- 'String of beads' sign on the erect AXR due to small gas pockets trapped between valvulae conniventes
- Absent or little air in the large bowel.

Differential diagnosis of dilated small bowel loops on AXR is paralytic ileus. Paralytic ileus may be generalized or localized. Localized ileus refers to dilated loops of bowel ('sentinel loops'), usually small bowel, overlying a local inflammation:
- Right upper quadrant: acute cholecystitis
- Left upper quadrant: acute pancreatitis
- Lower right abdomen: acute appendicitis.

Generalized ileus refers to non-specific dilatation of small and large bowel, which may occur postoperatively or with peritonitis. Scattered irregular fluid levels are seen on the erect X-ray (Fig. 4.8).

Causes of SBO that may occasionally be diagnosed on AXR include strangulated hernia and gallstone ileus.

4.4.2.2 Strangulated hernia

The term 'hernia' refers to abnormal protrusion of intra-abdominal contents, usually peritoneal fat and bowel loops. Inguinal hernia accounts for about 80 per cent of abdominal wall hernias. Femoral hernia is more common in females. Other types of external hernia include umbilical hernia and hernia related to previous surgery, either incisional or parastomal. Most hernias present with an inguinal or abdominal wall mass that increases in size when the patient stands or strains. Occasionally, hernias may become strangulated and present with localized pain and intestinal obstruction.

Radiographic signs of strangulated hernia (Fig. 4.9):
- Gas-containing soft tissue mass in the inguinal region may have a fluid level on the erect view
- Gas in the bowel wall within the hernia indicates incarceration and bowel wall infarction.

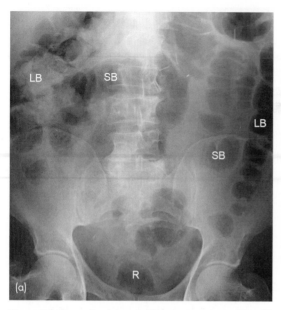
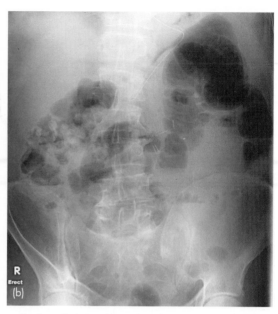

Figure 4.8 Generalized ileus. (a) Supine view shows dilated loops of both small (SB) and large bowel (LB). Gas is seen as far distally as the rectum (R) making a mechanical obstruction unlikely. (b) Erect view showing only scattered fluid levels.

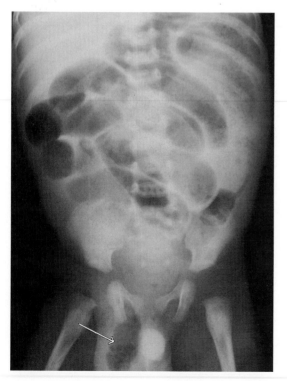

4.4.2.3 Gallstone ileus

Gallstone ileus refers to small bowel obstruction secondary to gallstone impaction. Gallstone ileus usually occurs in a setting of chronic cholecystitis where a large gallstone erodes through the inflamed gallbladder wall to enter the duodenum. The gallstone then becomes impacted in the distal small bowel causing small bowel obstruction.

Radiographic signs of gallstone ileus (Fig. 4.10):

- Small bowel obstruction
- Gas in the biliary tree seen as a branching pattern of gas density in the right upper quadrant
- Calcified gallstone lying in an abnormal position is occasionally seen.

Figure 4.9 Strangulated hernia. Multiple dilated small bowel loops indicating intestinal obstruction seen in an infant with abdominal distension. Note that in infants small and large bowel loops tend to be rather featureless making differentiation of small from large bowel difficult. The most reliable differentiating feature is the position, with small bowel loops tending to lie more centrally. Note the obstructed right inguinal hernia (arrow).

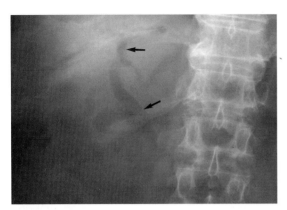

Figure 4.10 Gallstone ileus. Gas is seen outlining the bile ducts (arrows).

4.4.2.4 CT

CT is the investigation of choice for suspected SBO when clinical and AXR assessments are inconclusive. CT is highly accurate for establishing the diagnosis of small bowel obstruction, defining the location and cause of obstruction, and diagnosing associated strangulation. CT signs of SBO include dilated small bowel loops measuring >2.5 cm in diameter, with an identifiable transition from dilated to non-dilated or collapsed bowel loops (Fig. 4.11).

4.4.3 Suspected large bowel obstruction

Large bowel obstruction (LBO) may have a subacute to chronic presentation with abdominal pain and distension and constipation. The commonest cause for such a presentation is colorectal carcinoma. More acute presentations of LBO may be seen with sigmoid volvulus, caecal volvulus and diverticulitis. Most cases of LBO are diagnosed with clinical assessment and AXR.

Signs of large bowel obstruction on AXR (Fig. 4.12):
- Dilated large bowel loops, which have the following features
  - Peripheral location
  - Few in number
  - Large: above 5.0 cm diameter
  - Wide radius of curvature
  - Haustra, seen as thick white lines that are widely separated, and may or may not extend right across the bowel (compare these features with those of the small bowel valvulae conniventes described above)
  - Contain solid faeces
- Small bowel may also be dilated if the ileocaecal valve is 'incompetent'.

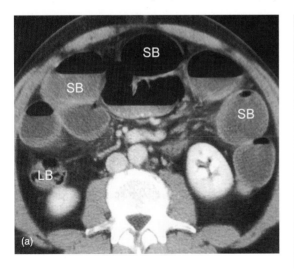

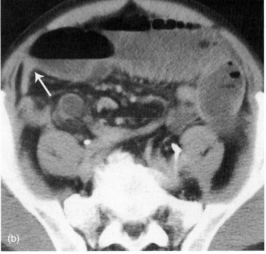

Figure 4.11 Small bowel obstruction: CT. (a) Note dilated loops of small bowel (SB) containing fluid levels and non-dilated large bowel (LB). (b) Abrupt transition from dilated to non-dilated small bowel (arrow) indicating mechanical small bowel obstruction.

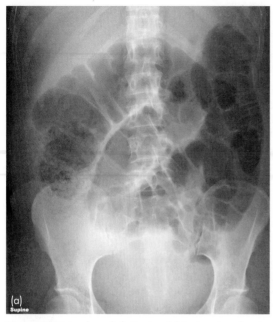
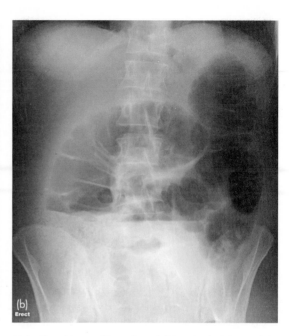

Figure 4.12 Large bowel obstruction. (a) Supine view showing multiple dilated loops of large bowel. Note the thick haustral folds and compare with the small bowel valvulae conniventes shown in Fig. 4.7. (b) Erect view showing fluid levels.

Depending on which large bowel loops are dilated, an approximate level of obstruction may be suggested on AXR. With respect to the cause of LBO, AXR appearances are generally non-specific and non-diagnostic. Cases where a specific diagnosis may be made with AXR include caecal volvulus and sigmoid volvulus.

4.4.3.1 Caecal volvulus

Caecal volvulus refers to twisting and obstruction of the caecum. Caecal volvulus occurs most commonly in patients aged 20–40 and is associated with an abnormally long mesentery and malrotation.

Radiographic signs of caecal volvulus (Fig. 4.13):
- Markedly dilated caecum containing one or two haustral markings
- The dilated caecum may lie in the right iliac fossa or left upper quadrant
- Attached gas-filled appendix
- Small bowel dilatation
- Collapse of left half of colon.

4.4.3.2 Sigmoid volvulus

Sigmoid volvulus refers to twisting of the sigmoid colon around its mesenteric axis with obstruction

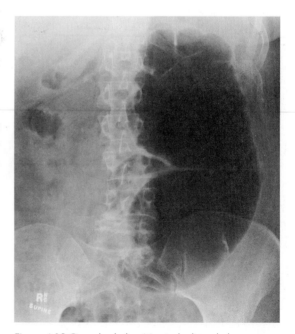

Figure 4.13 Caecal volvulus. Massively distended caecum passing across to the left. This is differentiated from sigmoid volvulus by its shape plus the absence of large bowel dilatation.

and marked dilatation. Sigmoid volvulus occurs in elderly and psychiatrically disturbed patients.

Radiographic signs of sigmoid volvulus (Fig. 4.14):

- Massively distended sigmoid loop in the shape of an inverted 'U', which can extend above T10 and overlap the lower border of the liver
- Usually has no haustral markings
- The outer walls and adjacent inner walls of the 'U' form three white lines that converge towards the left side of the pelvis
- Overlap of the dilated descending colon: 'left flank overlap' sign (good differentiating feature from caecal volvulus in which the remainder of the large bowel is not dilated).

4.4.3.3 Contrast enema

Contrast enema may be helpful to localize the location of LBO and to diagnose its cause, e.g. tumour or inflammatory mass (Fig. 4.2). Contrast enema will also differentiate true large bowel obstruction from pseudo-obstruction. Pseudo-obstruction (non-obstructive large bowel dilatation) occurs most commonly in elderly patients and may be indistinguishable on AXR from mechanical obstruction.

4.4.3.4 CT

CT may be used for the assessment of difficult or equivocal cases of large bowel obstruction (Fig. 4.15). In the majority of cases, CT will diagnose the location and cause of obstruction. CT may also diagnose other relevant findings, such as liver metastases in the case of an obstructing tumour.

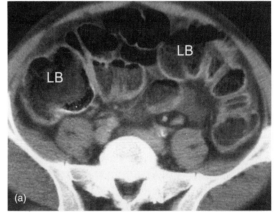

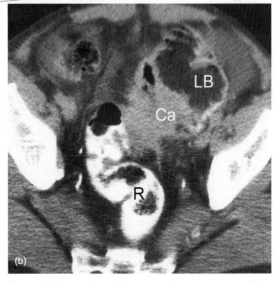

Figure 4.15 Large bowel obstruction due to carcinoma: CT. (a) Dilated loops of large bowel (LB). (b) Carcinoma (Ca) seen as a soft tissue mass in the sigmoid colon proximal to the rectum (R).

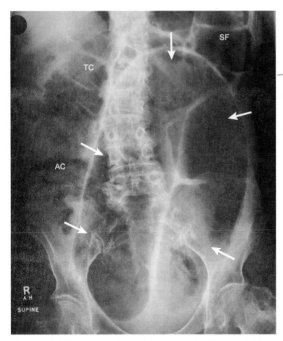

Figure 4.14 Sigmoid volvulus. Note the typical inverted 'U' appearance of sigmoid volvulus (arrows). Note also dilatation of ascending colon (AC), transverse colon (TC) and splenic flexure (SF). Note the characteristic overlap of dilated left colon and sigmoid loop below the splenic flexure.

4.4.4 Right upper quadrant pain

The primary diagnostic consideration in adult patients with right upper quadrant (RUQ) pain is acute cholecystitis.

4.4.4.1 US

US is the most sensitive investigation for the presence of gallstones and is therefore the investigation of choice for suspected acute cholecystitis. The diagnosis of acute cholecystitis is usually made by confirming the presence of gallstones in a patient with RUQ pain and fever (Fig. 4.16). Other signs of acute cholecystitis that may be seen with US include thickening of the gallbladder wall, fluid surrounding the gallbladder, and localized tenderness to direct probe pressure (Fig. 4.17).

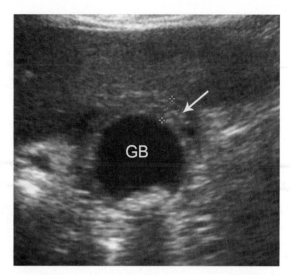

Figure 4.17 Acute cholecystitis: US. The gallbladder (GB) has a thickened wall (arrow) and contains multiple small gallstones.

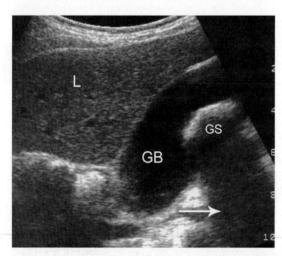

Figure 4.16 Gallstone: US. Note liver (L), gallbladder (GB), gallstone (GS) casting an acoustic shadow (arrow).

4.4.4.2 Scintigraphy

Scintigraphy with ^{99}mTc-labelled iminodiacetic acid (IDA) compounds has a limited role in difficult cases where clinical assessment and US are doubtful. Acute cholecystitis is diagnosed on IDA scan by non-visualization of the gallbladder with good visualization of the common bile duct and duodenum 1 hour after injection.

4.4.4.3 CT

CT may be used where US is negative and/or where alternative diagnoses are being considered.

CT is much less sensitive than US for the detection of gallstones. CT signs of gallbladder inflammation include thickening of the gallbladder wall with infiltrative streaking in adjacent fat.

4.4.5 Right lower quadrant pain

The commonest cause of acute right lower quadrant (RLQ) pain is acute appendicitis. Differential diagnosis includes inflammatory bowel disease, mesenteric adenitis, and gynaecological pathology in female patients. Although most cases of acute appendicitis are confidently diagnosed on clinical grounds, imaging may significantly lower the number of negative appendicectomies. Imaging is particularly useful in patients with atypical features on history and/or in young females where gynaecological pathologies, such as ectopic pregnancy or pelvic inflammatory disease, are suspected.

4.4.5.1 US

Where imaging is required, US is the initial investigation of choice in children, thin patients and women of childbearing age. Accuracy of US is increased by the use of compression and colour Doppler imaging and by concentrating the examination to the point of maximal tenderness as indicated by the patient (Fig. 4.18). Limitations of US

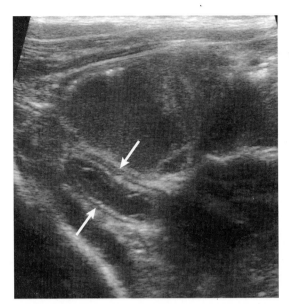

Figure 4.18 Acute appendicitis: US. Acutely inflamed appendix seen as a non-compressible blind ending tubular structure (arrows) in the right iliac fossa.

are that the normal appendix is often not visualized and retrocaecal appendicitis may be obscured. As such, the negative predictive value of a negative US examination is not as high as for CT.

4.4.5.2 CT

For most adult patients, excluding women of childbearing age, CT is the imaging investigation of choice in the assessment of RLQ pain (Fig. 4.19). Advantages of CT include its proven accuracy in the diagnosis of appendicitis and its ability to diagnose alternative causes of RLQ pain. The ability of CT to identify a normal appendix in the majority of patients plus its high level of sensitivity to inflammatory change mean that a negative CT has a very high negative predictive value.

4.4.6 Left lower quadrant pain

The primary diagnostic consideration for the patient with left lower quadrant (LLQ) pain is acute diverticulitis. The term 'acute diverticulitis' encompasses a range of inflammatory pathologies that occur secondary to diverticulosis, including bowel wall and pericolonic inflammation, perforation, abscess formation, and formation of sinus or fistula tracts.

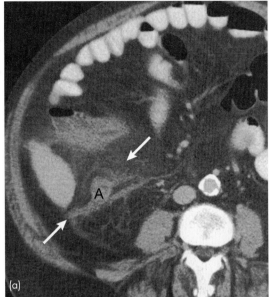

(a)

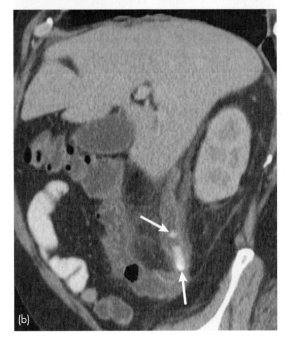

(b)

Figure 4.19 Acute appendicitis: CT. (a) CT shows a swollen appendix (A) with a soft tissue stranding pattern in adjacent fat (arrows). This stranding pattern is a highly useful sign on CT indicating oedema in fat adjacent to inflammation. (b) Oblique sagittal reconstruction shows the inflamed appendix extending superiorly. Note the large faecoliths at the base of the appendix (arrows).

US should be used in women of childbearing age in whom gynaecological pathology, such as ectopic pregnancy or pelvic inflammatory disease, would be more likely than acute diverticulitis.

CT is otherwise the investigation of choice for assessment of acute LLQ pain. CT is highly accurate for the diagnosis of acute diverticulitis (Fig. 4.20), and where diverticulitis is not present it may suggest alternative diagnoses, such as small bowel obstruction, pelvic inflammatory disease, renal colic, etc. CT signs of acute diverticulitis include localized bowel wall thickening and soft tissue stranding or haziness in pericolonic fat. Gas in the bladder may indicate formation of a colovesical fistula.

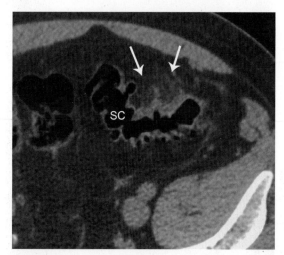

Figure 4.20 Acute diverticulitis: CT. Multiple gas filled diverticula arising from the sigmoid colon (SC). Note localized thickening of the bowel wall and adjacent fat stranding (arrow) indicating acute inflammation.

4.4.7 Renal colic and acute flank pain

Acute flank pain describes pain of the posterolateral abdomen from the lower thorax to the pelvis. The most common cause of acute flank pain is ureteral obstruction caused by an impacted renal calculus. For this reason, the terms 'acute flank pain' and 'renal colic' are often used interchangeably.

The term 'acute flank pain' more accurately reflects the fact that non-renal causes may produce similar symptoms to genuine renal colic. Non-renal causes of acute flank pain include appendicitis, torsion or haemorrhage of ovarian cyst, diverticulitis, inflammatory bowel disease and pancreatitis.

Other renal causes of acute flank pain include acute pyelonephritis, transitional cell carcinoma (TCC) of the ureter causing obstruction and 'clot colic', i.e. ureteric colic due to a blood clot complicating haematuria. In the patient with acute flank pain, initial assessment is directed towards confirming or excluding urinary tract obstruction secondary to a ureteric calculus.

4.4.7.1 CT

CT without contrast enhancement is the imaging test of choice for acute flank pain. Virtually all renal stones are identified on CT including cystine, urate, xanthine and matrix stones, which are generally not seen on AXR. The only exceptions are stones due to crystal precipitation in HIV patients on indinavir medication. The likelihood of a ureteric calculus passing spontaneously is largely related to size. A calculus of 5 mm or less will usually pass where a calculus of 10 mm or more is likely to become lodged. Stone position and size are accurately assessed on CT.

CT signs of urinary tract obstruction:
- Dilatation of the ureter above the calculus
- Dilatation of renal pelvis and collecting system
- Soft tissue stranding in the perinephritic fat due to distended lymphatic channels (Fig. 4.21).

A major advantage of CT is that non-renal causes of acute flank pain may also be diagnosed.

4.4.7.2 Radiograph of kidneys, ureters and bladder

Radiograph of kidneys, ureters and bladder (KUB) refers to a supine AXR done to diagnose and follow up renal or ureteric calculi. Where possible, follow-up of ureteric or renal calculi should be with KUB, as this will result in less radiation exposure than a repeat CT. KUB should generally be performed where an obstructing urinary tract calculus is diagnosed on CT, to confirm that the calculus is visible and therefore amenable to follow-up on plain film. KUB may then be used to confirm spontaneous passage of a calculus or to direct further management. KUB may also be performed after external shock wave lithotripsy or percutaneous calculus extraction to check for residual fragments in the urinary tract.

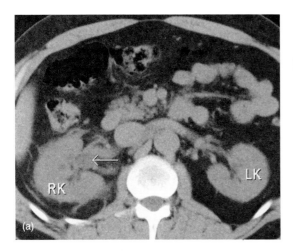

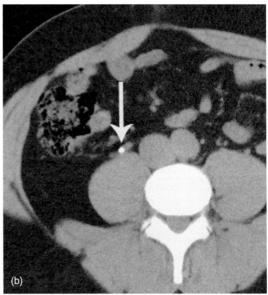

Figure 4.21 Ureteric calculus: CT. Non-enhanced CT performed in a patient with right renal colic. (a) Right kidney (RK), dilated right renal pelvis (arrow), left kidney (LK). (b) Ureteric calculus (arrow).

Ninety per cent of renal calculi contain sufficient calcium to be radio-opaque, i.e. visible on KUB (Fig. 4.22). Cystine stones (3 per cent) are faintly opaque and may be visualized on KUB with difficulty. Urate stones (5 per cent) are lucent, i.e. not visible on KUB. Rare xanthine and matrix stones are also lucent. Note that opacities seen on KUB/AXR thought to be renal or ureteric calculi need to be differentiated from other causes of calcification, such as arterial calcification, calcified lymph nodes and pelvic phleboliths. Phleboliths are small, round calcifications in pelvic veins. Phleboliths are extremely common, and are visible on AXR in most adults.

4.4.8 Acute pancreatitis

Acute pancreatitis usually presents with severe acute epigastric pain. Risk factors for the development of acute pancreatitis include heavy alcohol intake and the presence of gallstones. Initial evaluation for suspected pancreatitis consists of biochemical tests, including amylase and lipase levels.

CT is the imaging investigation of choice for the diagnosis of acute pancreatitis. CT signs in early pancreatitis may precede serum enzyme elevations. CT signs of acute pancreatitis include diffuse or focal pancreatic swelling with indistinct margins and thickening of surrounding fascial planes (Fig. 4.23). CT performed during infusion of contrast material can differentiate necrotic non-enhancing tissue from

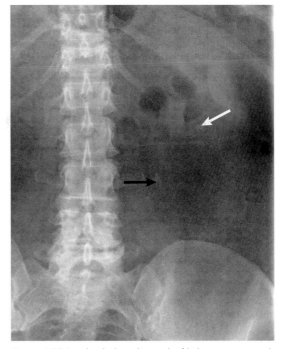

Figure 4.22 Renal calculi: radiograph of kidneys, ureters and bladder. Multiple left calculi, one in the lower pole of the kidney (white arrow) and the other at the pelviureteric junction (black arrow).

viable enhancing tissue; the presence of pancreatic necrosis is associated with a significantly increased mortality.

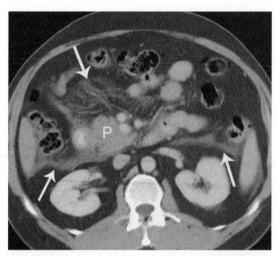

Figure 4.23 Acute pancreatitis: CT. Pancreas (P) is swollen with adjacent fat stranding and thickening of fascial planes (arrows).

Complications of pancreatitis, such as phlegmon, abscess and pseudocyst, are well shown on CT. CT can also be used to guide percutaneous aspiration and drainage procedures. Indications for percutaneous drainage of a fluid collection associated with acute pancreatitis include:

• Suspected abscess
• Enlarging cyst on follow-up imaging
• Symptoms due to mass effect on adjacent structures.

US is usually indicated in patients with acute pancreatitis, primarily to search for gallstones and to assess the biliary tree.

4.4.9 Acute mesenteric ischaemia

Acute mesenteric ischaemia (AMI) is caused by abrupt disruption of blood flow to the bowel. AMI usually presents with sudden onset of severe abdominal pain and bloody diarrhoea. The goal of diagnosis and therapy in AMI is prevention or limitation of bowel infarction. Prompt diagnosis requires a high index of suspicion and early referral for angiography in patients with clinical evidence of AMI. The most common causes of AMI are superior mesenteric artery (SMA) embolus, SMA thrombosis and non-occlusive SMA vasospasm. In the case of SMA embolus, the patient may have a history of cardiac disease, previous embolic event

or simultaneous peripheral artery embolus. SMA thrombosis is usually associated with an underlying stenotic atherosclerotic lesion in the SMA.

Depending on the cause and clinical situation, particularly the presence or absence of peritoneal signs, treatment will be immediate surgery or interventional radiology. Interventional radiology consists of thrombolysis via a selective catheter, which may be followed by angioplasty of any underlying stenosis or papaverine infusion for SMA vasospasm.

4.5 INFLAMMATORY BOWEL DISEASE

The two diseases included in this section are Crohn disease and ulcerative colitis. Patients with inflammatory bowel disease present with abdominal pain and diarrhoea. Extraintestinal manifestations may occur, including skin rashes, arthritis, ocular problems and sclerosing cholangitis. The clinical course after initial presentation usually consists of intermittent episodes of diarrhoea or intestinal obstruction, as well as complications such as infected sinus tracts and abscesses. The main roles of imaging at initial presentation are to confirm the diagnosis and assess the distribution of disease. Follow-up examinations are frequently required to assess the efficacy of therapy and to diagnose complications.

AXR is relatively insensitive and non-specific for the definitive diagnosis of inflammatory bowel disease. AXR is very useful however in patients with severe symptoms for the diagnosis of toxic megacolon (Fig. 4.24), perforation or obstruction. Barium studies and colonoscopy are contraindicated by these findings.

4.5.1 Crohn disease

Crohn disease is characterized by transmural granulomatous inflammation with deep ulceration, sinuses and fistula tracts. Crohn disease may involve any part of the gastrointestinal tract from mouth to anus with small bowel involvement alone in 30 per cent, large bowel in 30 per cent and both small and large bowel in 40 per cent. Involvement is discontinuous with normal bowel between diseased segments ('skip lesions').

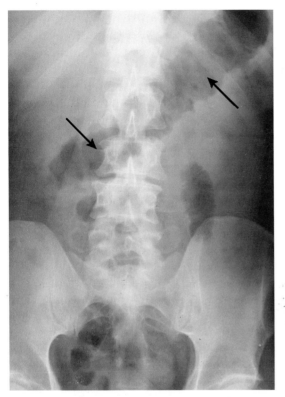

Figure 4.24 Toxic megacolon. AXR shows a dilated transverse colon (arrows) with thickening of the bowel wall.

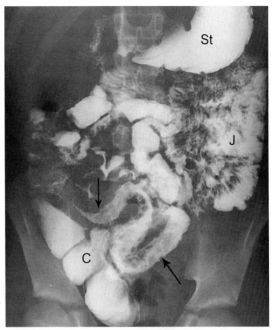

Figure 4.25 Crohn disease: small bowel study. Barium study of the small bowel shows the following: stomach (St), jejunum (J), segment of distal small bowel with irregularity of the mucosal surface indicating multiple deep ulcers (arrows), caecum (C).

Cross-sectional imaging techniques, CT enterography and MR enterography, are being used with increasing frequency in the diagnosis and follow-up of Crohn disease. Where CT enterography and MR enterography are unavailable, barium studies may be used to assess the small bowel, either small bowel follow-through or enteroclysis. Signs of Crohn disease on barium studies include:

- Ulcers
- Strictures
- 'Cobblestoning' due to fissures separating islands of intact mucosa
- Segmental distribution: diseased segments separated by normal bowel (Fig. 4.25).

Scintigraphy with ^{99m}Tc-HMPAO and ^{99m}Tc-labelled sucralphate may be useful for the following:

- Defining anatomical location of disease, particularly in acutely ill patients in whom barium studies are contraindicated

- Diagnosing relapse in patients with known inflammatory bowel disease.

4.5.1.1 CT enterography

CT enterography consists of CT abdomen following ingestion of a large volume (1–1.5 litres) of dilute contrast material, e.g. combination of Gastrografin and methylcellulose. CT enterography is highly accurate for the diagnosis of bowel wall inflammation, and for the demonstration of complications such as sinus tracts, abscesses and strictures. The major limitation of CT enterography is the radiation dose; this is particularly relevant in young patients requiring repeated follow-up examinations.

4.5.1.2 MR enterography

Where available, MR enterography (MR examination of the small bowel) is an excellent alternative to CT, particularly for follow-up examinations. MR enterography refers to MR of the abdomen following ingestion of fluid to distend the small bowel. Buscopan is often injected intravenously to temporarily paralyse the bowel. Intravenous gadolinium is also included to show abnormal enhancement of inflamed bowel wall (Fig. 4.26). Lack of ionizing radiation makes MR enterography particularly useful for diagnosis and follow-up of young patients with Crohn disease, and other chronic conditions of the small bowel that may require repeated follow-up examinations.

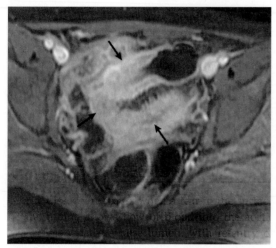

Figure 4.26 Crohn disease: MR enterography. Transverse T1-weighted contrast enhanced MRI of the lower abdomen shows an inflamed segment of small bowel. The inflamed segment shows irregular thickening and marked enhancement (arrows).

4.5.2 Ulcerative colitis

Ulcerative colitis is a disease of large bowel characterized by mucosal ulceration and inflammation.

The rectum is involved in virtually all cases with disease extending proximally in the colon. Distribution of disease is continuous with no 'skip lesions'. Initial diagnosis of inflammatory bowel disease involving the colon is usually by endoscopy, either sigmoidoscopy or colonoscopy, including biopsy. Where colonoscopy is unavailable or contraindicated, barium enema may be performed.

4.6 GASTROINTESTINAL BLEEDING

The goals of diagnosis and treatment of the patient with acute GIT bleeding are:

- Haemodynamic resuscitation
- Localization and diagnosis of the source of bleeding
- Control of blood loss either by endoscopic haemostatic therapy, interventional radiology or surgery.

4.6.1 Upper GIT bleeding

Upper GIT bleeding is defined as bleeding from the oesophagus to the ligament of Treitz. Acute upper GIT bleeding usually presents with haematemesis and/or malaena. It can usually be distinguished clinically from acute lower GIT bleeding, which presents with red blood loss per rectum. Causes of acute upper GIT bleeding include peptic ulcer disease, erosive gastritis, varices, Mallory–Weiss tear and carcinoma. An upper GIT source for GIT bleeding is diagnosed by emergency upper GIT endoscopy in the majority of cases. Endoscopic haemostatic therapies include injection of sclerosants, injection of vasoconstrictors, thermal coagulation and mechanical methods.

4.6.2 Lower GIT bleeding

Common causes of acute lower GIT bleeding are angiodysplasia and diverticular disease. Although colonic diverticula are more prevalent in the sigmoid colon, up to 50 per cent of bleeding from diverticular disease occurs in the ascending colon. Less common causes of lower GIT bleeding include inflammatory bowel disease, colonic carcinoma, solitary rectal ulcer and post-polypectomy.

Lower GIT bleeding is first investigated by sigmoidoscopy. If sigmoidoscopy is negative, scintigraphy, CT angiography and catheter angiography are used to further assess the patient. Scintigraphy and CT angiography are particularly useful in haemodynamically stable patients to diagnose and localize bleeding prior to catheter angiography.

4.6.2.1 Red blood cell scintigraphy

Red blood cell (RBC) scintigraphy with ^{99m}Tc-labelled RBCs shows a GIT bleeding point as an area of increased activity (Fig. 4.27). Scintigraphy is more sensitive than catheter angiography in that a lower rate of haemorrhage is required (0.1–0.2 mL/

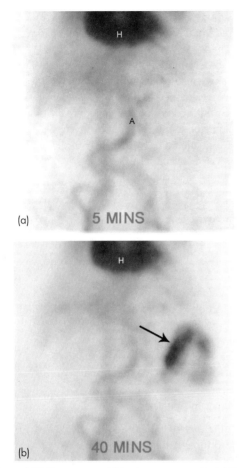

(a)   5 MINS

(b)   40 MINS

Figure 4.27 Gastrointestinal bleeding: scintigraphy. (a) The early phase of a labelled red blood cell study shows normal activity in the heart (H) and aorta (A). (b) A later scan shows accumulation of labelled red blood cells (arrow) in the left upper abdomen indicating bleeding into the large bowel. This was due to angiodysplasia.

min) to produce a positive result. Scintigraphy is less anatomically specific than angiography; for this reason surgery based on RBC scintigraphy alone is not recommended. RBC scintigraphy should be seen as a screening test used to direct further investigation:

- Positive scintigraphy will increase the accuracy of subsequent angiography.
- Negative scintigraphy implies that subsequent angiography is unlikely to identify a bleeding point; elective colonoscopy would be the next investigation in such cases.

4.6.2.2 CT angiography

CT angiography offers a sensitive and specific angiography method that is less invasive and time-consuming than catheter angiography. In many centres, CT angiography has replaced RBC scintigraphy as the initial investigation of choice for investigation of acute lower GIT bleeding. Identification of a bleeding source on CT angiography usually leads to treatment with surgery or interventional radiology (Fig. 4.28).

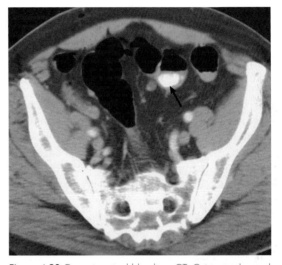

Figure 4.28 Gastrointestinal bleeding: CT. Contrast-enhanced CT shows extravasation of intravenous contrast material into the lumen of the sigmoid colon (arrow), immediately adjacent to a diverticulum. Subsequent surgery revealed a ruptured artery in the base of the diverticulum.

4.6.2.3 Angiography and interventional radiology

Catheter angiography is performed in acute GIT bleeding for two reasons:

- To locate a bleeding point
- To achieve haemostasis by infusion of vasoconstrictors, or embolization.

Extravasation of contrast material into the bowel will be seen if active bleeding of 0.5–1.0 mL/min or more is occurring at the time of injection. Diagnostic angiography may be followed by therapeutic options including selective infusion of vasoconstrictors such as vasopressin and embolization of small distal arterial branches following superselective catheterization. Therapeutic angiography may be used as a definitive treatment, or for stabilization of bleeding prior to surgery.

4.7 COLORECTAL CARCINOMA

4.7.1 Screening for colorectal carcinoma

Colorectal carcinoma (CRC) is the second leading cause of cancer death in Western society. CRC may present clinically with large bowel obstruction, GIT bleeding, or less specifically with weight loss or anaemia. A large percentage of CRC show locally invasive disease or distant metastases at the time of presentation.

The concept of the adenoma–carcinoma sequence describes the well-demonstrated fact that the vast majority of CRCs develop from small adenomatous polyps through a series of genetic mutations. The adenoma–carcinoma sequence is a slow process. On average, 5.5 years is required for large adenomas greater than 10 mm diameter to develop into CRC, with 10–15 years for small adenomas (<5 mm). Colonic polyps are very common; not all are adenomas and not all will develop cancer. Most polyps less than 5 mm are hyperplastic polyps or mucosal tags; these are not cancer precursors. Less than 1 per cent of adenomas up to 1 cm in diameter contain cancer, with cancer in small polyps (<5 mm) being extremely rare.

Given the above concepts, it would seem logical that screening for CRC be targeted at detecting larger, more advanced adenomas with a high malignant potential, rather than trying to identify every single polyp regardless of size, the majority of which will never develop cancer. Risk for the development of CRC may be stratified into three categories:

- Average risk: age >50
- Moderate risk: past personal history of large adenoma or CRC or first-degree relative with large adenoma or CRC
- High risk: inflammatory bowel disease; hereditary non-polyposis CRC syndromes; familial polyposis syndromes.

Various screening strategies are available and include faecal occult blood testing, barium enema (double contrast), CT colonography, sigmoidoscopy and colonoscopy. All have limitations including accuracy, patient reluctance and lack of community awareness:

- Faecal occult blood testing gives many false-positive results and will not detect adenomas or cancers that do not bleed.
- Sigmoidoscopy does not evaluate the entire colon.
- Barium enema has a relatively low sensitivity with detection rates of less than 50 per cent for polyps larger than 1 cm.

4.7.1.1 Colonoscopy

Colonoscopy provides the most complete and thorough examination and is the reference standard for evaluation of the colon.

Advantages of colonoscopy:
- Detection of polyps and cancers with a high degree of accuracy
- Direct visualization of the mucosal surface
- Able to diagnose the less common flat adenomas as well as inflammatory mucosal disease
- Biopsy and polypectomy.

Limitations of colonoscopy:
- Need for sedation
- Failure rate of 5–10 per cent due to colonic tortuosity or obstruction
- Complications such as perforation and bleeding are rare, with a slightly increased incidence where polypectomy has been performed.

4.7.1.2 CT colonography ('virtual colonoscopy')

CT colonography is a multidetector CT technique with the potential to play a role in screening for CRC. CT colonography consists of the following:
- Patient's colon thoroughly 'cleansed' prior to the procedure with commercially available preparation kits
- Faecal tagging: ingestion of contrast material prior to CT will cause any retained faecal material to be of high density and therefore easily distinguished from polyps
- Patient placed on CT table and rectal tube inserted
- Colon distended with room air or CO_2

- Two CT scans, first supine position and then prone, using a low radiation dose CT technique
- Images reviewed on computer workstation with software applications that allow instant multiplanar and 3D reconstructions, as well as specialized algorithms for viewing of the mucosal surface (Fig. 4.29).

CT colonography has a sensitivity of over 90 per cent for the detection of polyps measuring 10 mm or more (Fig. 4.30).

Limitations of CT colonography:

- Inability to reliably identify flat adenomas or mucosal inflammation
- Low reported sensitivities for the detection of small polyps (<5 mm)
- Biopsy and polypectomy are not able to be performed.

Due to these limitations, CT optical colonography cannot replace colonoscopy.

Indications for CT colonography include:

- Failed colonoscopy
- Evaluation of the colon proximal to an obstruction
- Where colonoscopy or sedation are contraindicated due to frailty or other factors.

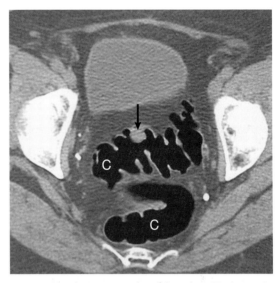

Figure 4.30 Adenomatous polyp of the colon: CT colonography. The colon (C) is distended with air. This transverse view shows a round polyp (arrow) arising in the sigmoid colon.

4.7.2 Staging of CRC

For principles of cancer staging, please see Chapter 14.

Staging of colorectal carcinoma may be summarized as follows:

- Stage I: tumour confined to the bowel wall
- Stage II: invasion through the full thickness of the bowel wall ± invasion of adjacent structures
- Stage III: metastasis to regional lymph node(s)
- Stage IV: metastasis to distant site(s) such as liver, non-regional lymph node(s), lung.

The two most critical factors influencing survival data in CRC are depth of invasion of the bowel wall and presence or absence of lymph node metastases. Unfortunately, two major limitations of imaging of CRC are assessment of depth of wall invasion and detection of microscopic metastases in non-enlarged lymph nodes. The exception to this is rectal CRC (see below). While accurate pretreatment staging of CRC is probably useful for planning of surgery, radiotherapy and chemotherapy, it remains controversial due to the limitations of imaging plus the fact that most patients with CRC will have surgery for either cure or palliation.

CT of the abdomen is the imaging investigation of choice for detection of locally invasive disease,

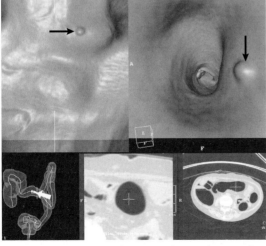

Figure 4.29 CT colonography: image showing the type of software used for reporting of CT colonography. Simultaneous display of cross-sectional and 3D images allows accurate appraisal of the mucosal surface of the colon. In this example there is a 5 mm polyp in the midtransverse colon (arrows).

lymphadenopathy and distant metastases in patients with CRC. CT is unable to assess the depth of wall invasion or detect small metastases in non-enlarged lymph nodes. Therefore, CT is accurate for advanced disease though less so for earlier non-invasive disease.

4.7.3 Staging of rectal carcinoma

Most rectal carcinomas are annular or polypoid tumours that invade the wall of the rectum. Tumour invasion occurs through the layers of the rectal wall, i.e. mucosal layer, submucosa and muscularis propria. Tumours that have invaded through the full thickness of the rectal wall may then extend into the surrounding mesorectal fat layer. Tumour may then invade adjacent structures such as bladder or seminal vesicles, or may perforate into the peritoneal cavity. Rectal carcinoma may also spread to regional lymph nodes in the pelvis or metastasize to distant sites, such as abdominal lymph nodes or liver.

Management options for rectal carcinoma include surgery, chemotherapy and radiotherapy. Surgery for rectal carcinoma is potentially curative and consists of complete removal of the rectum and surrounding mesorectal fat and lymphatics, i.e. total mesorectal excision (TME). TNM staging of rectal carcinoma may assist in directing management. TME may be used for tumours that have not invaded beyond the rectal wall, i.e. T1 or T2. For higher stage tumours, neoadjuvant chemotherapy or a combination of neoadjuvant chemotherapy and radiotherapy may be used prior to surgery. For advanced invasive disease or metastatic disease, non-curative surgery such as local excision and stoma may be used to palliate obstruction.

MRI and transrectal US (TRUS) are able to differentiate the layers of the rectal wall. These modalities are therefore able to assess accurately the depth of invasion of rectal tumour. Each modality has advantages and disadvantages. In general, TRUS is less widely available than MRI. Furthermore, a significant number of rectal tumours cannot be assessed with TRUS due to inablility to pass the US probe. For these reasons, MRI is more widely used for local staging of rectal carcinoma (Fig. 4.31).

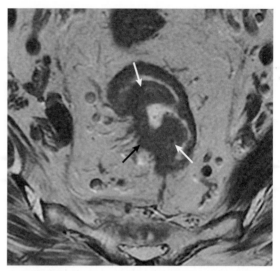

Figure 4.31 Carcinoma of the rectum: MRI. Transverse T2-weighted MRI of the rectum shows an annular tumour (white arrows). Note the nodular irregularity at the junction of tumour and mesorectal fat indicating tumour extension through the full thickness of the rectal wall (black arrow).

4.8 ABDOMINAL TRAUMA

Most patients who have suffered major trauma are assessed initially with an urgent 'trauma series' consisting of radiographs of the chest, lateral cervical spine and pelvis. Following the trauma series, the investigation path of a patient with suspected abdominal trauma depends largely on haemodynamic status and clinical presentation. Depending on varying factors, including the presence of other injuries and local expertise, haemodynamically unstable patients should undergo immediate surgery or may be assessed for intraperitoneal blood with a specialized US technique known as FAST. Focused abdominal sonography for trauma (FAST) consists of a rapid US assessment of the pelvis and abdomen looking for the presence of free fluid (Fig. 4.32). In many trauma and emergency centres, FAST has replaced peritoneal lavage, and is the initial imaging investigation in the patient with abdominal trauma. It may be used to help decide which patients require immediate laparotomy or to indicate further investigation with CT. Contrast-enhanced CT is the investigation of choice for suspected abdominal injuries in haemodynamically stable patients.

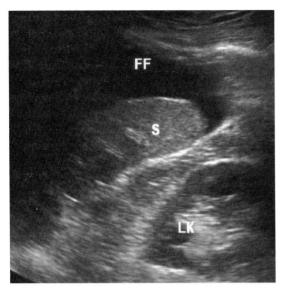

Figure 4.32 Free fluid: US (FAST). Free fluid (FF) is seen as anechoic material in the left upper abdomen adjacent to the spleen (S) and left kidney (LK).

- CT signs of bowel trauma
  - Free fluid between bowel loops or at the base of the mesentery
  - Free intraperitoneal and retroperitoneal gas
  - Bowel wall haematoma
- Active haemorrhage: localized 'puddle' or 'jet' of extravasated contrast material
  - This sign is an indication for immediate intervention, either surgery or angiography and embolization (see Fig. 3.20).

4.8.2 Angiography and embolization

Angiography and embolization may be used as a non-operative treatment option in the management of splenic, hepatic and renal injuries (see Fig. 3.20). Angiography and embolization may also be used as a substitute or adjunct to surgery to control active bleeding in association with mesenteric injuries or pelvic fractures.

4.8.1 CT in haemodynamically stable patients

CT provides excellent anatomical definition of intra-abdominal fluid collections and solid organ damage. CT for the assessment of abdominal trauma is usually performed with intravenous contrast material. In most cases, oral contrast material is not required for CT in abdominal trauma. Although free oral contrast material is a specific indicator of bowel perforation, it is not a sensitive sign. With multidetector CT, instant multiplanar reconstructions may be performed to provide rapid and accurate assessment of the spine and bony pelvis.

Signs of abdominal trauma that may be seen on CT:

- Free blood: hypodense material in more dependent parts of the peritoneal cavity, i.e. pelvis, hepatorenal pouch and paracolic gutters
- Solid organ injury: laceration, fracture, haematoma and contusion (Fig. 4.33)
- Lacerations involving the renal collecting system result in urine leak and urinoma
- Non-functioning kidney due to massive parenchymal damage, vascular pedicle injury or obstructed collecting system due to blood clot

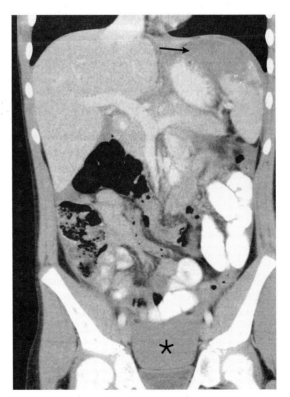

Figure 4.33 Splenic trauma: CT. Coronal reconstruction shows a laceration of the upper pole of the spleen and adjacent haematoma (arrow). Note also free fluid in the pelvis (*), above the bladder.

4.8.3 Urethrogram

Urethral injury complicates about 15 per cent of anterior pelvic fractures in males. Bladder catheterization should not be attempted prior to urethrogram in any patient with an anterior pelvic fracture or dislocation, or with blood at the urethral meatus following trauma. Urethrogram is a simple procedure that can be performed quickly in the emergency room (Fig. 4.34). The proximal bulbous urethra is the most common site of urethral injury.

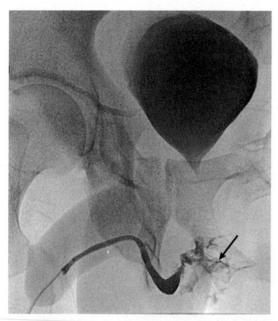

Figure 4.34 Urethral injury: urethrogram. Urethrogram outlines the bladder and urethra with leakage of contrast material (arrow) indicating a urethral tear.

4.8.4 CT cystogram

Bladder injury may be due to blunt, penetrating or iatrogenic trauma. About 10 per cent of pelvic fractures have an associated bladder injury. Radiographic signs suggestive of bladder trauma include fracture and/or dislocation of the pelvis, and soft tissue mass in the pelvis due to leakage of urine.

Contrast-enhanced CT of the abdomen and pelvis as performed for abdominal trauma has a poor sensitivity for the detection of bladder injuries. The accuracy of CT for the diagnosis and categorization

of bladder injuries may be enhanced with a CT cystogram, i.e. CT following direct injection of contrast material into the bladder via a catheter. If the urethra is normal on urethrogram, a catheter can be passed into the bladder and a cystogram performed.

Signs of bladder trauma on CT cystogram include bladder deformity and leakage of contrast material (Fig. 4.35). Leakage of contrast material may be extraperitoneal in 80 per cent and intraperitoneal in 20 per cent.

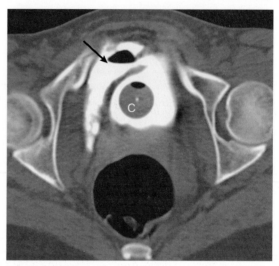

Figure 4.35 Bladder injury: CT cystogram. Transverse CT following infusion of contrast material into the bladder shows extraperitoneal leakage (arrow) through a tear in the lower anterior bladder. Note catheter balloon (C).

4.9 DETECTION AND CHARACTERIZATION OF LIVER MASSES

Liver masses may present clinically in a number of ways:

- Upper abdominal pain, often described as 'dragging' in nature
- Acute abdominal pain that may be caused by sudden haemorrhage
- Sudden deterioration in liver function due to hepatocellular carcinoma occurring in a cirrhotic liver.

Many liver masses are discovered as incidental findings during imaging investigation of unrelated symptoms. Liver masses may also be detected during imaging screening of the liver for metastases in a patient with a known primary malignancy. Characterization of liver masses, whether in the setting of a known malignancy or underlying cirrhosis, is an important goal of diagnostic imaging. Choice of imaging technique may vary depending on the clinical context, as well as local availability and expertise. Liver masses, listed in Table 4.1, usually have characteristic appearances on US, CT and MRI.

Table 4.1 Commonly encountered liver masses.

Benign	Malignant
Simple cyst	Metastases
Haemangioma	Hepatocellular carcinoma
Focal nodular hyperplasia	Cholangiocarcinoma
Adenoma	

4.9.1 Dynamic imaging studies

Dynamic imaging of the liver is possible due to fact that the liver receives a dual blood supply. The hepatic artery supplies 20 per cent of hepatic blood flow while the portal vein supplies the remaining 80 per cent.

Three phases of contrast enhancement occur following intravenous injection of a bolus of contrast material:

- Arterial phase: begins at around 25 seconds following commencement of injection
- Portal venous phase: begins at around 70 seconds, after blood has circulated through the mesentery, intestine and spleen
  - 80 per cent of the liver's blood supply is from the portal vein; therefore maximum enhancement of liver tissue occurs in the portal venous phase
- Equilibrium phase: several minutes after injection there is redistribution of contrast material to the extracellular space.

Most liver tumours receive their blood supply from the hepatic artery. Furthermore, most tumours are hypovascular, i.e. they receive less blood supply than surrounding liver. It follows then that maximum lesion conspicuity for most liver tumours including metastases will occur in the portal venous phase of contrast enhancement. Please note that this is due to liver enhancement, not enhancement of the tumour. Hypovascular tumours are seen as low-attenuation masses visualized against high-attenuation enhancing liver (Fig. 4.36).

Some liver tumours are hypervascular in that they receive more blood supply than surrounding liver. For these tumours, maximum lesion conspicuity occurs in the arterial phase of contrast enhancement (Fig. 4.37). Examples of hypervascular lesions best

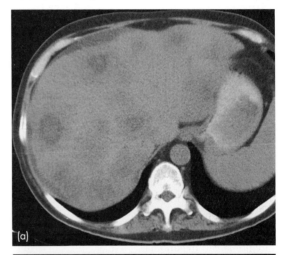

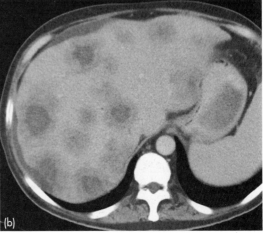

Figure 4.36 Hepatic metastases: CT. (a) Non-contrast CT of the liver shows multiple low density lesions throughout the liver. (b) CT during the portal venous phase of contrast enhancement shows multiple low attenuation metastases, more obvious than on the non-contrast scan.

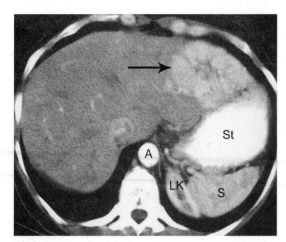

Figure 4.37 Focal nodular hyperplasia: CT. CT of the liver during the arterial phase of contrast enhancement shows the typical pattern of focal nodular hyperplasia with an intensely enhancing mass (arrow) containing a central non-enhancing scar. Note also aorta (A), left kidney (LK), spleen (S) and stomach (St).

seen in the arterial phase are small hepatocellular carcinoma (HCC), focal nodular hyperplasia (FNH) and hypervascular metastases. The arterial phase is particularly useful for detection of a small enhancing HCC in a cirrhotic liver; such lesions are often invisible in the portal venous phase. Hypervascular metastases are less common than hypovascular and may be seen with carcinoid tumour, renal cell carcinoma and melanoma.

Three methods are available for dynamic imaging of the liver: contrast-enhanced ultrasound (CEUS), multiphase CT with iodinated contrast material and MRI with gadolinium.

4.9.2 US

US is often the first investigation performed for a suspected liver mass as it is non-invasive and relatively inexpensive. Characterization of a lesion as a simple cyst on US usually means that further investigation is not required. A solid mass detected on US will in most circumstances require further characterization with dynamic imaging, i.e. CEUS, CT or MRI.

Other roles for US in hepatic masses:
- Follow-up of a known mass, e.g. suspected haemangioma where US is used to confirm lack of growth (Fig. 4.38)

- Intraoperative US: high frequency US probe directly applied to the surface of the liver during surgery to detect metastases.

Limitations of US in the detection of liver lesions:
- Less accurate for detection of lesions high in the liver near the diaphragmatic surface, particularly where the liver lies high up under the rib cage
- Hepatic steatosis (fatty liver): fatty infiltration produces an increasingly echogenic (bright) liver with deeper parts poorly seen on US.

4.9.3 CT

CT is generally the imaging investigation of choice for assessment of most liver masses. CT will reliably provide accurate anatomical localization and characterization of mass contents such as fluid, fat or calcification. Complications of HCC, such as invasion of the portal vein and arteriovenous shunting, are well demonstrated with CT.

As well as lesion detection, multiphase liver CT is often useful for liver mass characterization based on the contrast enhancement pattern. Common examples of this include differentiation of common benign masses, such as haemangioma and FNH, from more sinister lesions. Haemangioma and FNH are usually asymptomatic though large lesions may

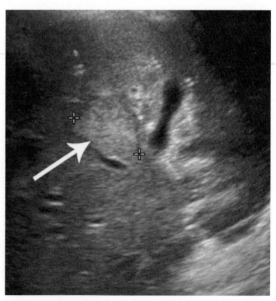

Figure 4.38 Haemangioma seen on US as a hyperechoic mass (arrow) in the liver.

produce pain. Characterization of these lesions is particularly important in patients with known primary malignancy, in whom metastatic disease is suspected. Most haemangiomas show a typical peripheral nodular enhancement pattern in the arterial phase, and this is usually adequate for diagnosis. FNH is usually isointense to liver on non-enhanced and portal venous phases, with intense enhancement on arterial phase plus a central scar. MRI may be used for atypical lesions.

4.9.4 MRI

MRI is being used more commonly for liver lesion detection and characterization, and in many centres has replaced CT as the primary investigation of choice. Fast imaging sequences allow imaging of the liver during a single breath-hold. As with CT, MRI may be performed during the arterial, portal venous and equilibrium phases of contrast enhancement following intravenous injection of gadolinium (Figs 4.39 and 4.40). The role of MRI for liver lesion detection and characterization has been expanded with the development and acceptance of gadolinium-based hepatobiliary contrast agents gadoxetic acid (Gd-EOB-DTPA) and gadobenate dimeglumine (Gd-BOPTA). Hepatobiliary contrast agents are taken up by functioning hepatocytes

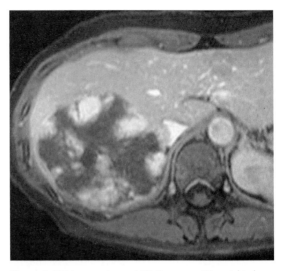

Figure 4.40 Haemangioma: MRI. Transverse T1-weighted MRI during the arterial phase of contrast enhancement shows peripheral nodular enhancement in a large liver mass indicating haemangioma.

and excreted in bile. On delayed imaging (10–60 minutes after injection for Gd-EOB-DTPA and 60–120 minutes for Gd-BOPTA), these agents produce increased signal of the liver and biliary tree, with increased conspicuity of small non-hepatocellular lesions including metastases. Furthermore, certain liver masses, such as FNH and cirrhotic dysplastic nodules, take up the hepatobiliary agents and therefore show increased signal on delayed imaging (Fig. 4.41).

4.10 IMAGING INVESTIGATION OF JAUNDICE

Causes of jaundice may be divided into two broad categories:
- Mechanical biliary obstruction
- Intrahepatic biliary stasis, also known as hepatocellular or non-obstructive jaundice.

Based on clinical findings, such as pain and stigmata of liver disease, plus biochemical tests of liver function, the distinction between these categories can be made in most patients. Imaging has no significant role in hepatocellular jaundice, other than US guidance of liver biopsy.

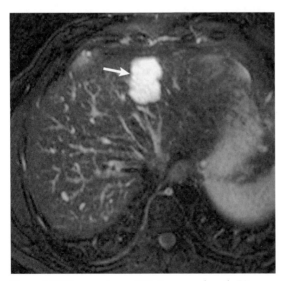

Figure 4.39 Haemangioma: MRI. Transverse heavily T2-weighted fat saturated MRI of the liver shows a well-defined high signal mass (arrow).

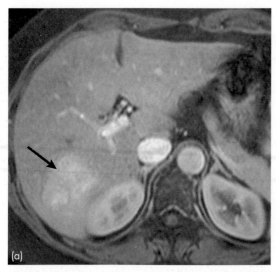 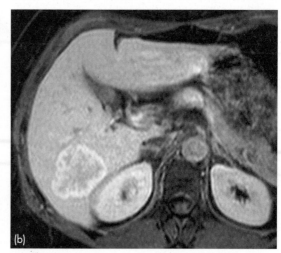

Figure 4.41 Focal nodular hyperplasia (FNH): MRI with hepatobiliary contrast agent (BOPTA). (a) Transverse T1-weighted MRI during the arterial phase of contrast enhancement shows an enhancing hypervascular mass (arrow). (b) Delayed (hepatobiliary) phase scan shows continued enhancement of the lesion, strongly favouring a diagnosis of FNH.

Mechanical biliary obstruction may occur at any level from the liver to the duodenum. Causes include gallstones in the bile ducts, pancreatic carcinoma, cholangiocarcinoma, carcinoma of the ampulla of Vater or duodenum, iatrogenic biliary stricture, chronic pancreatitis, liver masses and sclerosing cholangitis. The roles of imaging are to determine the presence, level and cause of biliary obstruction.

4.10.1 US

US is the first imaging investigation of choice for the jaundiced patient. Common bile duct diameter measurements are graded as follows: normal <6 mm; equivocal 6–8 mm; dilated >8 mm (Fig. 4.42). The site and cause of obstruction are defined on US in only 25 per cent of cases as overlying duodenal gas often obscures the lower end of the common bile duct (Fig. 4.43). Associated dilatation of the main pancreatic duct suggests obstruction at the level of the pancreatic head or ampulla of Vater. Depending on the results of US, further investigation may be directed as follows:

- Bile ducts not dilated: hepatocellular jaundice is considered and liver biopsy may be indicated
- Bile ducts dilated due to biliary calculus: endoscopic retrograde

cholangiopancreatography (ERCP) and sphincterotomy or surgery
- Bile ducts dilated due to soft tissue mass: CT for further characterization
- Bile ducts dilated without an obvious cause: CT may be performed as this has a higher rate of diagnosis of the cause of biliary obstruction than US (Fig. 4.44).

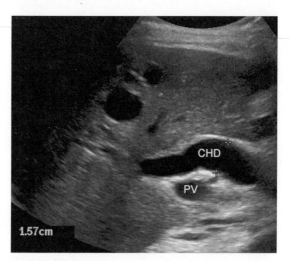

Figure 4.42 Biliary dilatation: US. Dilated common hepatic duct (CHD) seen as an anechoic tubular structure anterior to the portal vein (PV).

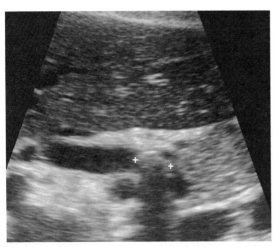

Figure 4.43 Choledocholithiasis: US. Biliary calculus seen as a hyperechoic focus (+) in the common bile duct.

Depending on the findings, US and CT may be followed by more definitive imaging of the biliary system with magnetic resonance cholangiopancreatography (MRCP), CT cholangiography, endoscopic ultrasound (EUS), ERCP or percutaneous transhepatic cholangiography (PTC).

4.10.2 Magnetic resonance cholangiopancreatography

Magnetic resonance cholangiopancreatography is non-invasive, does not involve ionizing radiation and does not require intravenous contrast material. MRCP uses heavily T_2-weighted images that show stationary fluids such as bile as high signal, with moving fluids and solids as low signal. The bile ducts and gallbladder are therefore seen as bright structures on a dark background (Fig. 4.45). MRCP is unaffected by bilirubin levels and may be combined with other sequences to provide more comprehensive imaging of the liver and pancreas.

Magnetic resonance cholangiopancreatography has largely replaced diagnostic ERCP as the investigation of choice for imaging of the biliary system, including assessment of jaundiced patients with dilated bile ducts on US. MRCP is commonly used prior to laparoscopic cholecystectomy to diagnose bile duct calculi and bile duct variants, and to avoid intraoperative exploration of the common bile duct.

Limitations of MRCP:

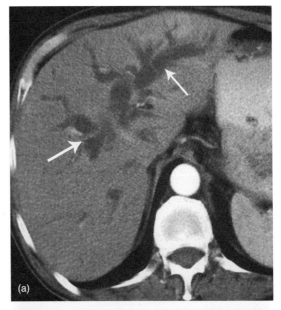

(a)

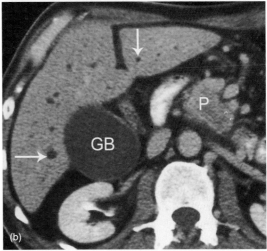

(b)

Figure 4.44 Biliary obstruction due to carcinoma of the head of the pancreas: CT. (a) Dilated bile ducts seen on CT as a low attenuation branching pattern (arrows) in the liver. (b) Note enlargement of head of pancreas (P) due to tumour and distended gallbladder (GB).

- Patients unsuitable for MRI, e.g. cardiac pacemakers, claustrophobia
- Limited spatial resolution, therefore difficulty visualizing stones <3 mm, tight biliary stenosis, small peripheral bile ducts and small side branches of the pancreatic duct
- No therapeutic applications, i.e. unable to perform sphincterotomy, insert stents, etc.

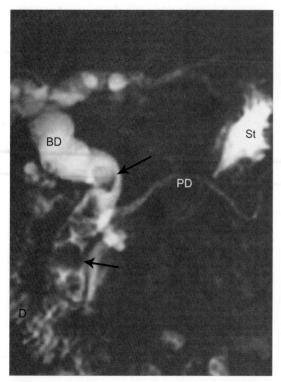

Figure 4.45 Choledocholithiasis: magnetic resonance cholangiopancreatography. Biliary calculi are seen as filling defects (arrows) within the dilated bile ducts (BD). Note also pancreatic duct (PD), stomach (St) and duodenum (D).

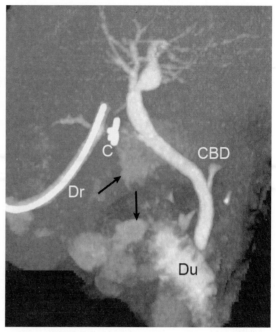

Figure 4.46 Bile leak post-laparoscopic cholecystectomy: CT cholangiogram. Note drain (Dr), surgical clips (C), common bile duct (CBD) and duodenum (Du). Contrast material lying outside biliary system (arrows) indicating bile leak.

4.10.3 CT cholangiography

CT cholangiography involves a slow intravenous infusion of an iodine containing cholangiographic agent (Biliscopin®) to opacify the bile ducts, followed by CT (Fig. 4.46). CT cholangiography is a reasonably reliable method of imaging the biliary system where MRCP and the other more invasive methods listed below are contraindicated or not available. Disadvantages of CT cholangiography include radiation exposure, allergy to contrast material, and non-visualization of the bile ducts in patients with high bilirubin.

4.10.4 Endoscopic US

As the name suggests, EUS combines a small US probe with an endoscope. EUS is highly sensitive in the detection of small biliary and pancreatic tumours. EUS may be used to guide biopsy of small masses or cyst aspiration. Limitations of EUS include limited availability, difficulty of interpretation following biliary stent placement or sphincterotomy, and technical difficulties following gastric surgery.

4.10.5 Endoscopic retrograde cholangiopancreatography

For ERCP, the ampulla of Vater is identified endoscopically and a small cannula passed into it under direct endoscopic visualization. Contrast material is then injected into the biliary and pancreatic ducts and images acquired (Fig. 4.47). Where MRCP is not available, ERCP is used to assess biliary obstruction diagnosed on US or CT. ERCP is the investigation of choice for suspected distal biliary obstruction that may require interventions such as sphincterotomy, basket retrieval of stones, biliary biopsy or biliary stent placement.

Disadvantages of ERCP include:

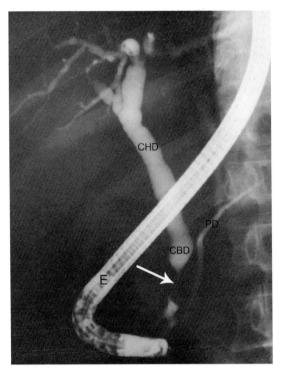

Figure 4.47 Cholangiocarcinoma: endoscopic retrograde cholangiopancreatography. Stricture (arrow) of the distal common bile duct (CBD) due to cholangiocarcinoma. Note also common hepatic duct (CHD), pancreatic duct (PD) and endoscope (E).

- Complications including pancreatitis (relatively uncommon though may be devastating when they do occur)
- Technical failure in up to 10 per cent.

4.10.6 Percutaneous transhepatic cholangiography

Percutaneous transhepatic cholangiography (PTC) is indicated for assessment of high biliary obstruction at the level of the porta and where biliary obstruction is unable to be outlined by ERCP due to previous biliary diversion surgery. PTC is performed under fluoroscopy with a fine needle passed into a peripheral bile duct in the liver and contrast material injected to outline the biliary system. PTC is often accompanied by biliary stent placement for relief of biliary obstruction. Patient preparation for PTC should include clotting studies and antibiotic cover to prevent septicaemia due to release of infected bile.

4.11 INTERVENTIONAL RADIOLOGY OF THE LIVER AND BILIARY TRACT

4.11.1 Liver biopsy

The two broad indications for guided liver biopsy are liver mass and diffuse liver disease. Liver biopsy may be performed under CT or US guidance. Core biopsy is often required, as fine needle aspiration may not provide sufficient material for diagnosis. Not all liver masses should undergo biopsy:

- Bleeding may complicate biopsy of haemangioma.
- Seeding of tumour cells may occur along the needle track following biopsy of hepatocellular carcinoma.
- Most liver masses are characterized with imaging as above and managed surgically or non-surgically without biopsy.

Biopsy of liver masses is restricted to a few specific indications:

- Liver metastases and an unknown primary tumour
- Known extrahepatic primary tumour and a liver mass not able to be characterized with imaging.

For liver biopsy in suspected diffuse liver disease imaging guidance is not strictly required, although it may increase safety and diagnostic yield. Use of a coaxial needle technique with placement of a gelfoam plug in the biopsy track may reduce the risk of haemorrhage.

4.11.2 Non-surgical management of bile duct stones

Non-surgical management of bile duct stones is normally done via ERCP, with widening of the lower end of the common bile duct (sphincterotomy) and removal of stones via a small wire basket. Occasionally, bile duct stones may be removed via a T-tube tract. This may be done via basket removal or flexible choledochoscope. The T-tube should be *in situ* for at least 4 weeks postsurgery to ensure a 'mature' tract able to accept wires and catheters. Complications are rare and may include pancreatitis, cholangitis and bile leak.

4.11.3 Non-surgical management of malignant biliary obstruction

A range of palliative procedures may be used to assist in the management of biliary obstruction caused by malignancies arising from the liver, bile ducts, pancreas and gallbladder. Indications are as follows:

- Symptomatic relief: relief of pruritis, pain or cholangitis
- Non-resectable tumour of bile ducts, head of pancreas or liver
- Medical risk factors which make surgery impossible.

Methods vary with the type of tumour and its location, plus local expertise and preferences:

- Endoscopic: 'from below' for mid to low biliary obstruction
- Percutaneous: 'from above' for high biliary obstruction or where the second part of duodenum is inaccessible to endoscopy due to tumour or prior surgery
- Combined percutaneous endoscopic.

Regardless of the approach to be used the basic technique is the same (see Fig. 14.6):

- Bile ducts opacified by ERCP or PTC
- Wire passed across the biliary obstruction
- Stent or internal–external drain inserted over the wire
- Internal biliary stents are made of plastic or self-expanding metal
- Stent is positioned with its upper end above the biliary obstruction and its lower end below, usually protruding into the duodenum.

Occasionally in severe obstruction, a two-stage procedure is required:

- Placement of a drainage tube above the obstruction for a few days
- After decompression of the biliary system, a wire is passed across the obstruction and a stent inserted.

Internal biliary stents are made of plastic or self-expanding metal and are better accepted by patients as they avoid the potential problems of external biliary drains, such as skin irritation, pain, bile leaks and risk of dislodgement.

4.11.4 Percutaneous cholecystostomy

Percutaneous cholecystostomy (drainage of the gallbladder) may be useful in the management of acute cholecystitis where the surgical risks are unacceptable. Percutaneous cholecystostomy is usually performed via US guidance. Gallbladder is punctured, a wire passed through the needle, and a drainage catheter placed in the gallbladder over the wire. Non-resolution of pyrexia within 48 hours may indicate gangrene of the gallbladder requiring surgery. A cholecystogram is performed once the acute illness has settled, with contrast material injected through the drainage catheter. Stones causing cystic duct obstruction may require surgery; otherwise the catheter is removed.

4.11.5 Transjugular intrahepatic portosystemic stent shunting (TIPSS)

A major cause of mortality and morbidity in patients with hepatic cirrhosis is haemorrhage from oesophageal varices. The transjugular intrahepatic portosystemic stent shunting (TIPSS) procedure is performed in the setting of portal hypertension for chronic, recurrent variceal haemorrhage not amenable to sclerotherapy. TIPSS is an interventional technique used to form a shunt from the portal system to the systemic venous circulation, thus lowering portal venous pressure. The liver is imaged with Doppler US prior to the procedure to exclude malignancy and confirm patency of the portal vein. TIPSS technique:

- Jugular vein puncture, often under US control
- Wire passed into the inferior vena cava (IVC) and catheterization of a hepatic vein
- Puncture device passed through this catheter
- Using US to select the most direct route the portal vein is punctured and a wire passed
- A tract from hepatic vein to portal vein is therefore formed
- Tract is dilated and stent inserted, usually a metallic prosthesis expanded by balloon.

Complications of TIPSS:

- Procedural complications: intraperitoneal haemorrhage, portal vein thrombosis
- Hepatic encephalopathy
- Renal failure
- Pulmonary oedema.

SUMMARY BOX

Clinical presentation	Investigation of choice	Comment
Dysphagia	Endoscopy where malignancy suspected Barium swallow for other indications	
Perforation of GIT	AXR	
Small bowel obstruction	AXR	CT in doubtful cases, or to define location and cause
Large bowel obstruction	AXR	Contrast enema to localize level of obstruction
Right upper quadrant pain	US	
Right lower quadrant pain	CT	US in children and women of childbearing age
Left lower quadrant pain	CT	US in children and women of childbearing age
Renal colic/flank pain	CT	AXR/KUB if ureteric calculus seen on CT
Acute pancreatitis	CT	US to search for gallstones
Acute mesenteric ischaemia	Catheter angiogram Interventional radiology	
Crohn disease	Colonoscopy CT or MR enterography	AXR in acute presentation
Ulcerative colitis	Colonoscopy	AXR in acute presentation
Upper GIT bleeding	Endoscopy	
Lower GIT bleeding	RBC scintigraphy CT angiography	Treat bleeding with interventional radiology or surgery
Abdominal trauma	US 'FAST' scan CT in haemodynamically stable	Interventional radiology for acute bleeding Urethrogram and CT cystogram
Liver mass: detection	US	CT or MRI following US
Liver mass: characterization	Dynamic contrast enhanced imaging: CT, MRI, CEUS	
Jaundice	US, MRCP	Other imaging/intervention as indicated: ERCP, PTC

CEUS, contrast-enhanced ultrasound; ERCP, endoscopic retrograde cholangiopancreatography; KUB, radiograph of kidneys, ureters and bladder; MRCP, magnetic resonance cholangiopancreatography; PTC, percutaneous transhepatic cholangiography; RBC, red blood cells.

5 | Urology

5.1 IMAGING INVESTIGATION OF THE URINARY TRACT

US and CT are the principal imaging investigations used for assessment of the urinary tract in both males and females. MRI is increasingly used as a problem-solving modality in the characterization of renal and adrenal masses, and in the staging of prostatic carcinoma. US, CT and MRI are discussed extensively throughout this chapter. Other imaging modalities and techniques used in the investigation of urinary tract disease are outlined below.

5.1.1 Scintigraphy

5.1.1.1 Renogram (renal scintigraphy)

Renal scintigraphy with ^{99}mTc-DTPA or ^{99}mTc-MAG3 is used to assess renal function and urodynamics, including calculation of the percentage of total renal function contributed by each kidney. Renal scintigraphy is used in renal transplant to assess transplant perfusion and function, diagnose rejection or acute tubular necrosis, and detect urinary leak or outflow obstruction.

For other specific indications, modifications to renal scintigraphy may be used as follows:
- Diuresis renogram
  - Renal scintigraphy with injection of furosemide
  - Indication: differentiation of mechanical urinary tract obstruction from non-obstructive hydronephrosis (Fig. 5.1)
- Angiotensin-converting enzyme (ACE) inhibitor renogram
  - Renal scintigraphy with injection of captopril

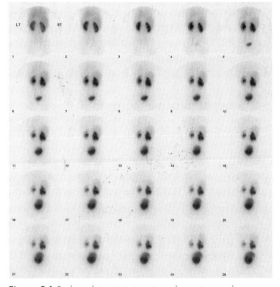

Figure 5.1 Right pelviureteric junction obstruction and hydronephrosis: MAG3 scan. Sequential series of images taken from 1 to 25 minutes following injection of ^{99}mTc-MAG3. Normal uptake and excretion of MAG3 by the left kidney. Increased accumulation of MAG3 in dilated right renal collecting system indicating mechanical obstruction. (Note images acquired posteriorly so left kidney shown on the left of image unlike most other cross-sectional imaging.)

  - Indication: screening test for renal artery stenosis in suspected renovascular hypertension.

5.1.1.2 Renal cortical scintigraphy

Indications for renal cortical scintigraphy with ^{99}mTc-DMSA:
- Acute pyelonephritis in infants and young children

- Renal scars complicating urinary tract infection in children (see Chapter 13).

5.1.2 Intravenous pyelogram

Intravenous pyelogram (IVP) is also known as intravenous urogram (IVU). IVP consists of a series of radiographs performed after intravenous injection of iodinated contrast material to show the kidneys, renal collecting systems, ureters and bladder. US, CT and scintigraphy have replaced IVP for most indications including renal colic, prostatism, urinary tract infection and renal cell carcinoma. In most centres, IVP is only rarely performed for very specific indications such as sorting out complex congenital anomalies or following surgical repair or reconstruction of the ureters.

5.1.3 Retrograde pyelogram

Retrograde pyelogram (RPG) is usually performed in the operating theatre, in conjunction with formal cystoscopy. At cystoscopy, the ureteric orifice is identified and a catheter passed into the ureter. Contrast material is then injected via this catheter to outline the collecting system and ureter.

Indications for RPG:
- To better define lesions of the upper renal tract identified by other imaging studies such as CT
- Haematuria where other imaging studies are normal or equivocal
- Guide for various interventional procedures including removal of ureteric calculus and ureteric stent placement.

5.1.4 Ascending urethrogram

For ascending urethrogram, a small catheter is passed into the distal urethra and contrast material injected. Radiographs are obtained in the oblique projection to show the urethra in profile.

Indications for ascending urethrogram:
- In the setting of trauma prior to urethral catheterization in a male patient with an anterior pelvic fracture or dislocation, or with blood at the urethral meatus (see Chapter 4)
- Suspected urethral stricture, which may be the result of previous trauma or inflammation.

5.1.5 Micturating cystourethrogram

Micturating cystourethrogram (MCU) is also known as voiding cystourethrogram (VCU). For MCU, the bladder is filled with contrast material via a urethral catheter. Images of the contrast-filled bladder are obtained. The catheter is then removed and radiographs are taken during micturition.

Indications for MCU:
- Assessment of urinary tract infection in children (see Chapter 13)
- Following radical prostatectomy to check the surgical anastomosis and the integrity of the bladder base
- Assess posterior urethral problems in male adults
- Stress incontinence in female adults.

5.2 PAINLESS HAEMATURIA

Painless haematuria may be classified clinically as macroscopic or microscopic. Initial clinical tests in the patient with haematuria consist of urine culture to exclude infection, examination of urine for protein and red cell casts, and measurement of blood pressure.

Over 70 per cent of cases of haematuria have no demonstrable cause. Demonstrable causes of haematuria include:
- Urinary tract infection
- Urinary calculi
- Tumour of urinary tract
- Trauma
- Glomerulonephritis
- Bleeding diathesis.

Other clinical symptoms and signs, such as acute flank pain and fever, usually accompany haematuria caused by urinary tract infection and ureteric calculi. Glomerulonephritis is suspected where haematuria is accompanied by heavy proteinuria and red cell casts. Glomerulonephritis is confirmed with renal biopsy, best done under imaging guidance, usually US. Patients with glomerulonephritis should have a CXR to search for cardiac enlargement and pulmonary oedema, plus a renal US to screen for underlying renal morphological abnormalities.

In the absence of compelling evidence of urinary tract infection or glomerulonephritis, painless haematuria should be considered to be due to urinary tract tumour until proved otherwise. The imaging workup of patients with painless haematuria is therefore directed at excluding or diagnosing renal cell carcinoma and urothelial carcinoma (transitional cell carcinoma or TCC). Urothelial carcinoma may occasionally produce a central renal mass. More commonly, urothelial carcinoma is a small, sometimes multifocal tumour arising in the renal collecting systems, ureters and bladder. Large or advanced bladder tumours may invade beyond the bladder wall and cause hydronephrosis due to obstruction of the distal ureters (Fig. 5.2). It follows from the above that the imaging assessment of painless haematuria requires visualization of the renal parenchyma to exclude a renal mass, plus visualization of the urothelium. This includes imaging of the collecting system, renal pelvis, ureters and bladder.

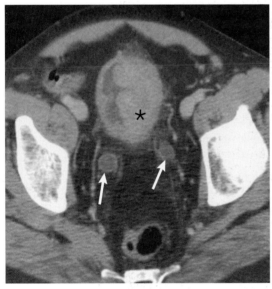

Figure 5.2 Urothelial tumour of the bladder: CT. Non-contrast-enhanced CT shows a large soft tissue mass arising from the bladder (*) and causing obstruction and dilatation of the distal ureters (arrows).

5.2.1 CT urography

CT urography is the investigation of choice for painless haematuria. CT urography is a term used to describe a contrast-enhanced CT technique designed to provide excellent delineation of the renal collecting systems, ureters and bladder, as well as cross-sectional images of the kidneys and adjacent structures. Although the precise method may vary, CT urography usually consists of a multiphase examination including scans performed with sufficient delay after contrast material injection to allow opacification of the collecting systems and ureters (Fig. 5.3).

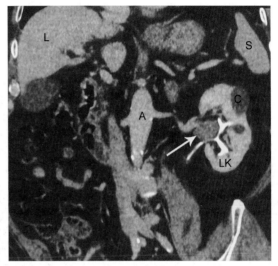

Figure 5.3 Urothelial tumour: CT urography. Urothelial tumour of the left kidney (LK) seen as a central mass (arrow) on a coronal CT image. Note also liver (L), aorta (A), spleen (S), left renal cyst (C).

5.2.2 Cystoscopy

Cystoscopy accompanied by ureteroscopy is the gold standard investigation for tumours of the lower urinary tract. Retrograde pyelography may also be performed at the time of cystoscopy where upper urinary tract tumour is suspected.

5.2.3 US

US of the urinary tract may supplement CT urography in selected cases.

Indications for US include:
- Characterization of complex cysts
- Differentiation of complex cysts from solid masses.

Limitations of US in this context include:
- Incomplete visualization of the kidneys due to obesity or intestinal gas
- Inability to visualize small urothelial tumours.

5.3 RENAL MASS

Goals of imaging a suspected renal mass include:
- Confirmation of presence and site of mass
- Classification into simple cyst, complicated cyst or solid mass
- Assessment of contents, such as the presence of fat
- Differentiation of benign from malignant
- Diagnosis of complications such as local invasion, venous invasion, lymphadenopathy and metastases.

Renal masses in children including hydronephrosis, multicystic dysplastic kidney and nephroblastoma (Wilm's tumour) are discussed in Chapter 13.

5.3.1 Classification of renal masses

Renal masses may be classified with imaging into simple cysts, complex cysts and solid masses. Simple renal cysts are extremely common in adults. They are usually small and asymptomatic, discovered incidentally on CT or US examinations of the abdomen. Occasionally, very large cysts may present with abdominal pain or a palpable abdominal mass. Simple cysts have thin walls and clear fluid contents.

A small percentage of benign cysts have more complex features and are classified as complex cysts. Causes of a complex cyst include a simple cyst complicated by haemorrhage or infection, benign cyst containing septations or calcifications, or a cystic tumour (see Table 5.1).

Most solid renal masses are malignant; renal cell carcinoma is the most common type. Renal cell carcinoma (RCC) may present clinically with haematuria or flank pain. Less commonly, RCC may present with pathological fracture or bone pain due to a skeletal metastasis. Increasingly, RCC and other renal masses or cysts are found incidentally on US and CT examinations performed for other reasons. Over 60 per cent of RCC are diagnosed incidentally. Uncommonly, urothelial carcinoma may produce a central mass centred in the collecting system and extending into the renal parenchyma. Other types of renal malignancy that may produce solid renal masses are lymphoma and metastases.

Angiomyolipoma (AML) is the commonest cause of a benign solid renal mass in adults. Eighty per cent of AML occur sporadically, and are usually small and asymptomatic. Twenty per cent of AML occur in association with tuberous sclerosis. Rarely, large AML may present as a palpable abdominal mass, or may be complicated by haemorrhage giving acute abdomen and haematuria. AMLs contain fat, giving them a characteristic appearance on US and CT; visible fat in a renal mass usually implies a benign aetiology.

Table 5.1 Bosniak classification of renal cysts.

Bosniak classification	CT features	Diagnosis	Management
I	Thin wall Low density Non-enhancing	Simple cyst	No follow-up
II	<3 cm; high density, thin septations, fine calcification	Benign complex cyst	No follow-up
IIF	>3 cm with same features as type 2; nodular calcification	Probably benign	Follow-up CT
III	Thick or irregular septations or calcification	Indeterminate; 50% malignant	Biopsy or surgery
IV	Enhancing soft tissue component	Malignant	Staging Surgery or other management as required

5.3.2 Imaging of renal masses

5.3.2.1 US

US is the initial investigation of choice for diagnosis of suspected renal mass, followed by CT. US will accurately characterize a renal mass as a simple cyst, complex cyst or a solid mass. A simple cyst appears on US as a round anechoic (black) structure with a thin or invisible wall (Fig. 5.4). No further imaging is required for simple renal cysts diagnosed with US.

The term 'complex cyst' refers to a cyst with internal echoes that may be due to haemorrhage or infection, soft tissue septations, calcifications, or an associated soft tissue mass (Fig. 5.5).

A solid mass on US may show areas of increased echogenicity due to calcification or fat, or areas of decreased echogenicity due to necrosis. Where renal cell carcinoma is suspected, US is also used to look for specific findings such as invasion of renal vein and inferior vena cava (IVC), lymphadenopathy, and metastases in the liver and contralateral kidney. Complex cysts or solid renal masses found with US usually require further assessment with CT or MRI.

US may also be used as a guide for various procedures including:
- Biopsy of solid lesions or complicated cysts
- Cyst aspiration for diagnostic and therapeutic purposes
- Cyst ablation by injection of ethanol
- Radiofrequency ablation of small tumours.

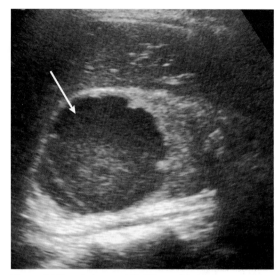

Figure 5.5 Renal abscess: US. US in a febrile patient with severe right flank pain shows a fluid collection in the upper pole of the right kidney (arrow). Note echogenic fluid contents and irregular wall indicating a complex cystic lesion. US-guided aspiration confirmed the diagnosis of abscess.

5.3.2.2 CT

Contrast-enhanced CT is used for further characterization of a solid lesion or complex cyst found on US. CT is more accurate than US for characterization of internal contents of a mass, in particular to show areas of fat confirming the diagnosis of AML (Fig. 5.6). Based on CT

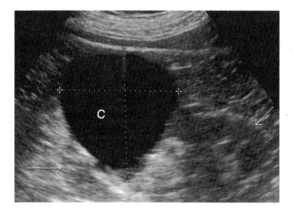

Figure 5.4 Simple renal cyst: Longitudinal US of left kidney (arrows). Note the US features of a simple cyst (C): anechoic contents, smooth wall, and no soft tissue components.

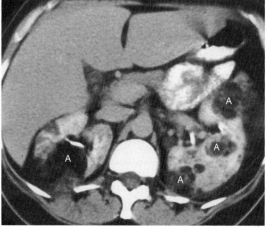

Figure 5.6 Angiomyolipoma: CT. Multiple angiomyolipomas (A) arising on both kidneys in a woman with tuberous sclerosis. Note the typical low attenuation fat content well shown on CT.

appearances, cystic renal lesions may be classified according to the Bosniak system (Table 5.1 and Figs 5.7 and 5.8).

The most common CT appearance of renal cell carcinoma is a heterogeneous soft tissue mass that enhances with intravenous contrast material (Fig. 5.9). CT is also used for staging of renal cell carcinoma. Factors relevant to staging of RCC include size of tumour, invasion of local structures such as adrenal gland, vascular invasion of renal vein or IVC, lymphadenopathy, and metastases in the liver and skeleton.

RCC is staged as follows:

- Stage I: tumour up to 7 cm confined to kidney
- Stage II: tumour >7 cm confined to kidney
- Stage III: invasion of adrenal gland, perinephric fat or IVC, and/or involvement of one regional lymph node
- Stage IV: local invasion beyond Gerota's fascia; spread to more than one lymph node; distant metastasis.

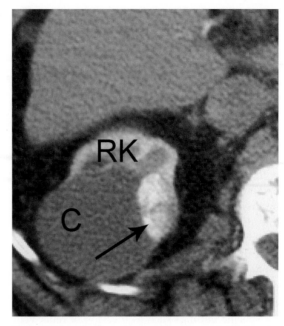

Figure 5.8 Renal cell carcinoma arising in a cyst: CT. A cyst (C) arising on the right kidney (RK) contains a soft tissue mass that enhances with intravenous contrast (arrow). This is the typical appearance of a Bosniak type IV cyst and indicates malignancy.

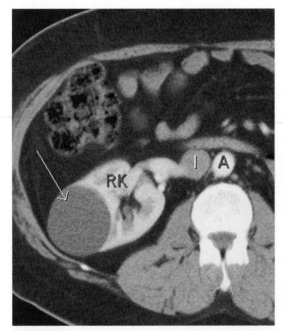

Figure 5.7 Simple renal cyst: CT. Note the CT features of a simple cyst (arrow) arising on the right kidney (RK): homogenous low attenuation contents, thin wall, and sharp demarcation from adjacent renal parenchyma. Note also inferior vena cava (I) and aorta (A).

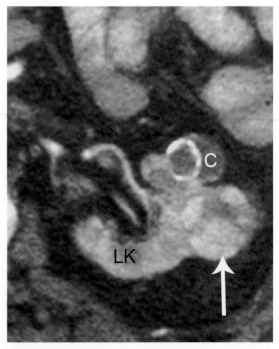

Figure 5.9 Renal cell carcinoma: CT. Renal cell carcinoma seen as a small mass (arrow) arising on the left kidney (LK). Note also the presence of a partly calcified cyst (C).

5.3.2.3 MRI

In some centres, MRI is used in preference to CT for the investigation and characterization of renal masses. MRI generally gives similar information to CT in the detection, classification and staging of renal cysts and tumours.

5.3.2.4 Biopsy

Biopsy of renal masses is not commonly performed, as tumour seeding may occur and histological interpretation is often difficult. The most common indication for renal mass biopsy is for management of a small mass (<3 cm), where a positive biopsy result would indicate a non-operative approach.

Other indications for biopsy of a renal mass include:
- High suspicion for lymphoma
- Known or previous primary carcinoma elsewhere, especially lung, breast or stomach.

5.4 IMAGING IN PROSTATISM

Prostatism refers to obstructive voiding symptoms due to prostatic enlargement. Nodular hyperplasia with enlargement of the central prostate is the commonest cause of symptomatic prostatic enlargement. Symptoms of prostatism include frequency, nocturia, poor stream, hesitancy and post-void fullness. The primary imaging investigation in the assessment of prostatism is urinary tract US. Urinary tract US includes assessment of prostate, bladder and upper urinary tracts. Prostate diameters are measured and approximate prostate volume calculated by a simple formula: height × width × length × 0.50 (Fig. 5.10). Bladder is assessed for morphological changes indicating bladder obstruction including bladder wall thickening and trabeculation, bladder wall diverticulum and bladder calculi. Bladder volume is measured pre- and post-micturition. Kidneys are examined for hydronephrosis, asymptomatic congenital anomalies and tumours, and renal calculi.

5.5 ADENOCARCINOMA OF THE PROSTATE

5.5.1 Diagnosis of adenocarcinoma of the prostate

Adenocarcinoma of the prostate is the second most common malignancy in males, its incidence increasing steadily with age. Adenocarcinoma of the prostate may be diagnosed in a number of ways:

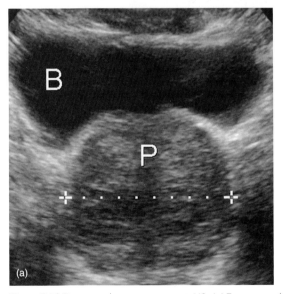
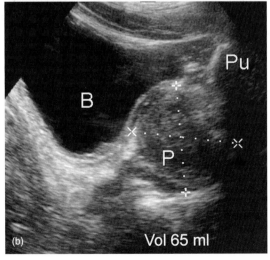

Figure 5.10 Prostate volume measurement: US. (a) Transverse plane. (b) Longitudinal plane. Note prostate (P), bladder (B), pubic bone (Pu).

- Urinary tract symptoms, e.g. haematuria, obstructive voiding symptoms
- Histological examination of tissue chips obtained by transurethral resection (TURP) for presumed benign prostatic enlargement
- Bone metastases may be the initial finding due to a specific presentation like bone pain or spinal cord compression
- Multiple sclerotic metastases are occasionally picked up as an incidental finding on a radiograph performed for unrelated reasons, e.g. pre-anaesthetic CXR or AXR for abdominal pain.

Most prostate carcinomas are now diagnosed through screening. Screening methods include digital rectal examination (DRE) and prostate specific antigen (PSA) blood assay. PSA screening is controversial for a number of reasons:

- PSA is non-specific and may be elevated in nodular hyperplasia and chronic prostatitis, as well as prostatic carcinoma.
- PSA is unable to differentiate those tumours that may remain small and confined to the prostate from those that may cause local invasion and metastases.

An increasing PSA level in an individual patient is considered more significant than a single reading. If either DRE or PSA are abnormal, prostate biopsy is performed. This is done under transrectal ultrasound (TRUS) guidance (Fig. 5.11). Less commonly, biopsies may be performed using a US-guided transperineal approach under general anaesthetic.

The peripheral zone of the prostate is targeted, as this is where most tumours arise. Most operators perform multiple biopsies including the upper, mid and lower parts of the peripheral zone on each side. Tumour is graded histologically using the Gleason scale from 2 (well differentiated) to 10 (anaplastic, highly aggressive).

In some specialized centres, MRI is used to assist in detection of prostate cancer. As outlined in Chapter 14, MRI is the imaging investigation of choice for local staging of prostate carcinoma. T_2-weighted scans are able to display the architecture of the prostate including differentiation of central and peripheral zones. Carcinoma is usually seen as a low signal mass in the peripheral zone. Spectroscopy

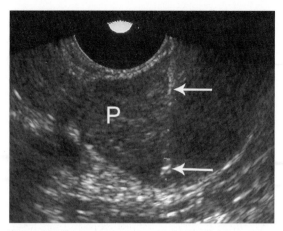

Figure 5.11 Prostate biopsy: transrectal US. Note the excellent visualization of the biopsy needle (arrows) within the prostate (P).

increases the accuracy of tumour detection with MRI, though has not replaced TRUS-guided biopsy.

Please see Chapter 14 for detailed notes on the staging of adenocarcinoma of the prostate.

5.6 INVESTIGATION OF A SCROTAL MASS

US with colour Doppler is the first investigation of choice for a scrotal mass. The primary role of US is to differentiate intratesticular from extratesticular masses; in most cases, this is sufficient to distinguish malignant and benign lesions.

5.6.1 Intratesticular masses

Most (over 90 per cent) intratesticular masses are malignant. Exceptions include testicular abscess, TB, sarcoidosis and benign tumour such as Sertoli-Leydig tumour.

On US, most intratesticular tumours are hypoechoic. Seminoma is usually seen as a localized hypoechoic mass outlined by surrounding hyperechoic testicular tissue (Fig. 5.12). Occasionally, with a large seminoma the entire testicle is replaced by abnormal hypoechoic tissue. Other tumour types, such as choriocarcinoma, embryonal cell carcinoma, teratoma and mixed tumours usually show a heterogeneous echotexture. Lymphoma of the testis is hypoechoic and homogeneous and may be focal or diffuse.

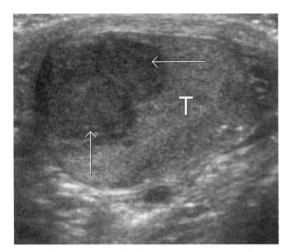

Figure 5.12 Seminoma: US. A seminoma is seen on US as a hypoechoic mass (arrow) arising in the testis (T).

Staging of testicular tumour incorporates four factors:
- Local growth within the testicle and invasion of adjacent structures including spermatic cord and scrotal skin
- Spread to regional lymph nodes
- Metastasis to distant lymph nodes or other organs, e.g. lung and brain
- Serum tumour marker levels
  - Lactate dehydrogenase (LDH)
  - Human chorionic gonadotropin (HCG)
  - Alpha-fetoprotein (AFP).

Imaging for staging of testicular tumours consists of scrotal US, abdomen CT for retroperitoneal lymphadenopathy, and chest CT for mediastinal lymphadenopathy and pulmonary metastases.

5.6.2 Extratesticular masses

Most (90 per cent) extratesticular lesions are benign. The most commonly encountered extratesticular masses are hydrocele, varicocele and epididymal cyst.

Hydrocele is seen on US as anechoic fluid surrounding the testicle. Hydrocele may be congenital, idiopathic, or secondary to inflammation, torsion, trauma or tumour.

Epididymal cyst, also known as spermatocele, is a common incidental finding on scrotal US, or may occasionally be large enough to present as a palpable mass. Epididymal cyst appears on US as a well-defined anechoic simple cyst in the head of the epididymis, i.e. posterolaterally at the superior pole of the testis.

Varicocele consists of dilated veins of the pampiniform plexus producing a tortuous nest of veins well seen on US. The vascular nature of the mass is confirmed with colour Doppler. Most varicoceles occur on the left and present with a clinically obvious mass or with infertility. Small asymptomatic varicoceles are common incidental findings on scrotal US. Varicoceles are caused by venous incompetence in most cases. Large varicoceles associated with infertility or discomfort may be amenable to therapeutic embolization of the testicular vein.

5.7 ACUTE SCROTUM

Acute scrotum is usually unilateral, and is defined as sudden, painful scrotal swelling. The main differential diagnosis in this situation is torsion versus acute epididymo-orchitis.

Common causes of acute epididymo-orchitis:
- Bacterial infection
- Mumps
- Scrotal haematoma, which is usually related to trauma
- Torsion of testicular appendages
- Strangulated hernia
- Haemorrhage into a testicular tumour.

The need for early surgical exploration in suspected torsion gives imaging a role only in doubtful cases and where it is quickly available. Where imaging is required, US with colour Doppler is the investigation of choice. US is quick, non-invasive and highly accurate at differentiating torsion from inflammation.

US signs of acute epididymo-orchitis:
- Enlarged hypoechoic epididymis with increased blood flow
- Enlarged hypoechoic testis with increased blood flow
- Surrounding fluid/hydrocele.

US signs of testicular torsion:
- Decreased spermatic cord Doppler signal and lack of blood flow in the testis

- Testis may be normal in appearance, or enlarged and hypoechoic.

5.8 INTERVENTIONAL RADIOLOGY IN UROLOGY

5.8.1 Percutaneous nephrostomy

Percutaneous nephrostomy refers to percutaneous insertion of a drainage catheter into the renal collecting system.

Indications for percutaneous nephrostomy include:

- Relief of urinary tract obstruction, which may be caused by ureteric calculus, carcinoma of the bladder, ureteric TCC or carcinoma of the prostate
- Pyonephrosis
- Leakage of urine from upper urinary tract secondary to trauma or postsurgery.

Technique of percutaneous nephrostomy:

- Antibiotic cover
- Local anaesthetic and intravenous conscious sedation; general anaesthetic in children
- Imaging guidance: US and fluoroscopy, or CT
- Renal collecting system punctured with a needle
- Passage of a guidewire
- Insertion nephrostomy catheter over the guidewire.

Complications may include haematuria, which is usually mild and transitory, and vascular trauma, which is very rare with imaging guidance.

5.8.2 Ureteric stent

Indications for ureteric stent insertion include:

- Malignant obstruction of urinary tract caused by carcinoma of the bladder, prostate or cervix
- Pelviureteric junction obstruction
- Other benign obstructions of the urinary tract, e.g. retroperitoneal fibrosis, radiotherapy
- Postureteric surgery
- Extracorporeal shock wave lithotripsy (ESWL) of large renal calculi, to promote passage of stone fragments and relieve ureteric obstruction by fragments.

Ureteric stent insertion may be either retrograde or antegrade. Retrograde insertion is done via cystoscopy.

Antegrade insertion is performed where the lower ureter is occluded making retrograde insertion impossible:

- Under imaging guidance, the renal collecting system is punctured with a needle and a guidewire passed through the needle down the ureter and into the bladder.
- The stent is then passed over the guide wire and pushed into position.
- The upper pigtail of the stent should lie in the renal pelvis or upper pole calyx.
- The lower pigtail should lie in the bladder (Fig. 5.13).

5.8.3 Shock wave lithotripsy

Shock wave lithotripsy uses highly focused sound waves to fragment renal or ureteric stones. Where

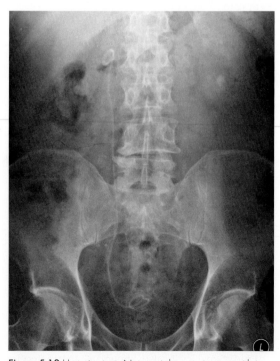

Figure 5.13 Ureteric stent. Note a right ureteric stent with its upper end in the right renal pelvis and its lower end in the bladder. Note also left renal calculi.

the shock waves are generated outside the body, the process is referred to as extracorporeal shock wave lithotripsy. Intracorporeal shock wave lithotripsy refers to shock waves generated inside the body through a ureteroscope. Shock wave lithotripsy is the technique of choice for the management of most renal stones.

5.8.4 Percutaneous nephrolithotomy

Indications for percutaneous nephrolithotomy (PCNL) include:

- Failed ESWL
- Staghorn calculus
- Cystine or matrix calculus.

Percutaneous nephrolithotomy is usually performed under general anaesthetic. A retrograde ureteric catheter is inserted via cystoscopy to opacify the renal collecting system with contrast material and to prevent calculus fragments passing down the ureter. The renal collecting system is then punctured with a needle followed by passage of a guidewire. A tract into the collecting system is made with a series of dilators and the renal stone extracted.

5.8.5 Renal artery embolization

For general notes on vascular embolization, please see Chapter 3.

Indications for renal artery embolization include:

- Control of urinary tract bleeding due to trauma (Fig. 4.33), surgery or biopsy
- Treatment of arteriovenous malformation (AVM) and arteriovenous fistula, which are most commonly seen as a complication of nephrostomy or biopsy
- Palliation or preoperative reduction of vascular renal tumour, either renal cell carcinoma or large angiomyolipoma.

5.8.6 Percutaneous tumour ablation

As stated above, over 60 per cent of RCCs are diagnosed incidentally. Most of these are small, early-stage tumours (<4 cm) amenable to minimally invasive, nephron-sparing treatment options. Such treatment options include open or laparoscopic partial nephrectomy and percutaneous tumour ablation. Percutaneous tumour ablation techniques are becoming widely available and include radiofrequency (RF) and cryoablation. Both techniques involve precise intratumoral placement of probes under imaging guidance. Ablation procedures may be performed with local anaesthesia and conscious sedation or general anaesthesia. Choice of imaging guidance technique (US, CT or MRI) depends on multiple factors including size and position of tumour, body habitus of patient, and local expertise and availability.

Patient preparation includes:

- Bleeding studies
- Biopsy: up to 25 per cent of small renal tumours are benign and do not require treatment.

Postprocedure follow-up includes:

- Observation for immediate complications, such as pain
- Imaging with contrast-enhanced CT or MRI to ensure ablation of the tumour and exclude complications such as haemorrhage.

SUMMARY BOX

Clinical presentation	Investigation of choice	Comment
Painless haematuria	CT urography and cystoscopy	US for further definition in selected cases
Renal mass	US CT	MRI in some centres Biopsy in selected cases
Prostatism	US	
Staging of adenocarcinoma of prostate	CT abdomen and pelvis Bone scintigraphy MRI prostate	
Scrotal mass	US	
Acute scrotum	US	

6 Obstetrics and gynaecology

US is by far the most common imaging technique in obstetrics and gynaecology. US is the investigation of choice at all stages of pregnancy. US may be used to confirm viability and dating of early pregnancy, and to assess placental position and fetal morphology in later pregnancy. Second and third trimester complications, such as placental abruption or suspected intrauterine growth retardation, are also assessed with US. US is also usually the investigation of choice for most gynaecological disorders, including pelvic mass, dysmenorrhoea and postmenopausal bleeding.

In obstetrics and gynaecology, transabdominal and/or transvaginal US may be performed. Transabdominal US has a wider field of view and requires a full bladder to visualize the pelvic organs. Transvaginal US (TVUS) utilizes a transvaginal probe and provides better anatomical detail of the uterus and ovaries. TVUS has a smaller field of view, and is not appropriate for very young or elderly patients. Apart from these constraints, TVUS is more accurate than transabdominal US in first trimester pregnancy and in most gynaecological conditions. TVUS may be used to guide interventional procedures, such as biopsy, cyst aspiration, abscess drainage and ovarian harvest.

MRI is used increasingly in obstetrics and gynaecology. Fetal MRI may be useful in second and third trimester pregnancy for sorting out complex fetal anomalies. MRI is used increasingly in gynaecology for diverse indications including suspected endometriosis, diagnosis of uterine pathology such as adenomyosis, and staging of gynaecological malignancies.

Interventional procedures used in gynaecology include recanalization of Fallopian tubes and embolization of uterine fibroids.

6.1 US IN OBSTETRICS

In Western society, virtually all women will have at least one US scan during pregnancy. US in pregnancy has multiple roles as follows:
- First trimester US
  - Confirmation of live pregnancy
  - Accurate assessment of dates
  - Management of complications, e.g. suspected ectopic pregnancy
- Nuchal thickness US at 11–14 weeks' gestation
- Fetal morphology scan at 19–21 weeks' gestation
- Third trimester US for a variety of indications, e.g. placenta praevia, suspected intrauterine growth retardation, follow-up of fetal anomalies.

6.1.1 First trimester bleeding

First trimester bleeding occurs in around 25 per cent of pregnancies. In most cases, it is a solitary event not accompanied by pain and is of no consequence. Initial assessment consists of physical examination, including speculum examination to visualize the cervix. First trimester bleeding accompanied by severe pain due to uterine contractions and a dilated cervix indicates a failed pregnancy and US is usually not indicated.

Transvaginal US may be helpful in threatened abortion, when bleeding and pain are mild and the cervix is closed. Differential diagnosis includes a normal pregnancy, missed abortion, blighted ovum, ectopic pregnancy and trophoblastic disease. The most important factors to establish on US are the presence and appearance of an intrauterine gestational sac. Knowledge of the human chorionic gonadotrophin (β-hCG) level may help to make sense of the findings. A gestational sac should become visible on TVUS at a β-hCG level of 1000 mIU/mL (Second International Standard). Yolk sac should become visible when the average diameter of the gestational sac is 8 mm; an embryo should be visible at 16 mm.

Measurement of the length of the embryo gives the crown-rump length (CRL) (Fig. 6.1). CRL correlates accurately with gestational age, especially if done at 6–10 weeks. Fetal heartbeat should be visible on TVUS when the CRL is 5 mm.

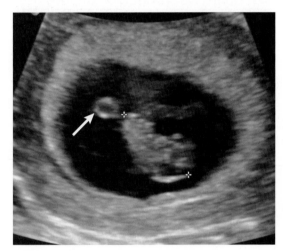

Figure 6.1 Early pregnancy: US. A gestational sac is seen as a round fluid-filled structure in the uterus. It contains a yolk sac (arrow) and a single fetus. Crown–rump length measurement (+) provides an accurate estimation of the stage of gestation, in this case 22 mm indicating 8 weeks and 5 days.

Signs of a failed pregnancy on TVUS include:
- Gestational sac >20 mm with no fetal pole identified
- Fetal pole >5 mm with no fetal heartbeat identified.

6.1.2 Suspected ectopic pregnancy

Clinical diagnosis of ectopic pregnancy is often difficult, with a history of a missed period present in only two-thirds of cases. The classic clinical triad of ectopic pregnancy consists of pain, vaginal bleeding and palpable adnexal mass. Like most classic triads, all three features occur in a minority of cases. Factors associated with an increased risk of ectopic pregnancy include increasing maternal age and parity, previous ectopic pregnancy and previous Fallopian tube surgery or infection.

Patients with suspected ectopic pregnancy who are haemodynamically unstable should be assessed laparoscopically. For all other patients with suspected ectopic pregnancy, TVUS correlated with serum β-hCG levels is the investigation of choice.

Signs of ectopic pregnancy on TVUS include:
- Empty uterus
- Free fluid in the pelvis
- Direct visualization of the ectopic gestation as a complex adnexal mass (Fig. 6.2)
- On rare occasions, fetal cardiac activity may be seen within the adnexal mass.

Note, however, that an adnexal mass may not be visualized and therefore a normal pelvic US examination does not exclude ectopic pregnancy. If a gestational sac cannot be identified in the uterus with TVUS despite a β-hCG level of 1000 mIU/mL or more, ectopic pregnancy should be considered.

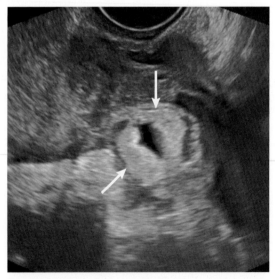

Figure 6.2 Ectopic pregnancy: US. Transvaginal US shows an echogenic adnexal mass (arrows).

6.1.3 Nuchal thickness scan

Towards the end of the first trimester, a thin hypoechoic layer can be observed in the posterior neck of the fetus, deep to the skin. This is known as the nuchal translucency (Fig. 6.3). Thickening of the nuchal translucency may be associated with Down

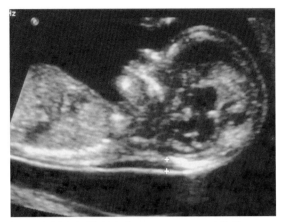

Figure 6.3 Nuchal fold thickness measurement: US. The nuchal fold is seen as a thin hypoechoic layer (+) at the back of the fetal neck.

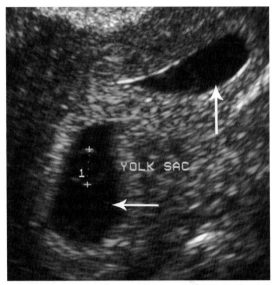

Figure 6.4 Twin gestation: US. US reveals two separate gestational sacs (arrows).

syndrome and other types of fetal aneuploidy. Nuchal thickness measurement is performed between 11 weeks and 13 weeks 6 days' gestation, by trained operators using standardized techniques. An accurate risk assessment for fetal aneuploidy is calculated based on:

- Maternal age
- Nuchal thickness
- Presence or absence of the fetal nasal bone
- Maternal levels of β-hCG and pregnancy-associated plasma protein A (PAPP-A).

A chromosomal abnormality can only be confirmed by amniocentesis or chorionic villous sampling (CVS). These tests are invasive and each carries a risk of subsequent miscarriage of about 1 per cent. In general, amniocentesis or CVS are recommended if the risk of aneuploidy, as calculated from the above, is 1 in 300 or more.

6.1.4 Multiple pregnancy

Multiple pregnancy occurs in 2 per cent of pregnancies, with a rate of about 10 per cent for assisted conceptions. It is important to recognize multiple pregnancy as early as possible as there are a number of associated risks, as well as social implications (Fig. 6.4). Risks to the fetuses include an increased incidence of congenital anomalies, intrauterine growth retardation and low birth-weight, and premature labour. Risks to the mother include hyperemesis, cholestasis, antepartum haemorrhage, polyhydramnios, hypertension and pre-eclampsia. Twin pregnancy, when recognized on US examination, may be classified as follows:

- Dichorionic diamniotic
  - May be dizygotic or monozygotic
  - Dizygotic may be different sex; monozygotic are same sex
  - Separating membrane seen between the fetuses
  - Separate placentas may be identified
  - Mortality rate 9 per cent
- Monochorionic diamniotic
  - Monozygotic, therefore same sex
  - Separating membrane between the fetuses may be seen
  - Single placenta
  - Mortality rate 26 per cent
- Monochorionic monoamniotic
  - Monozygotic, therefore same sex
  - No separating membrane
  - Single placenta
  - Mortality rate 44 per cent.

6.1.5 Fetal morphology scan

Obstetric US scan for assessment of fetal morphology is best performed at 19–21 weeks' gestation. The fetal morphology scan should only be performed when the referring doctor and patient have a clear view of the benefits and limitations of the technique. Potential implications of an abnormal finding should be understood prior to the examination. The fetal morphology scan provides an assessment of gestational age accurate to ±1 week, based on a number of measurements including:

- Biparietal diameter of the fetal skull
- Head circumference
- Abdomen circumference
- Femur length.

Placental position is documented, in particular the relationship of the lower placental edge to the internal os, i.e. diagnosis of placenta praevia. If low-lying placenta is diagnosed on the fetal morphology scan a follow-up scan is performed. Owing to increased growth of the lower uterine segment in later pregnancy, the majority of low-lying placentas will resolve spontaneously.

Amniotic fluid volume is assessed. Low amniotic fluid volume or oligohydramnios may be caused by intrauterine growth retardation secondary to placental insufficiency, chromosomal disorders, congenital infection and severe maternal systemic illness. Severe oligohydramnios may also indicate the presence of renal agenesis or obstruction of the fetal urinary tract. Common causes of increased amniotic fluid volume or polyhydramnios include maternal diabetes, multiple pregnancy, neural tube defect, fetal hydrops, and any disorder with impaired fetal swallowing such as oesophageal atresia. In many cases, polyhydramnios is idiopathic, with no underlying cause found.

A detailed assessment of fetal anatomy is performed. Most major fetal malformations are able to be diagnosed on US at this stage of pregnancy (Figs 6.5 and 6.6).

6.1.6 Second and third trimester

US may be indicated in later pregnancy for a variety of reasons.

6.1.6.1 Vaginal bleeding

Second or third trimester vaginal bleeding may be due to premature labour, or placental problems including placenta praevia, placental abruption and placenta accreta.

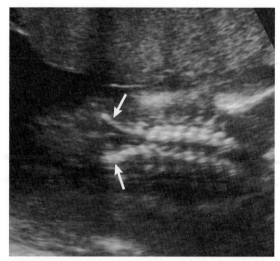

Figure 6.5 Spinal dysraphism: US at 19 weeks' gestation. Coronal view of the fetus shows separation of posterior ossification centres of the lower lumbar spine (arrow).

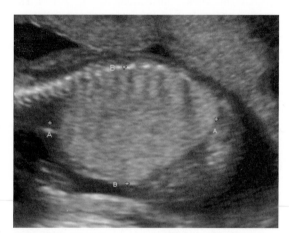

Figure 6.6 Fetal chest mass: US at 19 weeks' gestation. Longitudinal view of the fetus shows a large hyperechoic mass in the chest. Differential diagnosis would include congenital cystic adenomatoid malformation (CCAM), pulmonary sequestration and diaphragmatic hernia. Subsequently diagnosed as CCAM following delivery.

6.1.6.2 Follow-up of fetal abnormality

In some cases, a fetal abnormality diagnosed at the 19–21 week morphology scan may require follow up. Reasons for this may include monitoring of hydronephrosis or confirmation of anomaly suspected on an earlier scan (Fig. 6.7). Increasingly in modern practice, fetal MRI is used to provide further definition of fetal anomalies found on US.

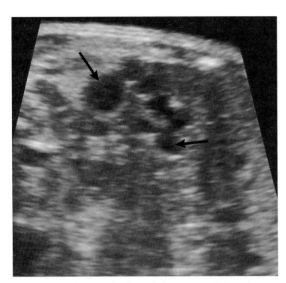

Figure 6.7 Multicystic dysplastic kidney: US at 34 weeks' gestation. Transverse view shows multiple non-communicating cysts in the expected position of the left kidney (arrows).

6.1.6.3 Suspected intrauterine growth retardation and fetal well-being

Clinical features suggestive of intrauterine growth retardation (IUGR) include small maternal size, slow weight gain, maternal hypertension, or a history of complications in previous pregnancies such as pre-eclampsia. IUGR may be confirmed by various US measurements of the fetus including measurements of biparietal diameter, head circumference, abdomen circumference and femur length, and estimation of fetal weight (EFW). A fetus is defined as being small for gestational age if the EFW is below the 10th centile. The most common cause of IUGR is placental insufficiency. In such cases, the IUGR is asymmetric, i.e. the abdomen is disproportionately small compared with the head. Symmetrical IUGR (head and abdomen reduced in size to an equal degree) may be caused by chromosomal disorders including trisomy 13 or 18.

Macrosomia refers to a fetus with EFW above the 90th centile for gestational age or EFW >4500 g. Macrosomia associated with maternal diabetes carries an increased risk of fetal demise. Macrosomia may also be associated with birth trauma. Management of placental insufficiency and other factors that may impact on fetal well-being is assisted by assessment of various US parameters including:

- Amniotic fluid volume
- Doppler analysis of umbilical artery, umbilical vein, ductus venosus and fetal middle cerebral artery
- Fetal breathing movements
- Fetal limb movements
- Fetal heart rate.

6.2 IMAGING IN GYNAECOLOGY

US is the primary imaging investigation of choice for assessment of gynaecological disorders. A variety of clinical presentations may occur, including pelvic mass, postmenopausal bleeding, irregular or painful periods in premenopausal women and chronic pelvic pain. MRI may be used for the diagnosis of uterine disorders including adenomyosis and endometriosis. MRI is also used for staging of gynaecological malignancies. Interventional radiology may also be used in gynaecology including:

- Biopsy
- Drainage of pelvic fluid collections
- Embolization of symptomatic uterine fibroids
- Recanalization of blocked Fallopian tubes in cases of infertility.

6.2.1 Pelvic mass

The first role of US in assessment of a pelvic mass is to ascertain the organ of origin. The majority of solid masses that arise from the uterus are fibroids. Fibroids are often multiple. Fibroids are usually seen on US as masses of variable echogenicity in the smooth muscle wall of the uterus (myometrium). Fibroids may project into the endometrial cavity or, alternately, may lie on the surface of the uterus or may even be attached by a stalk of tissue (pedunculated). Pedunculated fibroids may lie in the pelvis lateral to the uterus (adnexa) and may be difficult to distinguish from a solid ovarian tumour.

Most adnexal masses in women are ovarian in origin. Other possible causes of an adnexal mass would include bowel tumour, abscess or postoperative fluid collection.

Ovarian masses may be classified on US as simple cysts, complex cysts (cyst complicated by soft tissue septations or nodules) or solid. Other clinical data may be helpful in diagnosis, especially CA-125 (cancer antigen 125) levels.

6.2.1.1 Simple ovarian cysts

A cyst is classified as simple on US if it has anechoic fluid contents, a thin wall, and no soft tissue components. Most simple cysts in premenopausal women are follicular cysts (Fig. 6.8). Follicular cysts may measure up to 5 cm and if asymptomatic require no further assessment. Similarly, a simple cyst less than 5 cm in a postmenopausal woman may be regarded as benign. Occasionally, simple cysts may be associated with mild pain or discomfort, in which case review in a few weeks time may be useful. Usually, it is only those simple cysts that present with acute symptoms due to torsion or haemorrhage ('cyst accident') that require treatment.

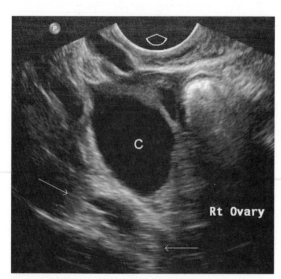

Figure 6.8 Simple ovarian cyst: US. Transvaginal US shows a simple cyst (C) arising on the right ovary and producing typical acoustic enhancement (arrows).

6.2.1.2 Polycystic ovarian syndrome

Polycystic ovarian syndrome (PCOS) is a common cause of chronic anovulation and infertility. PCOS refers to a spectrum of clinical disorders with the classic triad of oligomenorrhoea, obesity and hirsutism (Stein–Leventhal syndrome) being

the best known. The 'Rotterdam criteria' for the diagnosis of PCOS include:

- Anovulation
- Hyperandrogenism
- US findings of 12 or more follicles measuring 2–9 mm, and ovarian volumes of more than 10 cc
- Exclusion of other possible aetiologies such as Cushing's disease or androgen secreting tumour.

6.2.1.3 Complex ovarian cysts

Complex ovarian cysts include all cysts that do not fulfil the US criteria for a simple cyst, i.e. cysts with internal echoes or solid components such as soft tissue septations, wall thickening or associated soft tissue mass. In premenopausal women, the differential diagnosis of a complex ovarian cyst includes simple cyst complicated by haemorrhage giving echogenic fluid contents (Fig. 6.9). More complex cystic lesions may be caused by ectopic pregnancy (see Section 6.1.2), pelvic inflammatory disease, endometriosis and ovarian torsion.

The most common ovarian tumour in premenopausal women is benign cystic teratoma or 'dermoid cyst'. Dermoid cysts contain fat, hair and sometimes teeth, and are bilateral in 10 per cent

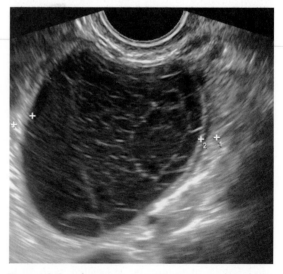

Figure 6.9 Complex ovarian cyst: US. Transvaginal US shows extensive complex echogenicity within an ovarian cyst due to haemorrhage.

of cases. Dermoid cysts are seen on US as complex cystic or solid lesions with markedly hyperechoic areas due to fat content (Fig. 6.10).

In postmenopausal women, a specialist gynaecologist should assess all complex cysts or simple cysts larger than 5 cm. Correlation with CA-125 levels may be helpful. Serous cystadenocarcinoma is the commonest type of ovarian malignancy. These are usually large (>15 cm) and seen on US as multiloculated cystic masses with thick, irregular septations and soft tissue masses (Fig. 6.11). US may also diagnose evidence of metastatic spread, such as ascites and liver metastases. Other ovarian tumours seen on US as complex, partly cystic ovarian masses include mucinous and serous cystadenoma, mucinous cystadenocarcinoma and endometroid carcinoma.

6.2.1.4 Solid ovarian masses

Causes of a solid ovarian mass include fibroma and Brenner tumour. A pedunculated fibroma may extend into the adnexa and mimic a solid ovarian mass.

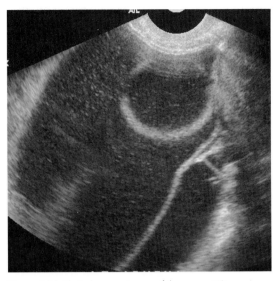

Figure 6.11 Cystadenocarcinoma of the ovary: US. Transvaginal US shows a multicystic ovarian mass with multiple septations and complex fluid contents.

6.2.2 Abnormal vaginal bleeding: premenopausal women

As described above, abnormal vaginal bleeding may be caused by complications of pregnancy. In non-pregnant premenopausal women, abnormal vaginal bleeding is usually caused by hormonal imbalance and anovulatory cycles (dysfunctional uterine bleeding), treated with hormonal therapy. If hormonal therapy does not control the bleeding, endometrial hyperplasia (precursor for endometrial carcinoma) or endometrial polyp are the primary diagnoses (Fig. 6.12). Factors associated with

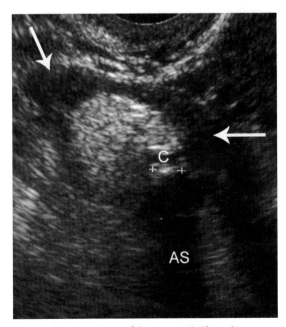

Figure 6.10 Dermoid cyst of the ovary: US. The right ovary (arrows) is enlarged due to the presence of a hyperechoic mass. The mass contains focal calcification (C) casting an acoustic shadow (AS).

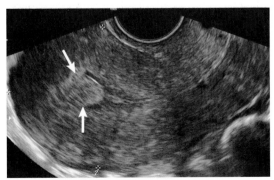

Figure 6.12 Endometrial polyp: US. Longitudinal transvaginal US shows an oval-shaped hyperechoic mass in the endometrial cavity of the uterus (arrows).

increased risk of endometrial pathology include age over 35 years, body weight over 90 kg and infertility.

Transvaginal US should be performed to measure endometrial thickness. Endometrial thickness varies with the phase of the menstrual cycle. The ideal time for TVUS is on days 4–6 of the menstrual cycle, when the endometrial echo should be at its thinnest. The likelihood of endometrial hyperplasia is low if the endometrial thickness measured with TVUS is <12 mm.

Saline infusion sonohysterography is a technique that enhances the accuracy of US assessment of the endometrium:

- A small catheter is placed in the uterus.
- Under direct visualization with TVUS, a small volume of sterile saline is injected to distend the uterine cavity.

Saline infusion sonohysterography produces excellent delineation of the two layers of endometrium and allows differentiation of endometrial masses from generalized endometrial thickening.

6.2.3 Postmenopausal bleeding

Postmenopausal bleeding is defined as spontaneous vaginal bleeding that occurs more than one year after the last menstrual period. In postmenopausal women, atrophic endometrium is the most common cause of abnormal vaginal bleeding. If bleeding persists despite a trial of hormonal therapy, endometrial carcinoma is the primary diagnosis and TVUS is indicated. The diagnostic sign of endometrial carcinoma on US is endometrial thickening. An endometrial thickness of more than 5 mm in a postmenopausal woman is an indication for further assessment with hysteroscopy and endometrial sampling.

6.3 STAGING OF GYNAECOLOGICAL MALIGNANCIES

For principles of cancer staging, please see Chapter 14. Malignancies of the female reproductive system are staged by the International Federation of Gynaecology and Obstetrics (FIGO). These classification systems are also converted into the TNM system and published by the American Joint Committee on Cancer (AJCC).

6.3.1 Ovarian carcinoma

Ovarian carcinoma is the leading cause of death from gynaecological malignancy. This is due to the high percentage of late stage tumours at the time of diagnosis, with over 75 per cent of patients having metastatic disease beyond the ovaries. The FIGO staging system for ovarian cancer is as follows:

- Stage I: tumour confined to the ovary
- Stage II: tumour involving one or both ovaries with pelvic extension
- Stage III: intraperitoneal metastases and/or regional lymphadenopathy
- Stage IV: distant metastases beyond the peritoneal cavity, e.g. liver metastases or malignant pleural effusion.

Most ovarian tumours are well seen with US (see above). CT of abdomen and pelvis is the investigation of choice for pretreatment staging of ovarian cancer. CT is used to search for signs of peritoneal spread, such as ascites and peritoneal masses, liver metastases, and lymphadenopathy (Fig. 6.13). Chest CT/CXR are also performed to detect pulmonary metastases and pleural effusion.

6.3.2 Carcinoma of the cervix

Cervical cancer is the third most common gynaecological malignancy. Mortality from cervical cancer has decreased over the last 40 years due to widespread use of the Papanicolaou (pap) smear. Histologically, most cervical carcinomas are squamous cell carcinoma. The mode of spread is by local invasion plus involvement of lymph nodes. The FIGO staging system for cervical carcinoma is as follows:

- Stage 0: carcinoma *in situ*
- Stage 1: confined to the uterus
- Stage 2: local invasion beyond the uterus not involving the lateral pelvic wall or lower third of vagina
- Stage 3: more extensive invasion with involvement of pelvic wall or lower vagina or causing hydronephrosis
- Stage 4: invasion of bladder or rectal mucosa or distant metastases, including pelvic and retroperitoneal lymph nodes.

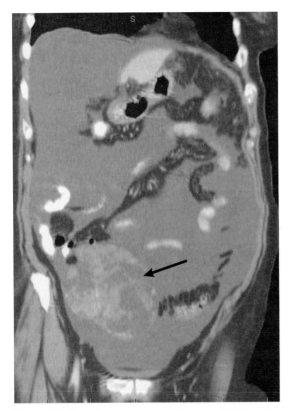

Figure 6.13 Cystadenocarcinoma of the ovary: CT. Coronal reconstruction CT abdomen shows a complex partly cystic mass in the right pelvis (arrow). Note extensive ascites due to peritoneal metastases.

Clinical assessment with examination under anaesthetic, colposcopy and ureteroscopy are used for initial diagnosis and assessment of carcinoma of the cervix. Imaging is used to differentiate stage 1 tumours that can be treated with surgery from more advanced disease. MRI is the investigation of choice for measuring tumour size and assessing depth of uterine invasion and local tumour extension in the pelvis. CT of abdomen and chest is usually also performed to search for retroperitoneal lymphadenopathy, liver metastases and lung metastases.

6.3.3 Endometrial carcinoma

Endometrial carcinoma is the most common gynaecological malignancy. Most tumours are adenocarcinomas, with a peak age of incidence of 55–65 years. The most common clinical presentation of endometrial carcinoma is postmenopausal

bleeding. Fifteen per cent of women with postmenopausal bleeding will have endometrial carcinoma. The FIGO staging system for endometrial carcinoma is as follows:

- Stage 0: carcinoma *in situ*
- Stage I: tumour limited to the uterus
  - Stage IA: tumour limited to the endometrium
  - Stage IB: invasion of less than 50 per cent of the myometrium
  - Stage IC: invasion of more than 50 per cent of the myometrium
- Stage II: invasion of the cervix with no extrauterine extension
- Stage III: extension beyond the uterus, but not outside the pelvis
- Stage IV: invasion of bladder or rectum, or distant metastases.

As can be seen from this staging system, the most important factor in early endometrial carcinoma is the degree of local invasion. MRI is the investigation of choice for early stage disease as it is more accurate than US in the assessment of depth of myometrial invasion and invasion of the cervix (Fig. 6.14).

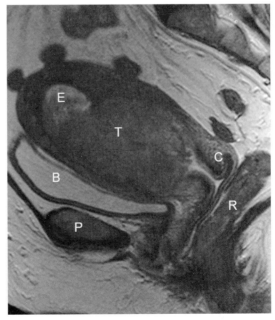

Figure 6.14 Endometrial carcinoma: MRI. Sagittal T2-weighted MRI shows a large endometrial tumour (T) confined to the body of the uterus. Note distended endometrial cavity (E) above the tumour, cervix (C), pubic symphysis (P), bladder (B), rectum (R).

7 Breast imaging

7.1 BREAST CANCER

Breast cancer is the commonest malignancy in women. Overall lifetime risk of development of breast cancer in women is 1 in 14 to 1 in 8. Factors associated with a higher risk of breast cancer include:

- First-degree relatives diagnosed with breast or ovarian cancer
- Genetic predisposition, most common mutation of *BRCA1/BRCA2* genes
- Cancer predisposition syndromes, e.g. Cowden syndrome, Li–Fraumeni syndrome
- Large-dose radiation exposure under the age of 30, most commonly radiotherapy of the chest for Hodgkin's lymphoma.

Most breast cancers arise from tissues in the terminal ductal/lobular units of the breast. The term '*in situ*' refers to tumours confined within the lumen of lobules or ducts. 'Invasive' or 'infiltrating' refers to tumours that have breached the basement membrane. Breast cancer is classified as follows:

- Ductal
  - Ductal carcinoma *in situ* (DCIS)
  - Invasive ductal carcinoma
  - Medullary
  - Mucinous/colloid
  - Rare types: papillary, apocrine, squamous
- Lobular
  - Lobular carcinoma *in situ* (LCIS)
  - Invasive lobular carcinoma
- Inflammatory carcinoma
  - Named for inflamed appearance of skin
  - Aggressive; poor prognosis.

Invasive ductal carcinoma is the most common type, accounting for about 70 per cent of cases of breast cancer. Breast cancer may present clinically as a palpable breast mass, or less commonly with other symptoms such as nipple discharge. Increasingly, breast cancer is detected in asymptomatic women through breast screening programmes. The main goal of breast imaging, whether it is in women with specific symptoms or in screening of asymptomatic women, is early diagnosis of breast cancer.

Consequences of diagnosis of breast cancer at an earlier stage include reduced risk of metastatic disease and local recurrence, and requirement for less radical therapy. Treatment of breast cancer consists of a combination of all or some of the following:

- Surgery for optimal tumour control in the breast and axillary lymph nodes
- Postoperative radiotherapy to reduce the risk of local recurrence
- Systemic chemotherapy and hormonal therapy to treat undetectable micrometastases.

The current trend towards less radical surgery requires accurate preoperative imaging to provide the following information:

- Precise site of tumour in the breast, including relationship to nipple and chest wall
- Presence of adjacent DCIS
- Presence of multifocal or contralateral disease.

7.2 BREAST IMAGING TECHNIQUES

7.2.1 Mammography

Mammography is a radiographic examination of the breast. Older mammography systems use standard X-ray film developed in a processor or darkroom. The newer technique of digital mammography (DM) is replacing conventional mammography in current clinical practice. DM uses digital radiographic systems as described in Chapter 1. Advantages of DM include the ability to manipulate the image plus the use of computer-aided detection (CAD). CAD is a refinement of DM in which a computer 'flags' potential abnormalities, which are then assessed by a radiologist. CAD has the potential to increase the sensitivity of mammography, although with reduced specificity.

Digital breast tomosynthesis (DBT) is a further extension of DM, in which multiple projection exposures are obtained from a mammographic X-ray source that moves over a limited arc. A series of cross-sectional images of the breast is obtained. DBT has the potential to increase sensitivity by removing overlying dense breast tissue that may otherwise obscure a mass. DBT currently has limited

availability, although with clinical acceptance its use may become more widespread.

Mammography is performed in two broad circumstances, diagnostic and screening. Diagnostic mammography is the first investigation of choice for a breast lump in women over 35 years of age. Diagnostic mammography may also be performed for other reasons, such as nipple discharge, or to search for a primary breast tumour where metastases are found elsewhere. Screening mammography is performed to search for early cancers in asymptomatic women.

The standard mammography examination consists of two views, craniocaudad (top to bottom) and mediolateral oblique (Fig. 7.1). A range of further views, including spot compression, magnification and angulated views, may be used to delineate an abnormality seen on the two standard views.

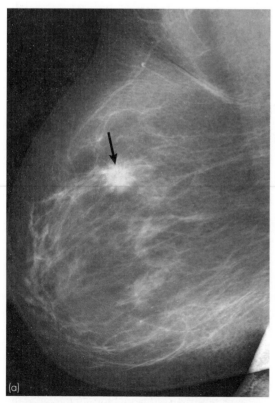
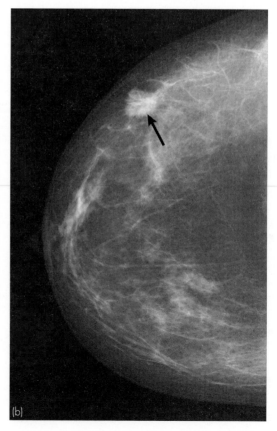

Figure 7.1 Mammogram: two standard views of the right breast. (a) Mediolateral oblique. (b) Craniocaudad. Note a small mass with a spiculated margin in the superior lateral aspect of the breast: invasive ductal carcinoma (arrow).

Abnormalities seen on mammography include soft tissue masses, asymmetric densities, calcifications, and secondary signs such as distortion of breast architecture and skin thickening.

Depending on their mammographic appearances, soft tissue masses may be categorized as benign, probably benign, malignant, probably malignant or indeterminate. A key mammographic finding in breast cancer is a stellate mass, i.e. a soft tissue density with irregular margins visible on both mammographic projections. Benign breast lesions including cyst, fibroadenoma, lipid cyst and galactocele tend to produce well-defined masses on mammography. Certain types of breast cancer, such as colloid and medullary cancers, may produce well-defined masses and therefore mimic benign pathology.

Calcification is a primary mammographic sign of early cancer, particularly DCIS. Most calcifications are small and therefore the term microcalcification is used. Malignant calcifications tend to occur in clusters, and are usually of variable size and density, often with a branching configuration. Causes of benign microcalcification include arterial calcification, calcification in cysts, and calcification of benign masses such as fibroadenoma (Fig. 7.2).

Mammography may be used to guide various procedures including:
- Biopsy of a mammographically visible mass
- Biopsy of microcalcification
- Hookwire localization of a non-palpable abnormality prior to surgical biopsy and removal (Fig. 7.3).

The principal disadvantage of mammography is its inherent false-negative rate. Overall sensitivity of mammography for detection of breast cancer is 85 per cent. In breasts that are composed primarily of fatty tissue, sensitivity of mammography may approach 95 per cent. In younger patients in whom dense breast tissue may obscure a focal abnormality, the sensitivity of mammography may be much lower. For this reason, US is generally preferred in women younger than 35. Another disadvantage is relatively poor specificity due to considerable overlap in appearances between malignant and benign pathologies. Fine needle aspiration (FNA), core biopsy or surgical removal are commonly required for assessment of mammographic

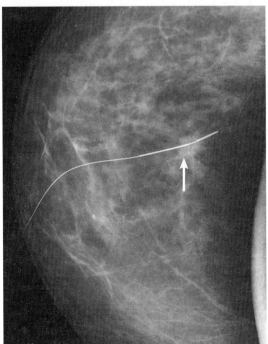

Figure 7.3 Hookwire localization: mammogram. Craniocaudad view showing a fine hookwire passing through a small mass: invasive ductal carcinoma.

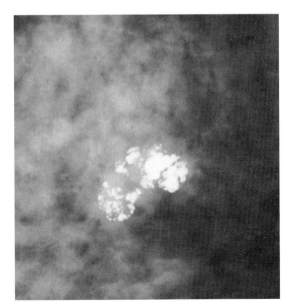

Figure 7.2 Fibroadenoma: mammogram. Small mass containing popcorn-like calcifications.

abnormalities. Breast MRI may be helpful in some instances.

7.2.2 US

US is the first investigation of choice for a palpable breast lump in a woman under 35 years of age, and in women who are pregnant or lactating. US may also be complementary to mammography, particularly for differentiating cysts from solid masses, and for assessment of mammographically dense breasts where small masses or cysts may be obscured by overlying breast tissue (Fig. 7.4). As well as diagnosing cysts, breast US is useful for providing further definition of solid masses, specifically for differentiating benign and malignant lesions. A major limitation of US is lack of sensitivity and specificity for the detection and characterization of microcalcifications.

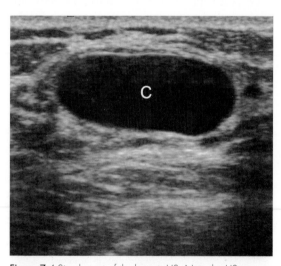

Figure 7.4 Simple cyst of the breast: US. Note the US features of a simple cyst (C): anechoic contents, smooth wall, no soft tissue components.

US may be used to guide various procedures including:
- Cyst aspiration
- FNA (Fig. 7.5)
- Core biopsy
- Guidewire localization
- Drainage of fluid collections, such as postoperative seroma or abscess complicating mastitis.

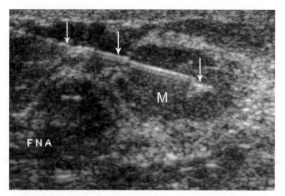

Figure 7.5 Fine needle aspiration of a breast mass under US guidance. The needle is seen as a hyperechoic line (arrows) passing into a hypoechoic mass (M). Cytology confirmed a fibroadenoma.

7.2.3 MRI

MRI using specifically designed breast coils and intravenous gadolinium injection is used for the detection and staging of breast cancer. MRI detection of breast cancer relies on malignant neovascularity, with 'leaky' capillaries allowing intense rapid enhancement with gadolinium, followed by rapid 'wash-out'. These contrast enhancement dynamics may be detected with rapid serial imaging of the breasts. MRI has high sensitivity for invasive cancer, with much lower sensitivity (approximately 40 per cent) for the detection of DCIS (Fig. 7.6). MRI is usually used as an adjunct to mammography and US.

Current roles for breast MRI include:
- Problem-solving for indeterminate findings on mammography or US
- Staging local tumour spread
- Assessment for tumour recurrence following lumpectomy
- Screening in high risk, young women
- Evaluation of nipple discharge
- Assessment of complications related to breast implants.

7.2.4 Lymphoscintigraphy (sentinel node detection)

Prognosis of breast cancer is greatly affected by axillary lymph node status at the time of diagnosis. Axillary lymph node dissection (ALND) is

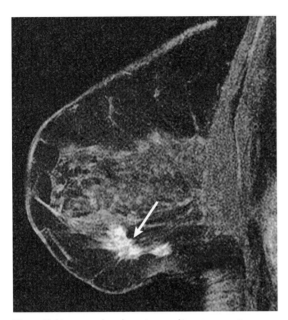

Figure 7.6 Invasive ductal carcinoma: breast magnetic resonance (MR). Sagittal T1-weighted, fat saturated, contrast-enhanced MR. Note in the inferior breast an intensely enhancing complex mass with a spiculated margin (arrow).

definitive in defining axillary node status, however is associated with a number of complications including lymphoedema, pain and reduced shoulder movement. Sentinel lymph node biopsy (SNLB) is much less traumatic than ALND. The sentinel lymph node is the first axillary lymph node on the lymphatic drainage pathway from the tumour, and therefore the first node to receive tumour cells if lymphatic metastatic spread has occurred. If the sentinel axillary lymph node can be identified and shown to be tumour free, then spread to any other axillary nodes is excluded with a high degree of accuracy.

For lymphoscintigraphy, ^{99m}Tc-labelled colloid particles are injected around the breast tumour prior to surgery. The accuracy of lymphoscintigraphy may be increased by injection of a combination of visible dye and radiopharmaceutical. The surgeon localizes the sentinel node in theatre with a hand-held gamma-detecting probe. The node is removed and examined by a pathologist:

- Sentinel node +ve = 40 per cent chance of spread to other axillary nodes and ALND is usually performed

- Sentinel node −ve = 98 per cent chance of no further lymph node spread and ALND not required.

7.2.5 Breast biopsy

Breast biopsy is usually performed under imaging guidance, either mammography or US. For most masses, US is the quickest and most accurate method (Fig. 10.9). Cyst aspiration under US control may be done to drain large cysts that are painful or to sample fluid from atypical cystic lesions. US is unable to accurately visualize microcalcification; therefore, for biopsy of microcalcification, mammographic guidance is required.

Several biopsy methods are used including FNA, core biopsy, vacuum-assisted core biopsy and open surgical biopsy requiring preoperative localization. FNA is usually performed with US guidance and is minimally invasive using 21–25 gauge needles. FNA requires an experienced cytopathologist for interpretation.

Core biopsy may be performed under US or mammographic guidance with 14–18 gauge cutting needles that obtain a core of tissue for histological diagnosis. A variation of core biopsy is vacuum-assisted core biopsy (Mammotome®). A Mammotome consists of an 11 gauge probe that is positioned under mammographic control. A vacuum pulls a small sample of breast tissue into the probe; this is cut off and transported back through the probe into a specimen chamber. This technique is particularly useful for microcalcification.

For open surgical biopsy, non-palpable masses may be localized under US or mammographic control prior to surgery. Suspicious microcalcifications may be localized under mammographic control. A needle containing a hook-shaped wire is positioned in or near the breast lesion. Once correct positioning is attained, the needle is withdrawn leaving the wire in place. US or mammography of the excised specimen is performed to ensure that the mass or calcifications have been removed.

7.3 INVESTIGATION OF A BREAST LUMP

Palpable breast masses may be discovered by self-examination or clinical examination. Prominent glandular tissue may commonly mimic a breast mass in younger women. Benign lesions tend to be mobile with well-defined smooth margins. Malignant masses tend to be firm to palpation with irregular margins and possible tethering to skin or deep structures.

7.3.1 Mammography

Mammography is the first investigation of choice for a breast lump in women over 35 years of age.

Mammographic features of a benign mass, e.g. cyst or fibroadenoma:

- Tend to compress but not invade adjacent tissue
- Round or oval in shape
- Well circumscribed, often with a surrounding dark halo due to compressed fat
- Calcification may occur in benign masses with various patterns seen:

- Large cyst: thin peripheral rim of wall calcification
- Fibroadenoma: dense coarse 'pop-corn' calcification (Fig. 7.2)
- Small cysts, adenosis and hyperplasia: multiple, tiny, pinpoint calcifications; milk of calcium in tiny cysts with multiple small fluid levels on the lateral view ('tea cupping').

Mammographic features of a malignant mass:
- Tend to invade adjacent tissue and often cause an irregular desmoplastic or fibrotic reaction
- Carcinomas therefore tend to have irregular or indistinct margins, often described as spiculated or stellate (Fig. 7.7)
- Distortion of surrounding breast tissue (architectural distortion)

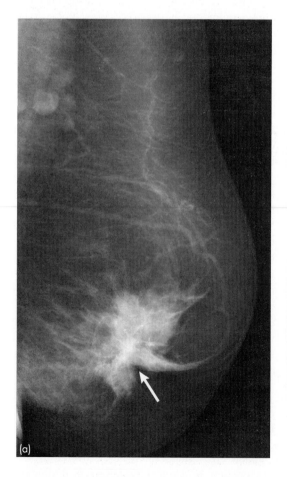

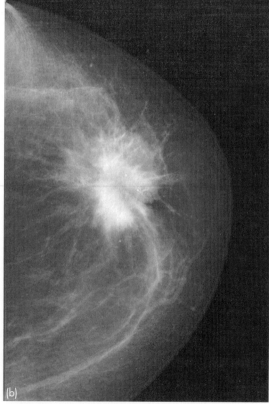

Figure 7.7 Invasive ductal carcinoma: mammogram. (a) Mediolateral oblique. (b) Craniocaudad. Large spiculated breast mass. Note the distorted margin of the mass on the mediolateral oblique view due to nipple retraction (arrow).

- Secondary signs, such as skin thickening and nipple retraction.

Malignant microcalcification is commonly seen in association with a mass, or without a mass in the case of DCIS (Fig. 7.8). Malignant microcalcification has the following features:
- Irregular
- Variable shape and size (pleomorphism)
- Branching, ductal pattern known as 'casting'
- Grouped in clusters
- Variable density.

US features of a benign mass, most commonly fibroadenoma (Fig. 7.9):
- Well-defined hypoechoic mass
- Ovoid in shape with long axis parallel to the chest wall.

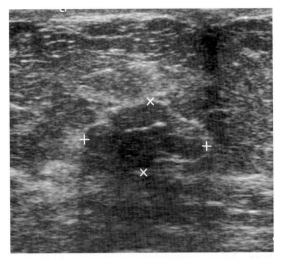

Figure 7.9 Fibroadenoma: US. Lobulated homogeneous hypoechoic mass, well-defined margin, long axis parallel to skin.

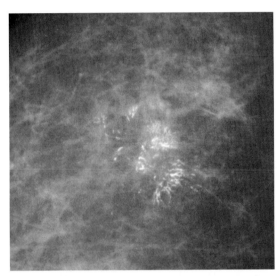

Figure 7.8 Ductal carcinoma *in situ*: mammogram. Note the typical features of malignant microcalcification: localized cluster of calcifications with an irregular branching pattern.

7.3.2 US

US is the investigation of choice for assessment of breast lumps in younger women. US may also be used for further characterization of a mass or localized density seen on mammography in older women. US features of a simple cyst (Fig. 7.4):
- Round with thin walls
- Anechoic contents
- Posterior acoustic enhancement.

Complicated cysts on US may have low-level internal echoes and slightly irregular walls due to infection, haemorrhage or cellular and proteinaceous debris.

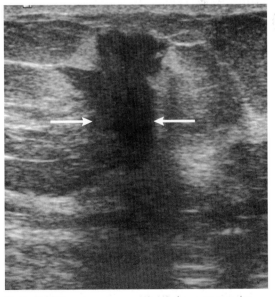

Figure 7.10 Breast carcinoma: US. US shows an irregular hypoechoic mass with an acoustic shadow (arrows). Note that the long axis of the mass is perpendicular to the skin.

US features of a carcinoma (Fig. 7.10):

- Focal mass with an irregular infiltrative margin and heterogeneous internal echoes
- Long axis perpendicular to chest wall
- Usually firm and non-compressible with posterior acoustic shadow
- Internal vascularity may be seen in high grade tumours.

7.4 INVESTIGATION OF NIPPLE DISCHARGE

Causes of nipple discharge include hormonal factors, infection, benign papilloma of a mammary duct, mammary duct ectasia and malignancy. Radiological investigation is particularly indicated for investigation of nipple discharge where various clinical factors indicate a greater likelihood of malignancy:

- Age over 60
- Discharge is unilateral, from a single duct
- Serous or bloodstained discharge
- Palpable mass.

Where imaging is indicated, mammography and US should be performed to exclude any obvious mass or suspicious microcalcification. High-resolution targeted US of the areolar region may also be able to diagnose papilloma or malignancy with visualization of a soft tissue mass associated with a prominent duct. If mammography and US are negative, MRI is the next investigation of choice. In centres where MRI is not available, galactography may be required.

Galactography is a procedure whereby the mammary duct orifice is gently cannulated and a small amount of contrast material injected, followed by radiographic images of the area of interest.

Findings on galactography include:

- Intraduct papilloma: smooth or irregular filling defect; these may be multiple
- Invasive carcinoma: irregular duct narrowing with distal dilatation.

In modern practice, MRI is replacing galactography in the investigation of suspicious nipple discharge.

7.5 STAGING OF BREAST CANCER

For principles of cancer staging, please see Chapter 14.

Lymph node status at the time of diagnosis is the most powerful predictor of long-term survival of breast cancer. Other less predictive factors include tumour size, histological grade, and hormone and HER2/neu receptor status. Techniques for assessing lymph node status include axillary lymph node dissection and sentinel lymph node biopsy (see Section 7.2.4). SLNB using a combination of visible dye and radiopharmaceutical injection carries less morbidity than ALND and is used widely in modern practice in the assessment of lymph node status.

Although metastatic disease is relatively common in breast cancer, this usually consists of undetectable micrometastases at the time of initial diagnosis. The incidence of macroscopically visible metastases at the time of initial diagnosis is low. Therefore, imaging for staging beyond assessment of regional lymph node status has limited benefit in otherwise asymptomatic women. Despite this, there is a tendency to perform staging at the time of diagnosis with various protocols including CT of neck, chest, abdomen and pelvis, radionuclide bone scan, and FDG-PET/CT. Common sites for metastases from breast cancer include lung, bone, distant lymph nodes (e.g. supraclavicular), liver, pleura, adrenal gland, brain and peritoneum. Specific imaging investigations may be indicated by symptoms, e.g. MRI of the brain for neurological symptoms.

7.6 BREAST SCREENING IN ASYMPTOMATIC WOMEN

Screening mammography refers to mammographic examination of asymptomatic women to diagnose early-stage breast cancers. Clinical trials have shown that screening mammography is of benefit in reducing mortality from breast cancer by up to 30 per cent in women aged 50–69 years. Women in this age group are actively recruited in countries that offer screening services. Practices vary for women aged 40–49 years. In Australia, women in this age group, as well as women aged over 70, may choose to be screened but are not actively recruited.

Owing to multiple factors, including reduced sensitivity of mammography in radiographically dense breasts, screening is generally less effective in younger women and not recommended below the age of 40. Exceptions to this include women at high risk of developing breast cancer, i.e. those with *BRCA1* or *BRCA2* gene mutations or history of chest radiotherapy before the age of 30. In these younger women, MR has greater sensitivity than mammography for breast cancer detection. Annual MR may be used for screening in high-risk asymptomatic women aged 30–49, after which annual mammography would be recommended. For women at intermediate risk, i.e. history of breast or ovarian cancer in first-degree relatives, annual mammography combined with clinical breast examination and US may be recommended.

Screening mammography in average-risk women is performed every two years. A dedicated team is essential to the screening process and includes radiographer, radiologist, surgeon, pathologist and counselling nurse. Mammography is the only validated screening test for breast cancer. Strict quality control over equipment, film processing and training of personnel is essential to provide optimum images and maximize diagnostic efficiency. An abnormality on initial screening leads to recall of the patient and a second stage of investigation comprising any or all of the following:

- US
- Further mammographic views including magnification
- Clinical assessment
- FNA or core biopsy.

If, after this second stage, a lesion is found to be malignant, the patient is referred for appropriate management. About 10 per cent of recalled women will be found to have a breast cancer. The overall rate of cancer diagnosis in screening programmes is about 0.5 per cent.

8 Musculoskeletal system

8.1 IMAGING INVESTIGATION OF THE MUSCULOSKELETAL SYSTEM

8.1.1 Radiographs

Radiographs are indicated in all fractures and dislocations. Radiographs are often sufficient for diagnosis in general bone conditions such as Paget's disease. Most bone tumours and other focal bone lesions are characterized by clinical history and plain radiographs. MRI and CT are used for staging or to assess specific complications of these lesions, but usually add little to the diagnostic specificity of radiographs. A major limitation of radiography is insensitivity for early bony changes in conditions such as osteomyelitis and stress fractures.

8.1.2 CT

Multidetector CT is used for further delineation of complex fractures. Common indications include depressed fracture of the tibial plateau, comminuted fracture of the calcaneus, and fractures involving articular surfaces. CT may also be used to diagnose complications of fractures such as non-union. CT may assist in staging bone tumours by demonstrating specific features, such as soft tissue extension and cortical destruction.

8.1.3 Scintigraphy

Bone scintigraphy, commonly known as 'bone scan', is performed with diphosphonate-based radiopharmaceuticals such as ^{99m}Tc-MDP. Bone scintigraphy is highly sensitive and therefore able to demonstrate pathologies such as subtle undisplaced fractures, stress fractures and osteomyelitis prior to radiographic changes becoming apparent. Scintigraphy is also able to image the entire skeleton and is therefore the investigation of choice for screening for skeletal metastases and other multifocal tumours. The commonest exception to this is multiple myeloma, which may be difficult to appreciate on scintigraphy. Skeletal survey (radiographs of the entire skeleton) or whole body MRI are usually indicated to assess the extent of multiple myeloma.

The major limitation of bone scintigraphy is its non-specificity. Areas of increased uptake are seen commonly in benign conditions, such as osteoarthritis. Correlative radiographs are often required for definitive diagnosis. Bone scintigraphy in combination with CT (SPECT–CT) reduces the rate of false-positive studies.

8.1.4 US

Musculoskeletal US (MSUS) is used to assess the soft tissues of the musculoskeletal system, i.e. tendons, ligaments and muscles. MSUS is able to diagnose muscle and tendon tears. MSUS is also used to assess superficial soft tissue masses and is able to provide a definitive diagnosis for common pathologies such as ganglion and superficial lipoma. MSUS is highly sensitive for the detection of soft tissue foreign bodies, including those not visible on radiographs, such as thorns, wood splinters and tiny pieces of glass. Limitations of MSUS include inability to visualize bone pathology and most internal joint derangements.

8.1.5 MRI

MRI is able to visualize all of the different tissues of the musculoskeletal system including cortical and medullary bone, hyaline and fibrocartilage, tendon, ligament and muscle. As such, MRI has a wide diversity of applications including internal derangements of joints, staging of bone and soft tissue tumours, and diagnosis of early or subtle bone changes in osteomyelitis, stress fracture and trauma.

8.2 HOW TO LOOK AT A SKELETAL RADIOGRAPH

8.2.1 Technical assessment

As is the case with CXR and AXR, a skeletal radiograph should be assessed for technical adequacy. This includes appropriate centring and projections for the area to be examined, plus adequate exposure. Features of a technically adequate radiograph of a bone or joint include:

- Fine bony detail, including sharp definition of bony surfaces and visibility of bony trabeculae
- Soft tissue detail, such as fat planes between muscles
- Where a joint is being examined, the articular surfaces should be visible with radiographs angled to show minimal overlap of adjacent bones.

Some bony overlap is unavoidable in complex areas such as the ankle and wrist, and multiple views with different angulations may be required to show the desired anatomy.

8.2.2 Normal radiographic anatomy

Viewing of skeletal radiographs requires knowledge of bony anatomy. This includes the ability to name bones and joints, plus an awareness of anatomical features common to all bones. Mature bones consist of a dense cortex of compact bone and a central medulla of cancellous bone. Cortex is seen radiographically as the white periphery of a bone. Central medulla is less dense. Cancellous bone that makes up the medulla consists of a sponge-like network of thin bony plates known as trabeculae.

Trabeculae support the bone marrow and are seen radiographically as a latticework of fine white lines in the medullary cavity. Cortex tends to be thicker in the shafts of long bones. Where long bones flare at their ends the cortex is thinner and the trabeculae in the medulla are more obvious.

Anatomical features of bones that may be recognized on radiographs are listed below. These include elevations and projections that provide attachments for tendons and ligaments and various holes and depressions (Figs 8.1 and 8.2):

- Head: expanded proximal end of a long bone, e.g. humerus, radius and femur
- Articular surface: synovial articulation with other bone(s); smooth bone surface covered with hyaline cartilage
- Facet: flat articular surface, e.g. zygo-apophyseal joints between vertebral bodies, commonly (though strictly speaking incorrectly) referred to as 'facet joints'
- Condyle: rounded articular surface, e.g. medial and lateral femoral condyles
- Epicondyle: projection close to a condyle providing attachment sites for the collateral ligaments of the joint, e.g. humeral and femoral epicondyles

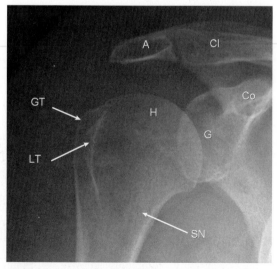

Figure 8.1 Normal shoulder. Note greater tuberosity (GT), lesser tuberosity (LT), surgical neck (SN), humeral head (H), glenoid (G), acromion (A), clavicle (Cl), coracoid process (Co).

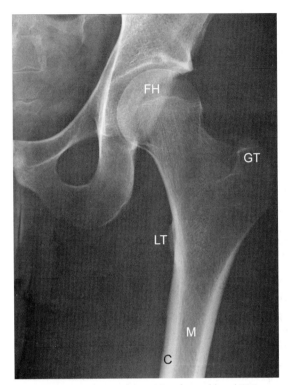

Figure 8.2 Normal upper femur. Note femoral head (FH), greater trochanter (GT), lesser trochanter (LT), cortex (C), medulla (M).

- Process: large projection, e.g. coracoid process of the scapula
- Tuberosity: rounded projection, e.g. lesser and greater tuberosities of the humerus
- Trochanter: rounded projection, e.g. greater and lesser trochanters of the femur
- Foramen: hole in a bone that usually transmits nerve and/or blood vessels, e.g. foramen ovale in the skull base
- Canal: long foramen, e.g. infraorbital canal
- Sulcus: long depression, e.g. humeral bicipital sulcus between lesser and greater tuberosities
- Fossa: wider depression, e.g. acetabular fossa.

Cartilage is not visible on plain radiographs; cartilage disorders are best assessed with MRI. Most cartilages in the body are hyaline or fibrocartilage. Hyaline cartilage covers the articular surfaces in synovial joints. The labrum is a rim of fibrocartilage that surrounds the articular surfaces of the acetabulum and glenoid. Fibrocartilage also forms the articular discs or menisci of the knee and temporomandibular joint, and the triangular fibrocartilage complex of the wrist.

8.2.3 Growing bones in children

Bones develop and grow through primary and secondary ossification centres (Fig. 8.3). Virtually all primary centres are present and ossified at birth. The part of bone ossified from the primary centre is termed the diaphysis. In long bones, the diaphysis forms most of the shaft. Secondary ossification centres occur later in growing bones, most appearing after birth. The secondary centre at the end of a growing long bone is termed the epiphysis. The epiphysis is separated from the shaft of the bone by the epiphyseal growth cartilage or physis. An apophysis is another type of secondary ossification centre that forms a protrusion from the growing bone. Examples of apophyses include the greater trochanter of the femur and the tibial

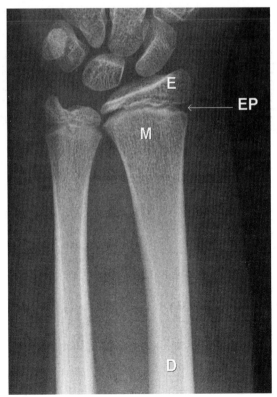

Figure 8.3 Normal wrist in a child. Note epiphysis (E), epiphyseal plate (EP), metaphysis (M), diaphysis (D).

tuberosity. The metaphysis is that part of the bone between the diaphysis and the physis. The diaphysis and metaphysis are covered by periosteum, and the articular surface of the epiphysis is covered by articular cartilage.

8.3 FRACTURES AND DISLOCATIONS: GENERAL PRINCIPLES

8.3.1 Radiography of fractures

- A minimum requirement for trauma radiography is that two views be taken of the area of interest
- Most trauma radiographs therefore consist of a lateral view and a front-on view, usually AP
- Where long bones of the arms or legs are being examined, the radiographs should include views of the joints at each end
  - For example, for fractures of midshaft radius and ulna, the elbow and wrist must be included
- For suspected ankle trauma three standard views are performed: AP, lateral and oblique
- In other areas, extra views may be requested depending on the clinical context
  - Acromioclavicular joint: weight-bearing views
  - Elbow: oblique view for radial head
  - Wrist: angled views of the scaphoid bone
  - Hip: oblique views of the acetabulum
  - Knee: intercondylar notch view; skyline view of the patella
  - Ankle: angled views of the subtalar joint; axial view of the calcaneus
- Stress views of the ankle may rarely be performed to diagnose ligament damage, though usually not in the acute situation.

8.3.2 Classification of fractures

Fractures may be classified and described by using terminology that incorporates a number of descriptors including fracture type, location and degree of comminution, angulation and deformity.

8.3.2.1 Fracture type

Complete fractures traverse the full thickness of a bone. Depending on the orientation of the fracture line, complete fractures are described as transverse, oblique or spiral. Incomplete fractures occur most commonly in children, as they have softer, more malleable bones. Incomplete fractures are classified as buckle or torus, greenstick, and plastic or bowing:

- Buckle (torus) fracture: bend in the bony cortex without an actual cortical break (Fig. 8.4)
- Greenstick fracture: only one cortex is broken with bending of the other cortex (Fig. 8.5)
- Plastic or bowing fracture: bending of a long bone without an actual fracture line (Fig. 8.6).

Other specific types of bone injury and fracture that may be seen include:
- Bone bruise
- Avulsion fractures
- Stress fractures
- Insufficiency fractures
- Pathological fractures.

Bone bruise or contusion is a type of bone injury due to compression. The term 'bone bruise' refers to bone marrow oedema in association with

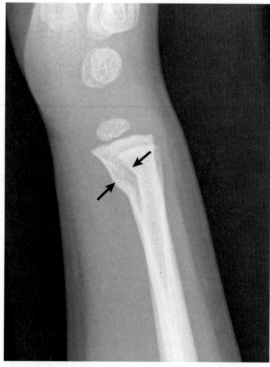

Figure 8.4 Buckle fracture distal radius and ulna.

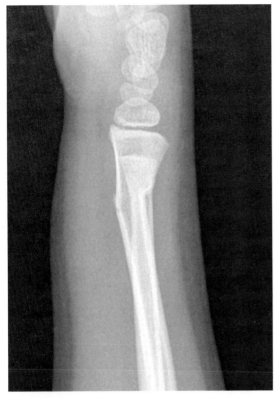

Figure 8.5 Greenstick fracture distal radius.

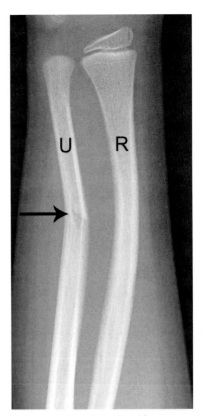

Figure 8.6 Bowing fracture. Undisplaced fracture (arrow) of the ulna (U), plus bowing of the radius (R).

microscopic fractures of bony trabeculae, without a visible fracture line. Bone bruises are seen on MRI, and are not visible on radiographs.

Avulsion fractures occur due to distraction forces at muscle, tendon and ligament insertions. Avulsion fractures are particularly common around the pelvis in athletes, such as the ischial tuberosity (hamstring origin) (Fig. 8.7) and anterior inferior iliac spine (rectus femoris origin). Avulsion fractures also occur in children at major ligament insertions, such as the insertion of the cruciate ligaments into the upper tibia. In children, the softer bone is more easily broken than the tougher ligament, whereas in adults the ligaments will tend to tear leaving the bony insertions intact.

Stress fractures occur due to repetitive trauma to otherwise normal bone, and are common in athletes and other active people. Certain types of stress fracture occur in certain activities, e.g. upper tibial stress fractures in runners, metatarsal stress fractures in marchers. Radiographs are often normal

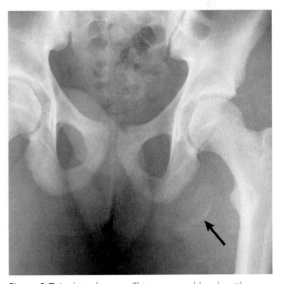

Figure 8.7 Avulsion fracture. Thirteen-year-old male with sudden onset of severe buttock pain after kicking a football. Frontal view of the pelvis shows a large curvilinear bone fragment below the ischial tuberosity (arrow). This is an avulsion of the hamstring origin.

at the time of initial presentation; after 7–10 days, a localized sclerotic line with periosteal thickening is usually visible (Fig. 8.8). MRI is usually positive at the time of initial presentation, as is scintigraphy with ^{99}mTc-MDP.

Insufficiency fracture is fracture of weakened bone that occurs with minor stress, e.g. insufficiency fracture of the sacrum in patients with severe systemic illnesses.

Pathological fracture is a fracture through a weak point in a bone caused by the presence of a bone abnormality. Pathological fractures may occur through benign bone lesions such as bone cysts or Langerhans cell histiocytosis (Fig. 8.9), or with primary bone neoplasms and skeletal metastases. The clue to a pathological fracture is that the bone injury is out of proportion to the amount of trauma.

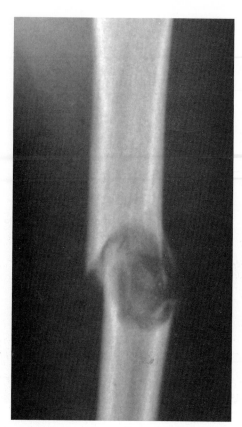

Figure 8.9 Pathological fracture: Langerhans cell histiocytosis. The history is of acute arm pain following minimal trauma in an eight-year-old child. Radiograph shows an undisplaced fracture through a slightly expanded lytic lesion in the humerus.

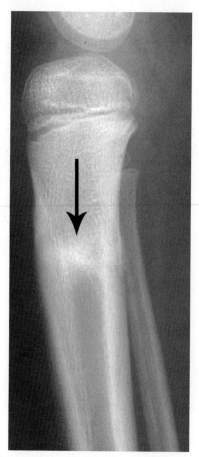

Figure 8.8 Stress fracture. A stress fracture of the upper tibia is seen as a band of sclerosis posteriorly (arrow).

8.3.2.2 Fracture location

Fracture description should include the name of the fractured bone(s), plus the specific part that is fractured, e.g. midshaft or distal shaft. Fracture lines involving articular surfaces are important to recognize as more precise reduction and fixation may be required.

Fractures in and around the epiphysis in children, also known as growth plate fractures, may be difficult to see and are classified by the Salter–Harris system as follows (Fig. 8.10):

- Salter–Harris 1: epiphyseal plate (cartilage) fracture
- Salter–Harris 2: fracture of metaphysis with or without displacement of the epiphysis (most common type) (Fig. 8.11)

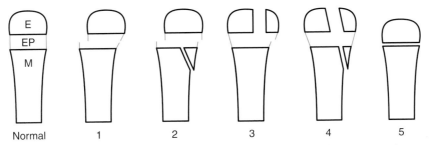

Figure 8.10 Schematic diagram illustrating the Salter–Harris classification of growth plate fractures. Note the normal anatomy: epiphysis (E), cartilage epiphyseal plate (EP) and metaphysis (M).

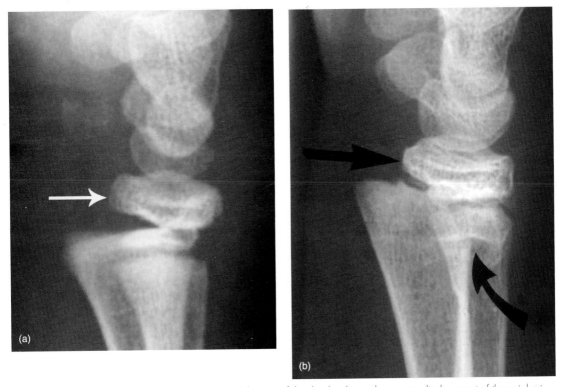

Figure 8.11 Salter–Harris fractures. (a) Salter–Harris 1 fracture of the distal radius with posterior displacement of the epiphysis (arrow). (b) Salter–Harris 2 fracture of the distal radius with fracture of the metaphysis (curved arrow) and posterior displacement of the epiphysis (straight arrow).

- Salter–Harris 3: fracture of epiphysis only
- Salter–Harris 4: fracture of metaphysis and epiphysis
- Salter–Harris 5: impaction and compression of the epiphyseal plate.

Salter–Harris types 1 and 5 are the most difficult to diagnose as the bones are intact and radiographic changes are often extremely subtle. Diagnosis of growth plate fractures is vital, as untreated disruption of the epiphyseal plate may lead to problems with growth of the bone.

8.3.2.3 Comminution

- Simple fracture: two fracture fragments only
- Comminuted fracture: fracture associated with more than two fragments.

Degree of comminution is important to assess as this partly dictates the type of treatment required. An example of this principle is fracture of the calcaneus.

Fractures with three or four major fragments are usually amenable to surgical reduction and fixation. A severely comminuted fracture of the calcaneus with multiple irregular fragments may be impossible to fix, the only option being fusion of the subtalar joint.

8.3.2.4 Closed or open (compound)

A compound or open fracture is usually obvious clinically. Where a bone end does not project through an open wound, air in the soft tissues around the fracture or in an adjacent joint may be a useful radiographic sign of a compound injury.

8.3.2.5 Degree of deformity

Types of deformity that may occur at fractures include displacement, angulation and rotation. Displacement refers to separation of bone fragments. Undisplaced fractures are often referred to as 'hairline' fractures. Undisplaced oblique fractures of the long bones can be especially difficult to recognize, particularly in paediatric patients, e.g. undisplaced fracture of the tibia in the one to three age group, the so-called 'toddler's fracture'. Undisplaced fractures through the waist of the scaphoid can also be difficult in the acute phase. Direction of angulation is classified according to the direction of the apex of the angle formed by the bone fragments. For example, Figure 8.12 shows a fracture of the distal radius. The apex of angulation points in a volar (anterior) direction; this is therefore referred to as volar angulation.

8.3.3 Fracture healing

Fracture healing is also known as fracture union, and occurs in three overlapping phases:
- Inflammatory phase: haematoma and swelling at the fracture site
- Reparative phase: proliferation of new blood vessels and increased blood flow around the fracture site. Collagen is laid down with early cartilage and new bone formation. This reparative tissue is known as callus

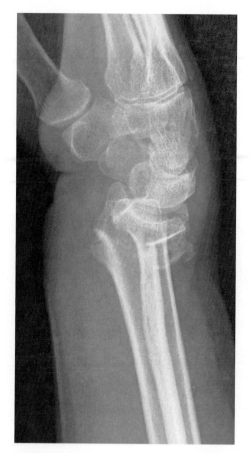

Figure 8.12 Colles' fracture. Fracture of the distal radius with impaction and volar angulation: apex of angle formed at the fracture site points in a volar direction.

- Remodelling phase: continued new bone formation bridging the fracture.

A major part of fracture management is assessing when union is sufficiently advanced to allow cessation of immobilization and resumption of unrestricted activity. The definition of 'complete union' may be quite difficult in individual cases and is usually made with a combination of clinical and radiographic assessments. Different stages of union are recognized.

Early union (incomplete repair) is indicated radiographically by densely calcified callus around the fracture with the fracture line still visible (Fig. 8.13). Clinical assessment will usually reveal an immobile fracture site, though with some tenderness with palpation and stress. Fracture immobilization

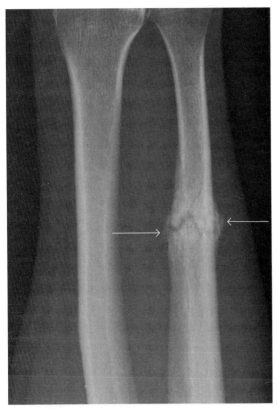

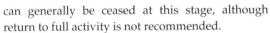

Figure 8.13 Early union. Subperiosteal new bone formation adjacent to the fracture (arrows).

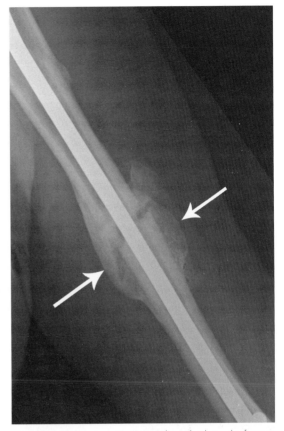

Figure 8.14 Late union. Dense new bone bridging the fracture margins (arrows).

can generally be ceased at this stage, although return to full activity is not recommended.

Late union (complete repair or consolidation) is indicated radiographically by ossification of callus producing mature bone across the fracture (Fig. 8.14). The fracture line may be invisible or faintly defined through the bridging bone. Clinically, the fracture is immobile with no tenderness. No further restriction of activity is necessary.

Due to variable biological factors, it is impossible to precisely predict fracture healing times in individual cases. A few basic principles of fracture healing are as follows:

- Spiral fractures unite faster than transverse fractures
- In adults, spiral fractures of the upper limb unite in 6–8 weeks
- Spiral fractures of the tibia unite in 12–16 weeks and of the femur in 16–20 weeks

- Transverse fractures take about 25 per cent longer to unite
- Union is much quicker in children, and generally slower in the elderly.

8.3.4 Problems with fracture healing

8.3.4.1 Delayed union

Delayed union is defined as union that fails to occur within the expected time as outlined above. Delayed union may occur in elderly patients, or may be caused by incomplete immobilization, infection at the fracture site, pathological fractures and vitamin C deficiency.

8.3.4.2 Non-union

The term 'non-union' implies that the bone will never unite without some form of intervention. Non-union is diagnosed radiographically with visualization of sclerosis (increased density) of the bone ends at the fracture site. The fracture margins often have rounded edges and the fracture line is still clearly visible (Fig. 8.15). A variation of non-union may be encountered in which there is mature bone formation around the edge of the fracture with failure of healing centrally. This may be difficult to recognize radiographically and CT may be required for diagnosis. This form of non-union may be suspected where there is ongoing pain despite apparently solid radiographic union.

8.3.4.3 Traumatic epiphyseal arrest

Traumatic epiphyseal arrest refers to premature closure of a bony growth plate due to failure of recognition or inadequate management of a growth plate fracture in a child. An example of this is fracture of the lateral epicondyle of the humerus leading to premature closure of the growth plate and alteration of the carrying angle of the elbow.

8.3.4.4 Malunion

Malunion refers to complete bone healing in a poor position leading to permanent bone or joint deformity, and often to early osteoarthritis (Fig. 8.16).

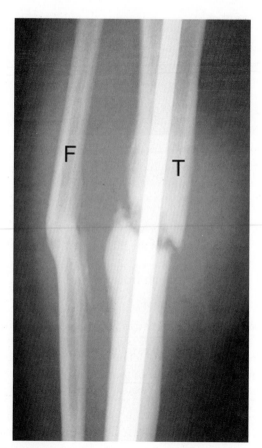

Figure 8.15 Non-union. Fracture of the tibia (T) six months previously. The fracture margins are rounded and sclerotic indicating non-union. The adjacent fracture of the fibula (F) has united.

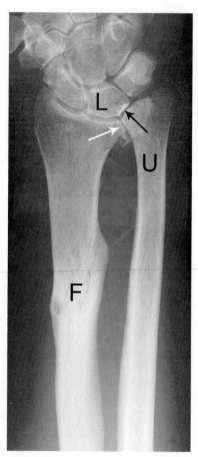

Figure 8.16 Malunion. A fracture of the radius (F) has united with shortening of the radius. As a result, the ulna is relatively longer than the radius (positive ulnar variance) and is contacting the lunate (black arrow). This is known as ulnar abutment and is a cause of wrist pain. There is also secondary osteoarthritis of the distal radio-ulnar joint (white arrow).

8.3.5 Other complications of fractures

8.3.5.1 Associated soft tissue injuries

Many examples exist of soft tissue injuries associated with fractures:

- Pneumothorax associated with rib fractures
- Bladder injury in association with fractures of the pelvis.

These soft tissue injuries may be of more urgent clinical significance than the bony injuries.

8.3.5.2 Complications of recumbancy

Complications such as pneumonia and deep vein thrombosis are common complications of recumbancy, especially in the elderly.

8.3.5.3 Arterial injury

Arterial laceration and occlusion causing acute limb ischaemia may be seen in association with displaced fractures of the femur or tibia, and in the upper limb with displaced fractures of the distal humerus and elbow dislocation.

8.3.5.4 Nerve injury

Nerve injury following fracture or dislocation is a relatively rare event; best known examples include:

- Shoulder dislocation: axillary nerve
- Fracture midshaft humerus: radial nerve
- Displaced supracondylar fracture humerus: median nerve
- Elbow dislocation: ulnar nerve
- Hip dislocation: sciatic nerve
- Knee dislocation: tibial nerve
- Fractured neck of fibula: common peroneal nerve.

8.3.5.5 Avascular necrosis

Traumatic avascular necrosis (AVN) occurs most commonly in three sites: proximal pole of scaphoid, femoral head and body of talus. In these sites, AVN is due to interruption of blood supply as may occur in fractures of the waist of the scaphoid, femoral neck and neck of talus. New bone is laid down on necrosed bone trabeculae causing the non-vascularized portion of bone to become sclerotic on radiographs over two to three months.

Due to weight-bearing, the femoral head and talus may show deformity and irregularity, as well as sclerosis.

8.3.5.6 Reflex sympathetic dystrophy

Reflex sympathetic dystrophy (RSD) (also known as Sudeck's atrophy) may follow trivial bone injury. It occurs in bones distal to the site of injury and is associated with severe pain and swelling. Radiographic changes of RSD include a marked decrease in bone density distal to the fracture site with thinning of the bone cortex. Scintigraphy shows increased tracer uptake in the limb distal to the trauma site.

8.3.5.7 Myositis ossificans

Myositis ossificans refers to post-traumatic non-neoplastic formation of bone within skeletal muscle, usually within 5–6 weeks of trauma. Myositis ossificans may occur at any site although the muscles of the anterior thigh are most commonly affected. It is seen radiographically as bone formation in the soft tissues; this bone has a striated appearance conforming to the structure of the underlying muscle.

8.4 FRACTURES AND DISLOCATIONS: SPECIFIC AREAS

In the following section, radiographic signs of the more common fractures and dislocations are discussed. Those lesions that may cause problems with diagnosis will be emphasized. Most fractures and dislocations are diagnosed with radiographs. Other imaging modalities will be described where applicable.

8.4.1 Shoulder and clavicle

8.4.1.1 Fractured clavicle

Fractures of the clavicle usually involve the middle third. Fractures are commonly angulated and displaced. When displaced, the outer fragment usually lies at a lower level than the inner fragment (Fig. 8.17).

Less commonly, fracture may involve the outer clavicle. In these cases, a small fragment of outer

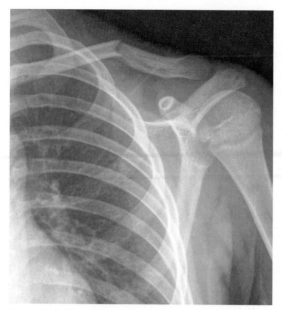

Figure 8.17 Superiorly angulated fracture midshaft clavicle.

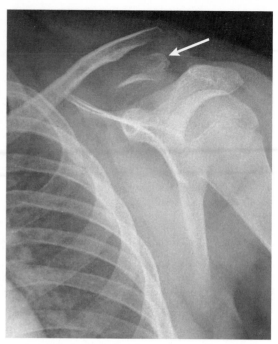

Figure 8.18 Outer clavicle fracture. Small clavicle fragment (arrow) maintains normal alignment with acromion. Outer end of medial fragment displaced upwards due to tear of coracoclavicular ligaments.

clavicle maintains normal alignment with the acromion. Due to tearing of the coracoclavicular ligaments, there is variable superior displacement at the fracture site (Fig. 8.18).

8.4.1.2 Sternoclavicular joint dislocation

Dislocation of the sternoclavicular joint is an uncommon injury usually caused by indirect trauma to the shoulder or a direct anterior blow. Anterior dislocation, in which the head of the clavicle lies anterior to the manubrium, is more common than posterior dislocation. In posterior dislocation the head of the clavicle may compress the trachea or underlying blood vessels including the brachiocephalic veins. Due to overlapping structures, the sternoclavicular joint is difficult to see on plain radiographs. CT is the investigation of choice where sternoclavicular joint injury is suspected.

8.4.1.3 Acromioclavicular joint dislocation

Acromioclavicular (AC) joint dislocation produces widening of the AC joint space and elevation of the outer end of the clavicle. The underlying pathology is tearing of the coracoclavicular ligaments, seen radiographically as increased distance between

the undersurface of the clavicle and the coracoid process. Radiographic signs may be subtle and a weight-bearing view may be useful in doubtful cases (Fig. 8.19).

8.4.1.4 Anterior dislocation of the shoulder

With anterior dislocation of the shoulder (gleno-humeral joint) the humeral head is displaced antero-medially. On the lateral radiograph, the humeral head lies anterior to the glenoid fossa. On the AP view, the humeral head overlaps the lower glenoid and the lateral border of the scapula. Associated fractures occur commonly (Fig. 8.20):

- Wedge-shaped defect in the posterolateral humeral head (Hill–Sachs deformity)
- Fracture of the inferior rim of the glenoid (Bankart lesion)
- Fracture of the greater tuberosity
- Fracture of the surgical neck of the humerus.

Recurrent anterior dislocation may be seen in association with fracture of the glenoid, tear of the anterior cartilagenous labrum, and laxity of the joint

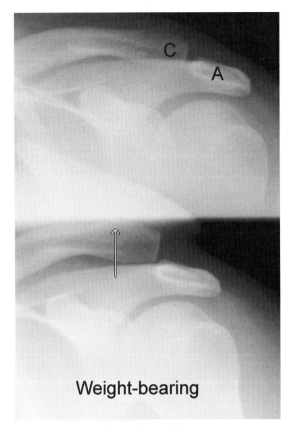

Weight-bearing

Figure 8.19 Acromioclavicular joint dislocation. At rest the acromioclavicular joint shows normal alignment. A radiograph performed with weight-bearing shows upward dislocation of the clavicle (arrow).

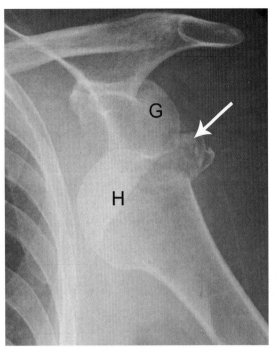

Figure 8.20 Anterior shoulder dislocation. The humeral head (H) lies anterior and medial to the glenoid (G). Associated fracture of greater tuberosity (arrow).

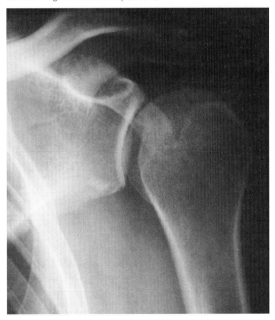

Figure 8.21 Posterior shoulder dislocation. In posterior dislocation, the humeral head is internally rotated with the articular surface of the humerus facing posteriorly. As a result, the humeral head has a symmetric round configuration likened to a light bulb or ice cream cone. Compare this with the normal appearance in Fig. 11.1.

capsule and glenohumeral ligaments. These injuries are diagnosed with MRI (see below).

8.4.1.5 Posterior dislocation of the shoulder

Posterior dislocation is a relatively uncommon injury, representing only 2 per cent of shoulder dislocations. It may easily be missed on radiographic examination. Signs on the AP film are often subtle (Fig. 8.21):

- Loss of parallelism of the articular surface of the humeral head and glenoid fossa
- Medial rotation of the humerus so that the humeral head looks symmetrically rounded like an ice cream cone or an electric light bulb.

On the lateral film, the articular surface of the humeral head is seen rotated posterior to the glenoid fossa.

8.4.2 Humerus

Fractures of the proximal humerus are common in the elderly. Proximal humeral fractures commonly involve the surgical neck, greater tuberosity, lesser tuberosity, and anatomical neck causing separation of the humeral head. Surgical neck fractures are often undisplaced, although significant angulation or impaction may occur. For the purposes of classification, the proximal humerus can be thought of as four parts or segments: humeral head including articular surface, greater tuberosity, lesser tuberosity, and humeral shaft. Displacement of upper femoral fractures is defined as >1 cm displacement of a segment, or >45° angulation. Proximal humeral fractures are classified according to the number of separate bone parts and the degree of displacement:

- 1 part fracture: no significant displacement or angulation of any segments
- 2 part fracture: displacement of one segment
- 3 part fracture: non-impacted fracture of surgical neck and displacement of two segments
- 4 part fracture: displacement of all four segments.

Humeral shaft fractures may be transverse, oblique, simple or comminuted.

8.4.3 Elbow

8.4.3.1 Elbow joint effusion

Fat pads lie on the anterior and posterior surfaces of the distal humerus at the attachments of the elbow joint capsule. On a lateral radiograph of the elbow, these fat pads are usually not visualized; occasionally, the anterior fat pad may be seen lying on the anterior surface of the humerus. In the presence of an elbow joint effusion, the fat pads are seen on lateral radiographs as dark grey triangular structures lifted off the humeral surfaces (Fig. 8.22); this is sometimes referred to as the 'fat pad' sign. There is a high rate of association of elbow joint effusion with fracture. Where an elbow joint effusion is present in a setting of trauma and no fracture can be seen on standard elbow radiographs, consider an undisplaced fracture of the radial head or a supracondylar fracture of the distal humerus. In this situation, either perform further oblique views, or treat and repeat radiographs in 7–10 days.

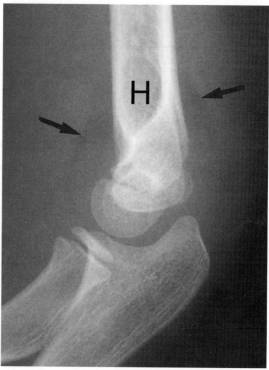

Figure 8.22 Elbow joint effusion. Elbow joint effusion causes elevation of the anterior and posterior fat pads producing triangular lucencies (arrows) anterior and posterior to the distal humerus (H).

8.4.3.2 Supracondylar fracture

Supracondylar fracture of the distal humerus is a common injury in children (Fig. 8.23). Supracondylar fracture may be undisplaced, or the distal fragment may be displaced anteriorly or posteriorly. Posterior displacement is the most common and when severe may be associated with injury to the brachial artery and median nerve (Fig. 8.24).

8.4.3.3 Fracture and separation of the lateral condylar epiphysis

Fracture of the lateral humeral condyle in children may be difficult to see on radiographs. Because the growth centre is predominantly cartilage, the bony injury may look deceptively small (Fig. 8.25). Adequate treatment is vital as this fracture may damage the growth plate and the articular surface leading to deformity.

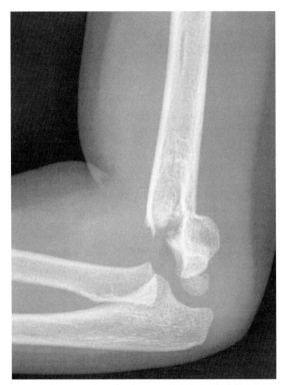

Figure 8.23 Supracondylar fracture distal humerus. The distal fragment is angulated though not displaced.

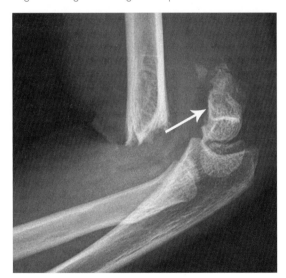

Figure 8.24 Supracondylar fracture distal humerus. The distal fragment is displaced posteriorly (arrow).

8.4.3.4 Fracture of the head of the radius

Three patterns of radial head fracture are commonly seen:

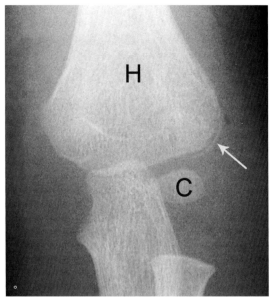

Figure 8.25 Lateral humeral condyle fracture. Note the normal appearance of the humerus (H) and growth centre for the capitulum (C) in an 18-month-old child. A fracture of the lateral humeral condyle is seen as a thin sliver of bone adjacent to the distal humerus (arrow).

- Vertical split (Fig. 8.26)
- Small lateral fragment
- Multiple fragments.

Radial head fracture may be difficult to visualize radiographically and elbow joint effusion may be the only radiographic sign on initial presentation. In such cases the arm is usually placed in a sling and radiographs repeated in a few days.

8.4.3.5 Fracture of the olecranon

Two patterns of olecranon fracture are commonly seen:
- Comminuted fracture
- Single transverse fracture line with separation of fragments due to unopposed action of the triceps muscle (Fig. 8.27).

8.4.3.6 Other elbow fractures

Other less commonly encountered elbow fractures include:
- 'T'- or 'Y'-shaped fracture of the distal humerus with separation of the humeral condyles

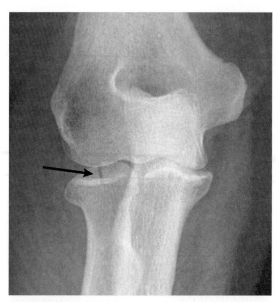

Figure 8.26 Radial head fracture. Vertically orientated split of the articular surface of the radial head (arrow).

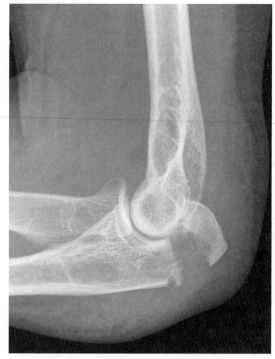

Figure 8.27 Olecranon fracture. Fracture through the articular surface of the olecranon with wide separation of bone fragments.

- Fracture and separation of the capitulum usually results in the capitulum being sheared off vertically
- Fracture and separation of the medial epicondylar apophysis may occur in children and may be difficult to recognize (Fig. 8.28).

8.4.4 Radius and ulna

8.4.4.1 Midshaft fractures

Midshaft fractures of radius and ulna usually involve both bones and may be transverse or oblique with varying degrees of angulation and displacement.

Isolated fracture of the midshaft of either radius or ulna is commonly associated with disruption of wrist or elbow joint:

- Monteggia fracture: anteriorly angulated fracture of upper third of the shaft of the ulna associated with anterior dislocation of the radial head (Fig. 8.29)
- Galeazzi fracture: fracture of the lower third of the shaft of the radius associated with subluxation or dislocation of the distal radio-ulnar joint.

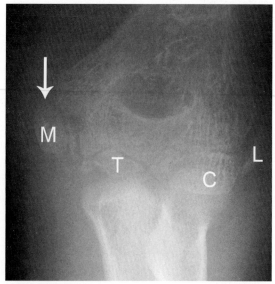

Figure 8.28 Medial humeral epicondyle fracture. Note the normal growth centres in a 12-year-old child: capitulum (C), trochlea (T), lateral epicondyle (L). The growth centre for the medial epicondyle (M) is displaced with a small adjacent fracture fragment. Although subtle, this represents a significant elbow injury.

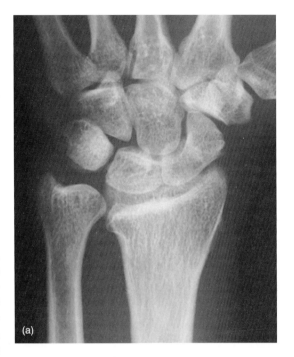

Figure 8.29 Monteggia fracture–dislocation. Fracture of the ulna. The head of the radius (R) is displaced from the capitulum (C) indicating dislocation.

8.4.4.2 Fracture of the distal radius

The distal radius is the most common site of radial fracture. The distal radius is a common fracture site in children with buckle, greenstick or Salter–Harris type 2 fractures particularly common (Figs 8.4, 8.5 and 8.6). Distal radial fractures are also common in elderly patients, particularly those with osteoporosis. Classical Colles' fracture consists of a transverse fracture of the distal radius with volar angulation (Fig. 8.12). The distal fragment is angulated and/or displaced posteriorly, often with a degree of impaction. Distal radial fractures are commonly associated with avulsion of the tip of the ulnar styloid process. Dorsally angulated fracture of the distal radius, commonly known as Smith's fracture, is less common than Colles' fracture.

Comminuted fracture of the distal radius is a common injury in adults. Fracture lines may extend into the articular surfaces of the radiocarpal and distal radio-ulnar joints. CT may be used for planning of surgical fixation of these complex fractures.

8.4.5 Wrist and hand

8.4.5.1 Scaphoid fracture

Two types of scaphoid fracture are encountered commonly:
- Transverse fracture of the waist of the scaphoid
- Fracture and separation of the scaphoid tubercle.

Undisplaced fracture of the waist of the scaphoid may be difficult to see on radiographs at initial presentation, even on dedicated oblique views (Fig. 8.30). Further investigation may be required

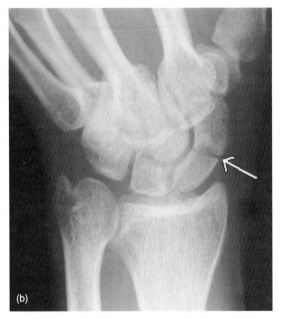

Figure 8.30 Scaphoid fracture. (a) Frontal radiograph of the wrist shows no fracture. (b) Oblique view of the scaphoid shows an undisplaced fracture (arrow). This example demonstrates the need to obtain dedicated scaphoid views where scaphoid fracture is suspected.

to confirm the diagnosis. This usually consists of a repeat radiograph after 7–10 days of immobilization. If immediate diagnosis is required, MRI is the investigation of choice.

8.4.5.2 Lunate dislocation

Lunate dislocation refers to anterior dislocation of the lunate. This may be difficult to appreciate on the frontal film, though it is easily seen on the lateral view with the lunate rotated and displaced anteriorly (Fig. 8.31).

8.4.5.3 Perilunate dislocation

In perilunate dislocation the lunate articulates normally with the radius, and other carpal bones are displaced posteriorly. On the frontal radiograph, there is abnormal overlap of bones, with dissociation of articular surfaces of the lunate and capitate. The lateral film shows minimal, if any, rotation of the lunate and posterior displacement of the remainder of the carpal bones (Fig. 8.32). Perilunate dislocation may be associated with scaphoid fracture (trans-

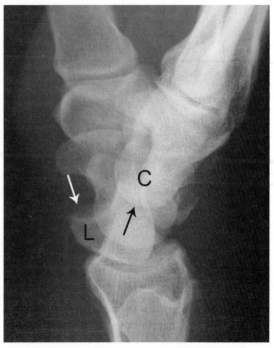

Figure 8.32 Perilunate dislocation. Lateral radiograph of the wrist showing the lunate (L) in normal position with the capitate (C) and other carpal bones displaced posteriorly. Note the separation of the distal articular surface of the lunate (white arrow) from the proximal articular surface of the capitate (black arrow).

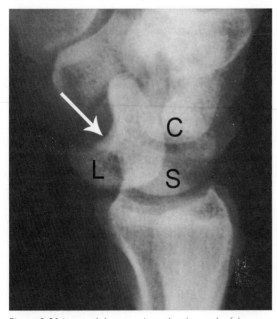

Figure 8.31 Lunate dislocation. Lateral radiograph of the wrist showing the capitate (C) and scaphoid (S) in normal position with the lunate (L) displaced anteriorly. Note the distal articular surface of the lunate (arrow). This would normally articulate with the capitate.

scaphoid perilunate dislocation), or fracture of the radial styloid.

8.4.5.4 Other carpal fractures

Avulsion fracture of the triquetral is seen on the lateral view as a small fragment of bone adjacent to the posterior surface. Fracture of the hook of hamate is a common injury in golfers and tennis players. Due to overlapping structures, this fracture is difficult to diagnose on radiographs unless dedicated views are performed. CT or MRI may be required to confirm the diagnosis.

8.4.5.5 Hand fractures

Fractures of the metacarpals and phalanges are common. Fracture through the neck of the fifth metacarpal is the classic 'punching injury'. Fractures of the base of the first metacarpal are usually unstable.

Two types of proximal first metacarpal fracture are seen:

- Transverse fracture of the proximal shaft with lateral bowing
- Oblique fracture extending to the articular surface at the base of the first metacarpal (Fig. 8.33).

Avulsion fracture of the distal extensor tendon insertion at the base of the distal phalanx may result in a flexion deformity of the distal interphalangeal joint (mallet finger) (Fig. 8.34).

8.4.6 Pelvis

8.4.6.1 Pelvic ring fracture

Pelvic ring fractures are most commonly the result of significant trauma, such as motor vehicle and cycling accidents. In general, fractures of the pelvic ring occur in two separate places, although there are exceptions. Isolated fractures of the ischium and pubic rami may occur due to minor falls in elderly patients.

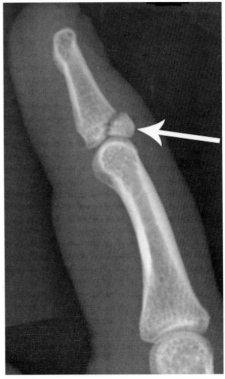

Figure 8.34 Mallet finger. Lateral radiograph shows an avulsion fracture (arrow) at the dorsal base of the distal phalanx at the distal attachment of the extensor tendon. As a result, the distal interphalangeal joint cannot be extended.

Three common patterns of anterior pelvic injury are seen:

- Separation of the pubic symphysis
- Bilateral fractures of the pubic rami
- Unilateral fractures of the pubic rami.

These anterior fractures are often associated with posterior injuries:

- Widening of sacroiliac joint
- Unilateral vertical sacral fracture
- Fracture of iliac bone
- Combinations of the above.

Pelvic ring fractures have a high rate of association with urinary tract injury (see Chapter 4), and with arterial injury causing severe blood loss. Angiography and embolization may be required in such cases. Due to overlapping structures, pelvic ring fractures may be difficult to define accurately with plain films and CT is often indicated (Fig. 8.35).

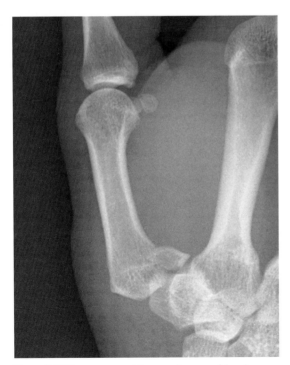

Figure 8.33 First metacarpal fracture. Fracture of the ulnar side of the base of the first metacarpal; fracture involves articular surface.

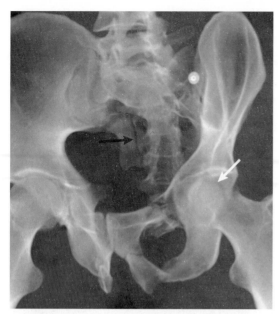

Figure 8.35 Pelvis fractures: CT. Obliquely orientated 3D CT reconstruction demonstrates multiple pelvic fractures including bilateral superior and inferior pubic rami, left acetabulum (white arrow) and right sacrum (black arrow).

8.4.6.2 Avulsion fractures

Multiple large muscles attach to the pelvic bones. Sudden applied stress to the muscle insertion may result in avulsion, i.e. separation of the bony attachment. Commonly avulsed muscle insertion sites include:

- Anterior inferior iliac spine: rectus femoris
- Anterior superior iliac spine: sartorius
- Ischial tuberosity: hamstrings (Fig. 8.7)
- Lesser trochanter: iliopsoas
- Greater trochanter: gluteus medius and minimis.

8.4.6.3 Hip dislocation

Anterior hip joint dislocation is a rare injury easily recognized radiographically and usually not associated with fracture.

Posterior dislocation is the most common form of hip dislocation. Femoral head dislocates posteriorly and superiorly. Posterior dislocation is usually associated with fractures of the posterior acetabulum, and occasionally fractures of the femoral head.

8.4.6.4 Fractures of the acetabulum

Three common acetabular fracture patterns are seen:
- Fracture through the anterior acetabulum associated with fracture of the inferior pubic ramus
- Fracture through the posterior acetabulum extending into the sciatic notch associated with fracture of the inferior pubic ramus
- Horizontal fracture through the acetabulum.

Combinations of the above fracture patterns may be seen, as well as extensive comminution and central dislocation of the femoral head. Acetabular fractures are difficult to define radiographically owing to the complexity of the anatomy and overlapping bony structures (Fig. 8.36). CT is useful for definition of fractures and for planning of operative reduction (Fig. 8.37).

8.4.7 Femur

8.4.7.1 Upper femur ('hip fracture')

Fractures of the upper femur (also known as hip fractures) are particularly common in the elderly and have a strong association with osteoporosis. Fractures are generally classified anatomically as femoral neck, intertrochanteric and subtrochanteric.

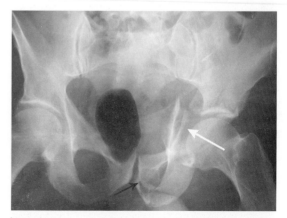

Figure 8.36 Acetabulum fracture. A comminuted fracture of the acetabulum with central impaction of the femoral head (white arrow). Note also a fracture of the pubic bone (black arrow).

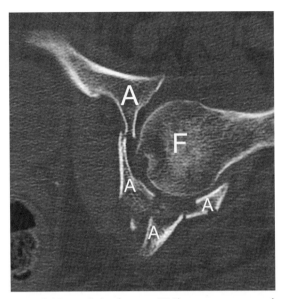

Figure 8.37 Acetabulum fracture: CT. The precise anatomy of an acetabular fracture is demonstrated with CT. Note multiple acetabular fragments (A) and the femoral head (F).

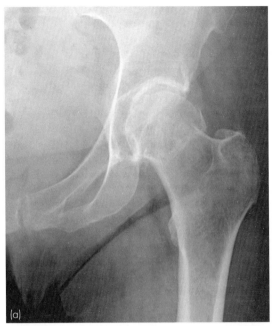

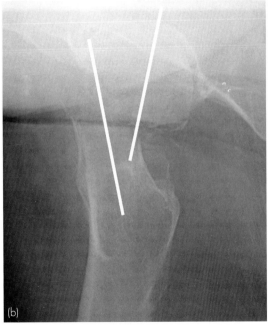

(a)

(b)

Figure 8.38 Subcapital neck of femur fracture. (a) Frontal view underestimates degree of deformity. (b) Lateral view shows considerable angulation and displacement. Lines show axes of femoral neck and head.

Femoral neck fractures are classified according to location:

- Subcapital: junction of femoral neck and head
- Transcervical: middle of femoral neck
- Basilar: junction of femoral neck and intertrochanteric region.

Femoral neck fractures display varying degrees of angulation and displacement. These may be underestimated on a frontal view and a lateral view should be obtained where possible. The lateral view may be difficult to obtain due to pain, and difficult to interpret due to overlapping soft tissue density. Despite these limitations, the lateral view often provides invaluable information in the setting of femoral neck fracture (Fig. 8.38). Undisplaced or mildly impacted femoral neck fracture may be difficult to recognize radiographically. These fractures may be seen as a faint sclerotic band passing across the femoral neck (Fig. 8.39).

Fracture of the femoral neck is complicated by avascular necrosis in 10 per cent of cases, with a higher incidence in severely displaced fractures.

Intertrochanteric fractures involve the greater and lesser trochanters and the bone in between. Intertrochanteric fractures vary in appearance from undisplaced oblique fractures to comminuted fractures with displacement of the lesser and greater trochanters (Fig. 8.40).

Subtrochanteric fractures involve the upper femur below the lesser trochanter (Fig. 8.41).

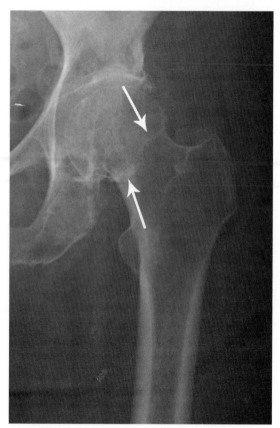

Figure 8.39 Subcapital neck of femur fracture. Undisplaced minimally impacted fracture seen as a sclerotic line (arrows).

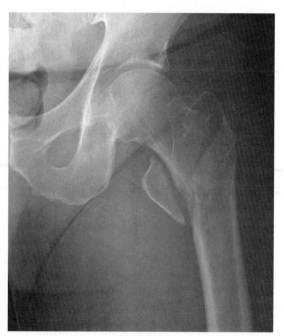

Figure 8.40 Intertrochanteric fracture. Complex intertrochanteric fracture that includes separation of the lesser trochanter.

8.4.7.2 Shaft of the femur

Fractures of the femoral shaft are easily recognized radiographically. Common patterns include transverse, oblique, spiral and comminuted fractures with varying degrees of displacement and angulation. Femoral shaft fractures are often associated with severe blood loss, and occasionally with fat embolism.

8.4.8 Knee

8.4.8.1 Lower femur

Three types of distal femoral fracture are seen:
- Supracondylar fracture of the distal femur usually consists of an anteriorly angulated transverse fracture above the femoral condyles
- Isolated fracture and separation of a femoral condyle

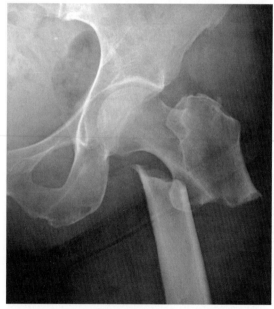

Figure 8.41 Subtrochanteric fracture.

- 'T'- or 'Y'-shaped distal femoral fracture with a vertical fracture line extending upwards from the articular surface causing separation of the femoral condyles.

8.4.8.2 Patella

Three types of patellar fracture are seen:
- Undisplaced simple fracture
- Displaced transverse fracture (Fig. 8.42)
- Complex comminuted fracture.

Fracture of the patella should not be confused with bipartite patella. Bipartite patella is a common anatomical variant with a fragment of bone separated from the superolateral aspect of the patella. Unlike an acute fracture, the bone fragments in bipartite patella are corticated (well-defined margin) and rounded.

8.4.8.3 Tibial plateau

Common patterns of upper tibial injury include:
- Crush fracture of the lateral tibial plateau (Fig. 8.43)

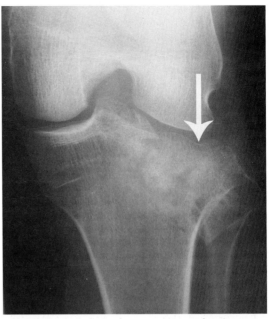

Figure 8.43 Tibial plateau fracture. Note an inferiorly impacted fracture of the lateral tibial plateau (arrow).

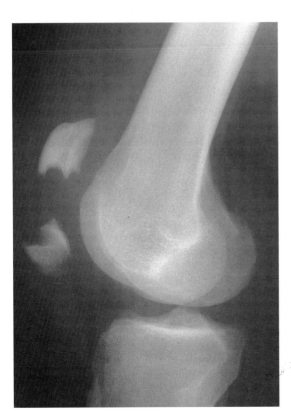

Figure 8.42 Transverse fracture of patella. Bone fragments markedly displaced due to unopposed action of quadriceps muscle.

- Fracture and separation of one or both tibial condyles
- Complex comminuted fracture of the upper tibia.

Minimally crushed or displaced fractures of the upper tibia may be difficult to recognize radiographically. Often the only clue is the presence of a knee joint effusion or lipohaemarthrosis. Knee joint effusion is best recognized on a lateral view. Fluid distension of the suprapatellar recess of the knee joint produces an oval-shaped opacity between the quadriceps tendon and the anterior surface of the distal femur (Fig. 8.44). With lipohaemarthrosis, a fluid-fluid level may be seen in the distended suprapatellar recess due to low-density fat 'floating' on blood in the knee joint (Fig. 8.45). Lipohaemarthrosis is due to release into the knee joint of fatty bone marrow, and is almost always associated with an intra-articular fracture. Oblique views may be required to diagnose subtle fractures. CT is often performed to assist in the planning of surgical management. In particular, 3D CT views are used to assess the degree of comminution and depression of the articular surface.

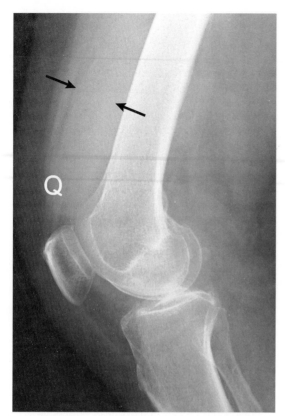

Figure 8.44 Knee joint effusion. Lateral radiograph shows fluid distending the suprapatellar recess of the knee joint (arrows) between the quadriceps tendon (Q) and the femur.

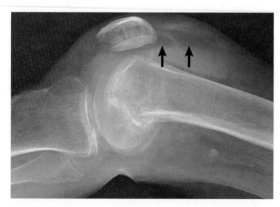

Figure 8.45 Lipohaemarthrosis. Lateral radiograph obtained with the patient supine shows a fluid level (arrows) in the distended suprapatellar recess of the knee joint. Lipohaemarthrosis is virtually always associated with a fracture, in this case an undisplaced supracondylar fracture of the distal femur.

8.4.9 Tibia and fibula

Fracture of the tibial shaft is often associated with fracture of the fibula. Fractures may be transverse, oblique, spiral and comminuted with varying degrees of displacement and angulation. Fractures of the tibia are often open (compound) with an increased incidence of osteomyelitis. Displaced upper tibial fractures may be associated with injury to the popliteal artery and its major branches, requiring emergency angiography and treatment.

Isolated fracture of the tibia is a relatively common injury in children aged one to three (toddler's fracture). These fractures are often undisplaced and therefore very difficult to see. They are usually best seen as a thin oblique lucent line on the lateral radiograph (Fig. 8.46). Scintigraphic bone scan or MRI may be useful in difficult cases.

Isolated fracture of the shaft of the fibula may occur secondary to direct trauma. More commonly, fracture of the upper fibula is associated with disruption of the syndesmosis between the distal tibia and fibula (Maisonneuve fracture).

8.4.10 Ankle and foot

8.4.10.1 Common ankle fractures

Ankle injuries may include fractures of the distal fibula (lateral malleolus), medial distal tibia (medial malleolus) and posterior distal tibia; talar shift and displacement; fracture of the talus; separation of the distal tibiofibular joint (syndesmosis injury); ligament rupture with joint instability. Salter–Harris fractures of the distal tibia and fibula are common in children.

The types of fracture seen radiographically depend on mechanism of injury:

- Adduction (inversion): vertical fracture of the medial malleolus, avulsion of the tip of the lateral malleolus, medial tilt of the talus
- Abduction (eversion): fracture of the lateral malleolus, avulsion of the tip of the medial malleolus, separation of the distal tibiofibular joint
- External rotation: spiral or oblique fracture of the lateral malleolus, lateral shift of the talus (Fig. 8.47)
- Vertical compression: fracture of the distal tibia posteriorly or anteriorly, separation of the distal tibiofibular joint.

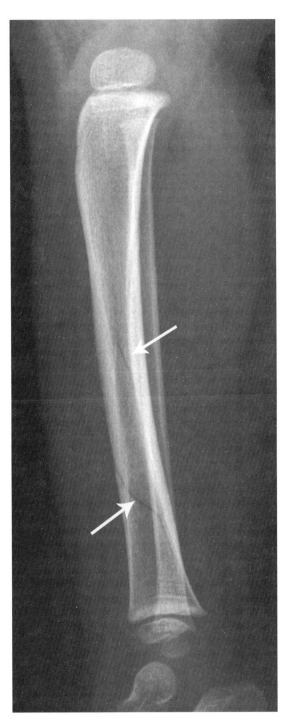

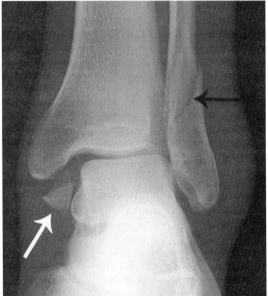

Figure 8.47 Ankle fracture due to external rotation. Note spiral fracture of distal fibula (black arrow), avulsion of medial malleolus (white arrow), lateral shift of talus, widening of the space between distal tibia and fibula indicating syndesmosis injury.

8.4.10.2 Fractures of the talus

Small avulsion fractures of the talus are commonly seen in association with ankle fractures and ligament damage.

Osteochondral fracture of the upper articular surface of the talus (talar dome) is a common cause of persistent pain following an inversion ankle injury. Osteochondral fractures of the medial talar dome tend to be rounded defects in the cortical surface, often with loose bone fragments requiring surgical fixation. Osteochondral fractures of the lateral talar dome are usually small bone flakes. Osteochondral fractures may be difficult to see on radiographs and often require CT or MRI for diagnosis (Fig. 8.48).

Fracture of the neck of the talus may be widely displaced, associated with disruption of the subtalar joint, and complicated by avascular necrosis.

8.4.10.3 Fractures of the calcaneus

Fractures of the calcaneus may show considerable displacement and comminution, and may involve the subtalar joint. Boehler's angle is the angle formed by a line tangential to the superior extra-articular

Figure 8.46 Toddler's fracture. Undisplaced spiral fracture of the tibia (arrows).

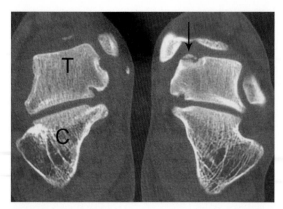

Figure 8.48 Osteochondral fracture talus: coronal CT of both ankles. Note the normal appearance of right talus (T) and calcaneus (C). A defect in the cortical surface of the left talar dome is associated with a loose bone fragment (arrow).

portion of the calcaneus and a line tangential to the superior intra-articular portion. Boehler's angle normally measures 25–40°. Reduction of Boehler's angle in a setting of trauma is a useful sign of a displaced intra-articular fracture of the calcaneus; these fractures may otherwise be difficult to see on radiographs (Fig. 8.49).

CT is useful for the assessment of calcaneal fractures and to assist in planning of surgical reduction. Calcaneal fractures, particularly when bilateral, have a high association with spine and pelvis fractures.

8.4.10.4 Other fractures of the foot

Any of the tarsal bones may be fractured. With major trauma, dislocation of intertarsal or tarsometatarsal joints may occur. Lisfranc fracture/dislocation refers to disruption of the Lisfranc ligament, with midfoot instability. Lisfranc ligament joins the distal lateral surface of the medial cuneiform to the base of the second metatarsal, and is a major stabilizer of the midfoot. Radiographic signs of Lisfranc ligament disruption may be difficult to appreciate, and include widening of the space between the bases of the first and second metatarsals and associated fractures of metatarsals, cuneiforms and other tarsal bones (Fig. 8.50). CT or MRI may be required to confirm the diagnosis.

Metatarsal fractures are usually transverse. The growth centre at the base of the fifth metatarsal lies parallel to the shaft and should not be mistaken for a fracture; fractures in this region usually lie in the transverse plane (Fig. 8.51).

Stress fractures of the foot are common, particularly involving the metatarsal shafts, and less commonly the navicula and talus.

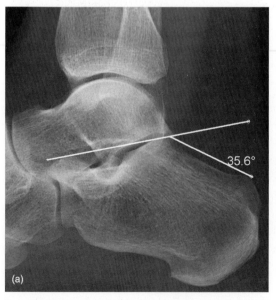

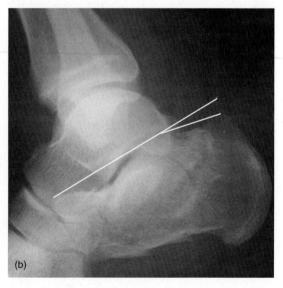

Figure 8.49 Calcaneus fracture. (a) Note the method of drawing Boehler's angle. (b) In this example, there is reduction of Boehler's angle associated with multiple fractures of the calcaneus.

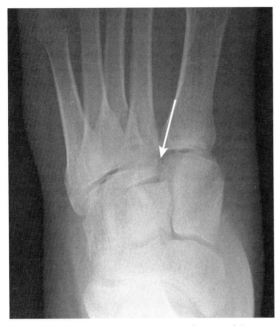

Figure 8.50 Lisfranc ligament tear. Severe foot pain following major trauma. No obvious fracture on initial inspection of radiographs. Note widening of gap between base of second metatarsal and medial cuneiform (arrow) and malalignment of second tarsometatarsal joint. These signs indicate a tear of the Lisfranc ligament.

8.5 INTERNAL JOINT DERANGEMENT: METHODS OF INVESTIGATION

Internal joint derangements refer to disruption of supporting structures such as ligaments and articular cartilages, and fibrocartilage structures such as the menisci of the knee and the hip and shoulder labra. Causes of internal joint derangements are:
- Trauma including sporting injuries
- Overuse syndromes as may occur in occupational or athletic settings
- Secondary to degenerative or inflammatory arthropathies.

8.5.1 Wrist

The wrist is an anatomically complex area with several important ligaments and cartilages supporting the carpal bones. Persistent wrist pain following trauma or post-traumatic carpal instability may be due to ligament or cartilage tears. The two most commonly injured internal wrist structures are the scapholunate ligament and the triangular fibrocartilage complex (TFCC):

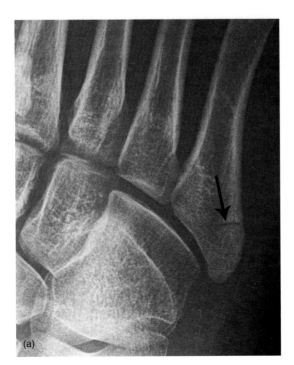

(a)

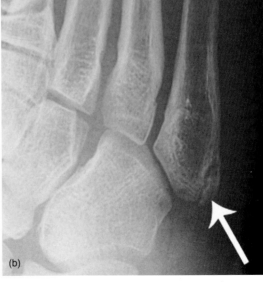

(b)

Figure 8.51 Fifth metatarsal fracture. (a) Transverse fracture of the base of the fifth metatarsal (arrow). (b) Normal growth centre at the base of the fifth metatarsal (arrow). This is aligned parallel to the long axis of the bone and should not be confused with a fracture.

- Scapholunate ligament: strong 'C'-shaped ligament that stabilizes the joint between scaphoid and lunate
- TFCC: fibrocartilage disc and adjacent ligaments joining distal radius to base of ulnar styloid; major stabilizer of ulnar side of wrist joint.

Radiographs of the wrist including stress views may be useful to confirm carpal instability, in particular widening of the space between the scaphoid and lunate with disruption of the scapholunate ligament. MRI is the investigation of choice to confirm tears of internal wrist structures (Fig. 8.52).

8.5.2 Shoulder

8.5.2.1 Rotator cuff disease

Two types of rotator cuff disorder are common causes of shoulder pain:
- Calcific tendonosis
- Degenerative tendonosis and rotator cuff tear.

Calcific tendonosis due to hydroxyapatite crystal deposition is particularly common in the supraspinatus tendon, and occurs in young to middle-aged adults. Calcific tendonosis usually presents with acute shoulder pain accentuated by abduction.

Tears of the rotator cuff most commonly involve the supraspinatus tendon, and are usually caused by tendon degeneration ('wear and tear') seen in elderly patients. Clinical presentation is with persistent shoulder pain worsened by abduction. The pain is often worse at night, with interruption of sleep a common complaint.

For suspected rotator cuff disease, radiographs of the shoulder are used to diagnose calcific tendonosis (Fig. 8.53) and to exclude underlying bony pathology as a cause of shoulder pain. US is the investigation of choice for suspected rotator cuff tear (Fig. 8.54). MRI is used as a problem-solving tool for difficult or equivocal cases.

8.5.2.2 Glenohumeral joint instability (recurrent dislocation)

Dislocation of the glenohumeral (shoulder) joint is a common occurrence and in most cases recovery is swift and uncomplicated. In a small percentage of cases, tearing of stabilizing structures, such as the labrum and glenohumeral ligaments, may cause glenohumeral instability and recurrent dislocation. MRI is the investigation of choice for assessment of glenohumeral instability. The accuracy of MRI may be enhanced by the intra-articular injection of a dilute

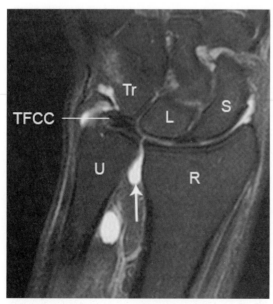

Figure 8.52 Triangular cartilage complex tear: MRI of the wrist, coronal plane. Fluid is seen passing into the distal radio-ulnar joint (arrow) through a perforation of the radial insertion of the triangular fibrocartilage complex (TFCC). Note also triquetral (Tr), lunate (L), scaphoid (S), ulna (U), radius (R).

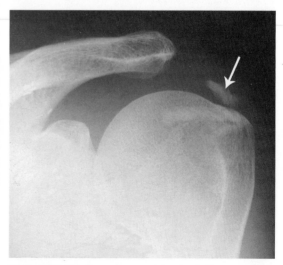

Figure 8.53 Calcific tendonosis. A focal calcification is seen above the humeral head (arrow) in the supraspinatus tendon.

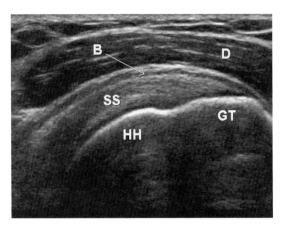

Figure 8.54 Normal rotator cuff: US. A US scan of the shoulder in an oblique coronal plane shows the following: deltoid muscle (D), subdeltoid bursa (B), supraspinatus tendon (SS), humeral head (HH) and greater tuberosity (GT).

solution of gadolinium (MR arthrogram); this is done under fluoroscopic or US guidance (Fig. 8.55).

8.5.3 Hip

Hip pain is a common problem and may occur at any age. (Hip problems in children are discussed in Chapter 13.) In young active adults, a tear of the fibrocartilagenous labrum may present with hip pain plus an audible 'clicking'. MR arthrogram is the investigation of choice for suspected labral tear. In elderly patients, osteoarthritis is a common cause of hip pain. Radiographs are usually sufficient for the diagnosis of osteoarthritis of the hip. Less commonly, hip pain may be due to bone disorders such as avascular necrosis (AVN), and a history of risk factors such as steroid use may be relevant. MRI is the investigation of choice for suspected AVN.

8.5.4 Knee

Radiographs are performed for the assessment of most causes of knee pain. MRI is the investigation of choice in the assessment of most internal knee derangements, including meniscus injury (Fig. 8.56), cruciate ligament tear, collateral ligament tear, osteochondritis dissecans, etc. MSUS is useful in the assessment of periarticular pathology such as popliteal cysts and patellar tendonopathy. MSUS is not able to reliably diagnose other internal derangements.

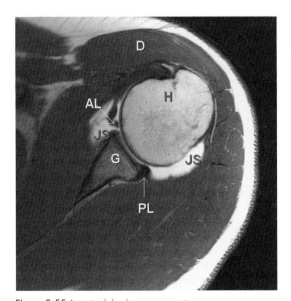

Figure 8.55 Anterior labral tear: magnetic resonance arthrogram of the shoulder, transverse plane. Note the following: deltoid muscle (D), humerus (H), glenoid (G), posterior labrum (PL), joint space distended with dilute gadolinium (JS) and anterior labrum (AL). Joint fluid is seen between the base of the anterior labrum and the glenoid indicating an anterior labral tear.

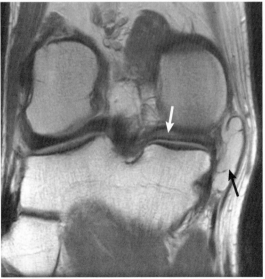

Figure 8.56 Meniscus tear: coronal proton density MRI of the knee. A horizontal tear of the medial meniscus, seen as a high signal line (white arrow), is associated with formation of a meniscal cyst (black arrow).

8.5.5 Ankle

Persistent ankle pain post-trauma may be due to delayed healing of ligament tears or osteochondral fracture of the articular surface of the talus. MRI is the investigation of choice in the assessment of persistent post-traumatic ankle pain. Tendonopathy and tendon tears are common around the ankle joint. The most commonly involved tendons are the Achilles tendon, tibialis posterior, and peroneus longus and brevis. These tendons are well assessed with US and MRI.

8.6 APPROACH TO ARTHROPATHIES

In the diagnosis of arthropathies, it is probably most useful to decide first whether there is involvement of a single joint (monoarthropathy), or multiple joints (polyarthropathy). This is fine as long as one remembers that a polyarthropathy may present early with a single painful joint.

Polyarthropathies may be divided into three large categories:

- Inflammatory
- Degenerative
- Metabolic.

Various clinical features and biochemical tests may be used for further assessment of arthropathies. Biochemical tests may include:

- Erythrocyte sedimentation rate (ESR); C-reactive protein (CRP)
- Rheumatoid factor
- Antinuclear antibody
- Uric acid
- HLA-B27.

Radiographs are usually sufficient for the imaging assessment of suspected arthropathy. Certain radiographic features of affected joints may assist in diagnosis:

- Distribution
  - Symmetrical or asymmetrical
  - Small joints or large weight-bearing joints
- Erosions
- Joint space narrowing
- Osteophytes.

Occasionally, MRI may be useful to detect early signs of joint inflammation where radiographs are normal or equivocal. MRI is able to detect synovial inflammation, as well as bone changes such as marrow oedema and small erosions.

Outlined below is a summary of radiographic manifestations of the more commonly encountered arthropathies.

8.6.1 Monoarthropathy

A common cause for a single painful joint is trauma. In most cases, diagnosis is obvious from the clinical history, and radiographs are usually sufficient for diagnosis. In cases of septic arthritis, the affected joint may be radiographically normal at the time of initial presentation. After a few days, radiographic signs such as periarticular bone erosions and destruction may occur. MRI or scintigraphy with ^{99}mTc-MDP are usually positive at the time of presentation.

The other major category of monoarthropathy is polyarthropathy presenting initially in a single joint, e.g. osteoarthritis, gout and rheumatoid arthritis.

8.6.2 Inflammatory polyarthropathy

Inflammatory arthropathies present with painful joints and associated soft tissue swelling. Inflammatory joint pain is usually non-mechanical in nature, i.e. not related to movement and not relieved by rest. Pain is often worse on waking, and 'morning stiffness' is a common complaint. Inflammatory polyarthropathies are classified into seropositive and seronegative arthropathies. The term 'seropositive' means that rheumatoid factor (RhF) is present in the blood. RhF is an autoantibody against the Fc portion of immunoglobulin G (IgG). It is present in the blood of most, though not all, patients with rheumatoid arthritis (RA) and other seropositive arthropathies associated with connective tissue disorders.

8.6.2.1 Rheumatoid arthritis

The fundamental pathological process in RA is inflammation of synovium. Synovial inflammation leads to joint swelling and formation of synovial inflammatory masses (pannus). Pannus may cause bone erosions and lead to joint deformity. RA is usually symmetrical in distribution, and affects predominantly the small joints, especially metacarpophalangeal, metatarsophalangeal, carpal, and proximal interphalangeal joints. Spinal involvement is rare, apart from erosion of the odontoid peg.

Radiographic signs of RA (Fig. 8.57):

- Soft tissue swelling overlying joints
- Bone erosions occur in the feet and hands, best demonstrated in the metatarsal and metacarpal heads, articular surfaces of phalanges and carpal bones
- Reduced bone density adjacent to joints (periarticular osteoporosis)
- Abnormalities of joint alignment with subluxation of metacarpophalangeal joints causing ulnar deviation of fingers, and subluxation of metatarsophalangeal joints producing lateral deviation of toes.

8.6.2.2 Other connective tissue (seropositive) arthropathies

Other ('non-RA') seropositive arthropathies include SLE, systemic sclerosis, CREST, mixed connective tissue disease, polymyositis and dermatomyositis. These arthropathies tend to present with symmetrical arthropathy involving the peripheral small joints, especially the metacarpophalangeal and proximal interphalangeal joints. Radiographic signs of non-RA seropositive arthropathies may be subtle and include:

- Soft tissue swelling
- Periarticular osteoporosis
- Soft tissue calcification is common, especially around joints
- Bone erosions are less common than with RA
- Resorption of distal phalanges and joint contractures are prominent features of systemic sclerosis.

8.6.2.3 Seronegative spondyloarthropathy

The seronegative spondyloarthropathies (SpA) are asymmetrical polyarthropathies, usually involving only a few joints. SpAs have a predilection for the spine and sacroiliac joints. Five subtypes of SpA are described with shared clinical features including association with HLA-B27:

- Ankylosing spondylitis
- Reactive arthritis
- Arthritis spondylitis with inflammatory bowel disease
- Arthritis spondylitis with psoriasis
- Undifferentiated spondyloarthropathy (uSpA).

Clinical features of SpA may include inflammatory back pain, positive family history, acute anterior uveitis, and inflammation at tendon and ligament insertions (enthesitis).

Enthesitis most commonly involves the distal Achilles tendon insertion and the insertion of the plantar fascia on the undersurface of the calcaneus. Features of inflammatory back pain include insidious onset, morning stiffness and improvement with exercise. Ankylosing spondylitis is the most common SpA.

Radiographic findings of ankylosing spondylitis (Fig. 8.58) are:

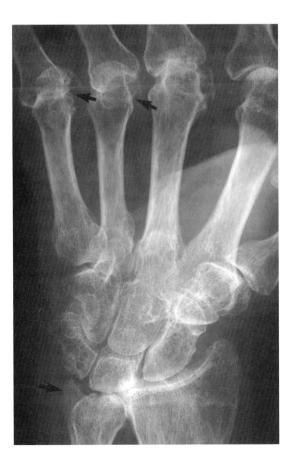

Figure 8.57 Rheumatoid arthritis of the hand and wrist. Bone erosions are seen involving the metacarpals and the ulnar styloid process (arrows).

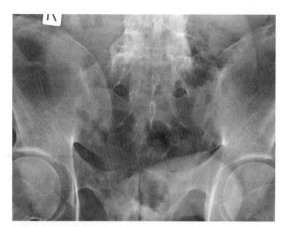

Figure 8.58 Ankylosing spondylitis. Frontal view of the pelvis showing fused sacroiliac joints.

- Vertically orientated bony spurs arising from vertebral bodies (syndesmophytes)
- Fusion or ankylosis of the spine giving the 'bamboo spine' appearance
- Sacroiliac joint changes including erosions producing an irregular joint margin
- Sclerosis and fusion of sacroiliac joints later in the disease process.

Psoriatic arthropathy is an asymmetrical arthropathy, predominantly affecting the small joints of the hands and feet. Radiographic changes of psoriatic arthropathy include periarticular erosions and periosteal new bone formation in peripheral joints.

8.6.3 Degenerative arthropathy: osteoarthritis

Primary osteoarthritis (OA) refers to degenerative arthropathy with no apparent underlying or predisposing cause. Primary OA is an asymmetric process involving the large weight-bearing joints, hips and knees, lumbar and cervical spine (see Chapter 13), distal interphalangeal, first carpometacarpal and lateral carpal joints. Secondary OA refers to degenerative change complicating underlying arthropathy, such as RA, trauma or Paget's disease. The fundamental pathological process in OA is loss of articular cartilage. Loss of articular cartilage results in joint space narrowing and abnormal stresses on joint margins; these abnormal stresses lead to the formation of bony spurs (osteophytes) at the joint margins.

Radiographic changes of OA (Fig. 8.59) are:
- Joint space narrowing
- Osteophytes
- Sclerosis of joint surfaces
- Periarticular cyst formation
- Loose bodies in joints due to detached osteophytes and ossified cartilage debris.

8.6.4 Metabolic arthropathies

8.6.4.1 Gout

Gout is caused by uric acid crystal deposition in soft tissues and articular structures. Acute gout refers to soft tissue swelling, with no visible bony changes. Chronic gouty arthropathy occurs with recurrent acute gout. Gouty arthropathy is usually asymmetric in distribution and often monoarticular. Gouty arthropathy involves the first metatarsophalangeal joint in 70 per cent of cases. Other commonly affected joints include ankles, knees and intertarsal joints.

Radiographic features of gouty arthropathy (Fig. 8.60) are:
- Bone erosions: usually set back from the joint surface (para-articular)
- Calcification of articular cartilages, especially the menisci of the knee
- Tophus: soft tissue mass in the synovium of joints, the subcutaneous tissues of the lower leg, Achilles tendon, olecranon bursa at the elbow, helix of the ear
- Calcification of tophi is an uncommon feature.

8.6.4.2 Calcium pyrophosphate deposition disease

Also known as pseudogout, calcium pyrophosphate deposition disease (CPPD) may occur in young adults as an autosomal dominant condition, or sporadically in older patients. CPPD presents clinically with intermittent acute joint pain and swelling. CPPD may affect any joint, most commonly knee, hip, shoulder, elbow, wrist and ankle. Radiographic signs of CPPD include calcification of intra-articular cartilages, especially the menisci of the knee and the triangular fibrocartilage complex of the wrist (Fig. 8.61). Secondary OA may occur with subchondral cysts and joint space narrowing.

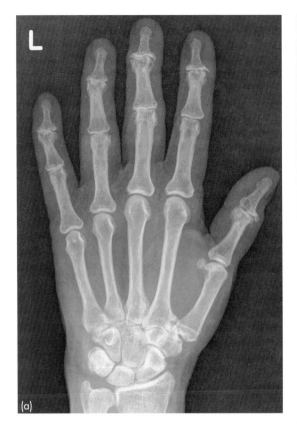

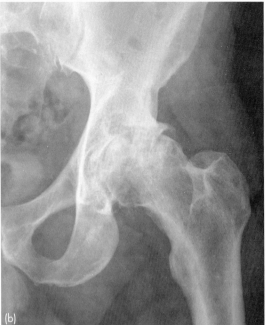

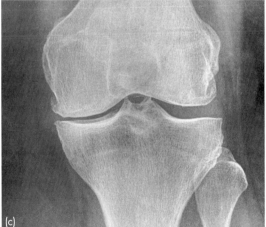

Figure 8.59 Osteoarthritis. (a) Hands: joint space narrowing, articular surface irregularity and osteophyte formation involving interphalangeal joints. (b) Hip: joint narrowing, most marked superiorly; articular surface sclerosis and irregularity; lucencies in acetabulum and femoral head due to subcortical cyst formation. (c) Knee: narrowing of the medial joint compartment due to thinning of articular cartilage.

8.6.4.3 Calcium hydroxyapatite crystal deposition disease

Calcium hydroxyapatite crystal deposition usually manifests with calcific tendonosis of the supraspinatus tendon (Fig. 8.53). Clinical presentation consists of severe shoulder pain and limitation of movement in patients aged 40–70. Virtually any other tendon in the body may be affected, although much less commonly than supraspinatus. The classical radiographic sign of calcium hydroxyapatite deposition is calcification in the supraspinatus tendon. In acute cases, the calcification may be semiliquid and difficult to see radiographically. Calcific tendonosis may also be diagnosed with US. US-guided aspiration of calcification and steroid injection may be curative.

8.7 APPROACH TO PRIMARY BONE TUMOURS

Primary bone tumours are relatively rare, representing less than 1 per cent of all malignancies.

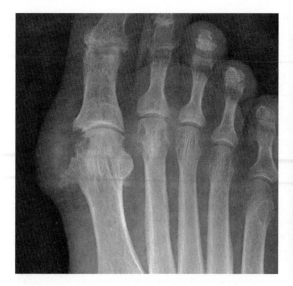

Figure 8.60 Chronic gouty arthropathy of first metatarsophalangeal joint. Bone erosions adjacent to, but not directly involving articular surfaces (juxta-articular). Faint calcification in overlying soft tissue swelling.

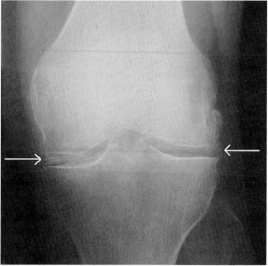

Figure 8.61 Chondrocalcinosis of the knee. Calcification of the lateral and medial menisci of the knee (arrows) due to calcium pyrophosphate deposition.

Imaging, particularly radiographic assessment, is vital to the diagnosis and delineation of bone tumours and a basic approach is outlined here, along with a summary of the roles of the various modalities. Remember that in adult patients, a solitary bone lesion is more likely to be a metastasis than a primary bone tumour.

Remember also that in children and adults, several conditions may mimic bone tumour (Table 8.1) including:
- Benign fibroma (fibrous cortical defect)
- Simple (unicameral) bone cyst
- Osteomyelitis
- Fibrous dysplasia
- Langerhans cell histiocytosis.

Clinical history may be extremely helpful:
- Age of the patient
- Location.

On examination of the radiograph, a number of parameters are assessed:
- Location of tumour within the bone, for example
  - Diaphysis: Ewing sarcoma
  - Metaphysis: osteogenic sarcoma
  - Epiphysis: chondroblastoma and giant cell tumour

- Matrix of lesion, i.e. appearance of material within the tumour
  - Lytic, i.e. lucent or dark
  - Sclerotic, i.e. dense or white
- Zone of transition, i.e. the margin between the lesion and normal bone
  - Thin, sclerotic rim: more likely benign
  - Wide and irregular: more likely malignant
- Effect on surrounding bone
  - Expansion and thinning of cortex: more likely benign
  - Penetration of cortex: more likely malignant
  - Periosteal reaction and new bone formation: osteogenic sarcoma, Ewing sarcoma
- Associated features
  - Soft tissue mass
  - Pathological fracture.

Most diagnostic information as to tumour type comes from clinical assessment and radiographic appearances (Fig. 8.62). Other imaging modalities add further, often complementary information on staging and complications. MRI is used to assess tumour extent within the marrow cavity of the bone and associated soft tissue mass (Fig. 8.63). CT is more sensitive than MRI in the detection of calcification; it may be used in specific instances

Table 8.1 Features of common bone tumours and 'mimics'.

Diagnosis	Age	Site	Matrix	Margin	Effect on bone
Simple bone cyst	5–15	Proximal metaphysis femur and humerus	Lucent	Thin, sclerotic	Mild expansion, thin cortex
Fibroma	10–20	Femur and tibia	Lucent	Thin, sclerotic	Mild expansion of cortex
Osteoid osteoma	10–30	Femur, tibia	Lucent nidus	Thick, sclerotic	Mild eccentric expansion
Osteosarcoma	10–25	Metaphysis femur, tibia, humerus	Lytic or mixed lytic and sclerotic	Wide	Eccentric expansion, cortical destruction, spiculated periosteal new bone
Enchondroma	10–50	Hands; metaphysis humerus and femur	Lytic with focal calcifications	Thin, sclerotic	Mild expansion, thin cortex
Chondrosarcoma	30–60	Pelvis and shoulder; metaphysis humerus and femur	Lytic with focal calcifications	Irregular, sclerotic	Expansion and cortical destruction
Giant cell tumour	20–40	Subarticular ends of long bones	Lucent	Thin, ill-defined	Eccentric expansion, thin or destroyed cortex
Ewing sarcoma	5–15	Diaphysis of femur; pelvis	Lytic	Wide	Layered or spiculated periosteal new bone

where accurate characterization of the tumour matrix may be diagnostic, such as suspected cartilage tumour. Scintigraphy with ^{99m}Tc-MDP (bone scan) may be used to assess the activity of the primary bone lesion and to detect multiple lesions. In modern practice, bone tumours are commonly treated with chemotherapy or radiotherapy prior to surgery. MRI and/or PET/CT may be used to assess response to therapy.

8.8 MISCELLANEOUS COMMON BONE CONDITIONS

8.8.1 Skeletal metastases

Almost any primary tumour may metastasize to bone. The most common primary sites associated with skeletal metastases are:

- Breast
- Prostate
- Kidney
- Lung
- Gastrointestinal tract
- Thyroid
- Melanoma.

Bone metastases are often clinically occult, or they may present with bone pain, pathological fracture or hypercalcaemia. Radiographically, skeletal metastases are most commonly lytic, with focal lesions of bone destruction seen (Fig. 8.62c). Sclerotic metastases occur with prostate, stomach and carcinoid tumour.

Skeletal metastases most commonly involve spine, pelvis, ribs, proximal femur and proximal humerus, and are uncommon distal to the knee and elbow.

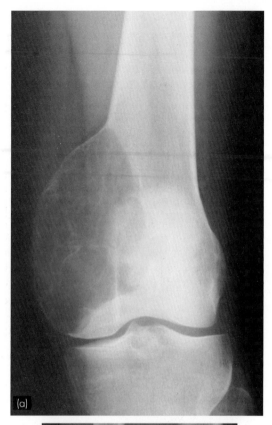

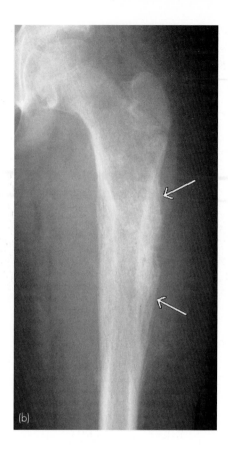

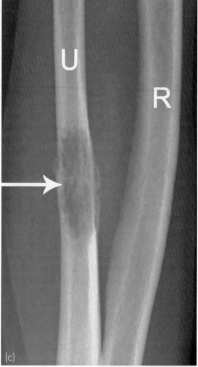

Figure 8.62 Bone tumours; three examples. (a) Giant cell tumour of the distal femur seen as an eccentric lytic expanded lesion with a well-defined margin. (b) Osteosarcoma of the upper femur. Note irregular cortical thickening with new bone formation beneath elevated periosteum (arrows). (c) Metastasis (from non-small cell carcinoma of the lung) in the ulna (arrow) seen as a lytic lesion with irregular margins.

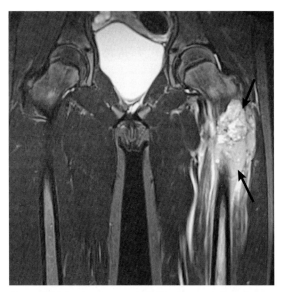

Figure 8.63 Ewing sarcoma: MRI. Thigh pain and swelling in a 13-year-old female. Coronal STIR images of the thighs and pelvis show a lesion with a large soft tissue component (arrows) arising from the left femur.

Scintigraphy with ^{99}mTc-MDP (bone scan) is used in staging those tumours that are known to metastasize commonly to bone, e.g. prostate or breast. Skeletal metastases usually show on bone scan as multiple areas of increased tracer uptake (Fig. 8.64).

8.8.2 Multiple myeloma

Multiple myeloma is a common malignancy of plasma cells characterized by diffuse bone marrow infiltration or multiple nodules in bone. It occurs in elderly patients, and is rare below the age of 40. Multiple myeloma may present clinically in a number of non-specific ways including bone pain, anaemia, hypercalcaemia or renal failure. Unlike most other bone malignancies, bone scintigraphy is relatively insensitive in the detection of multiple myeloma. Radiography is therefore the investigation of choice in the detection and staging of multiple myeloma. Alternatively, whole-body MRI may be used. MRI

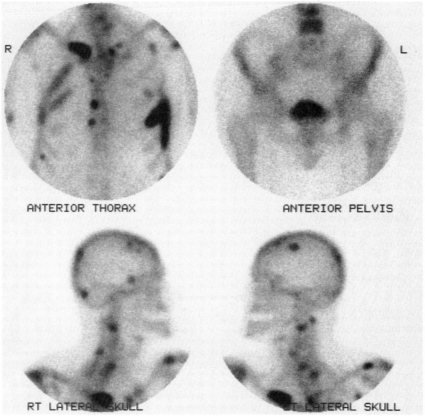

ANTERIOR THORAX

ANTERIOR PELVIS

RT LATERAL SKULL

LT LATERAL SKULL

Figure 8.64 Skeletal metastases, seen on scintigraphy as multiple areas of increased activity.

has equal sensitivity to radiography in the detection of multiple myeloma. Common sites of involvement include spine, ribs, skull (Fig. 8.65), pelvis and long bones. Several different radiographic patterns may be seen with multiple myeloma including:

- Generalized severe osteoporosis
- Multiple lytic, punched-out defects
- Multiple destructive and expansile lesions.

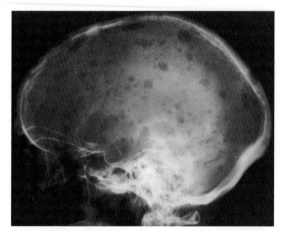

Figure 8.65 Multiple myeloma. Note the presence of multiple lucent 'punched-out' defects throughout the skull.

8.8.3 Paget's disease

Paget's disease is a common bone disorder, occurring in elderly patients, and characterized by increased bone resorption followed by new bone formation. The new bone thus formed has thick trabeculae, and is softer and more vascular than normal bone. Common sites include the pelvis and upper femur, spine, skull, upper tibia and proximal humerus. Paget's disease is often asymptomatic and seen as an incidental finding on radiographs performed for other reasons. Clinical presentation may otherwise be quite variable and falls into three broad categories:

- General symptoms: pain and fatigue
- Symptoms related to specific sites
  - Cranial nerve pressure; blindness, deafness
  - Increased hat size
  - Local hyperthermia of overlying skin
- Complications
  - Pathological fracture

- Secondary osteoarthritis
- Sarcoma formation (rare).

Radiographic changes of Paget's disease are variable depending on the phase of the disease process:

- Early active phase of bone resorption
  - Well-defined reduction in density of the anterior skull: osteoporosis circumscripta
  - V-shaped lytic defect in long bones extending into the shaft of the bone from the subarticular region
- Later phase of sclerosis and cortical thickening, or mixed lytic and sclerotic change
  - Thick cortex and coarse trabeculae with enlarged bone (Fig. 8.66)
  - Bowing of long bones.

8.8.4 Fibrous dysplasia

Fibrous dysplasia is a common condition characterized by single or multiple benign bone lesions composed of islands of osteoid and woven

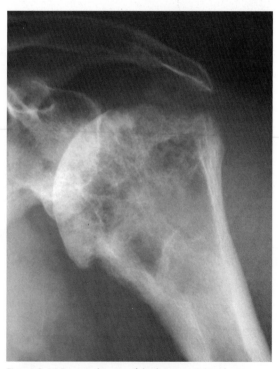

Figure 8.66 Paget's disease of the humerus. Note the coarse trabecular pattern in the humeral head and thickening of the bony cortex.

bone in a fibrous stroma. Fibrous dysplasia may occur up to the age of 70, although peak age of incidence is from age 10 to 30. It most commonly involves the lower extremity or skull and presents with local swelling, pain or pathological fracture. Bone lesions are solitary in 75 per cent of cases.

Radiographic features of fibrous dysplasia (Fig. 8.67) are:

- Expansile lytic lesion
- Cortical thinning
- Areas of homogeneous grey hazy density, usually described as 'ground glass'; a characteristic radiographic feature that differentiates fibrous dysplasia from other pathologies.

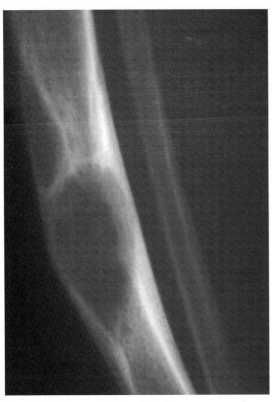

Figure 8.67 Fibrous dysplasia of the tibia seen as a well-defined lucent lesion expanding the midshaft of the tibia.

CT in fibrous dysplasia shows an expansile lesion with ground glass density, based in the medullary cavity of the affected bone.

Associated syndromes are:

- McCune–Albright syndrome: polyostotic fibrous dysplasia, patchy cutaneous pigmentation and sexual precocity
- Leontiasis ossea ('lion's face'): asymmetric sclerosis and thickening of skull and facial bones.

Cherubism, a rare condition characterized clinically by symmetrical swelling of the face, is often described incorrectly as a form of fibrous dysplasia. Cherubism is an autosomal disorder presenting in early childhood. Facial swelling increases to puberty followed by spontaneous regression. Imaging with radiography and CT shows symmetrical expansion of mandible and maxilla with multiloculated osteolytic lesions.

8.8.5 Osteochondritis dissecans

Osteochondritis dissecans is a traumatic bone lesion that affects males more than females, most commonly in the 10–20 year age group. The knee is most commonly affected; other less common sites include the dome of the talus and the capitulum. In the knee, the lateral aspect of the medial femoral condyle is involved in 75–80 per cent of cases, with the lateral femoral condyle in 15–20 per cent and the patella in 5 per cent. Trauma is thought to be the underlying cause in most cases. Subchondral bone is first affected, then overlying articular cartilage. Subsequent revascularization and healing occur, although a necrotic bone fragment may persist. This bone fragment may become separated and displaced as a loose body in the joint.

Radiographs show a lucent defect on the cortical surface of the femoral condyle, often with a separate bone fragment (Fig. 8.68). MRI is the investigation of choice to further define the bone and cartilage abnormality. MRI helps to establish prognosis, guide management, and confirm healing.

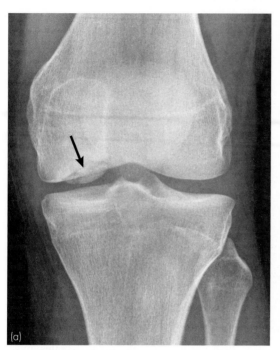
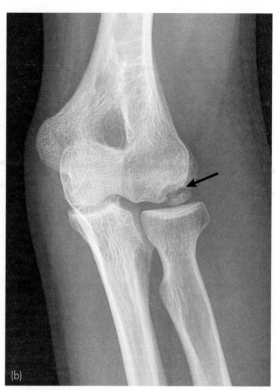

Figure 8.68 Osteochondritis dissecans: concave defect in the articular surface with a loose bone fragment. (a) Knee: medial femoral condyle (arrow). (b) Elbow: capitulum (arrow).

SUMMARY BOX

Clinical presentation	Investigation of choice	Comment
Trauma: suspected fracture or dislocation	Radiography	CT in selected cases for further definition of anatomy MRI in selected cases for detection of subtle fractures not shown on radiographs, e.g. scaphoid
Arthropathy/painful joint(s)	Radiography	MRI in selected cases to detect synovial or bony inflammation
Primary bone tumour	Radiography	Bone scintigraphy, CT, MRI for further characterization and staging
Skeletal metastases	Bone scintigraphy	
Multiple myeloma	Radiography (skeletal survey)	Increasing role for whole body MRI
Paget's disease	Radiography	
Fibrous dysplasia	Radiography	CT for complex areas, e.g. craniofacial
Osteochondritis dissecans	Radiography MRI	

9.1 RADIOGRAPHIC ANATOMY OF THE SPINE

Anatomical features of each vertebral body that can be identified radiographically (Figs 9.1, 9.2 and 9.3) include:
- Anterior vertebral body
- Posterior arch formed by pedicles and lamina, enclosing the spinal canal
- Pedicles: posterior bony projections from the posterolateral corners of the vertebral body
- Laminae curve posteromedially from the pedicles and join in the midline at the base of the spinous process to complete the bony arch of the spinal canal
- Spinous process projects posteriorly
- Transverse processes project laterally from the junction of pedicle and lamina.

Articulations between adjoining vertebrae include intervertebral disc, zygapophyseal joints and uncovertebral joints.
- Intervertebral disc
  - Occupies the space between each vertebral body
  - Composed of central nucleus pulposus enclosed by annulus fibrosis

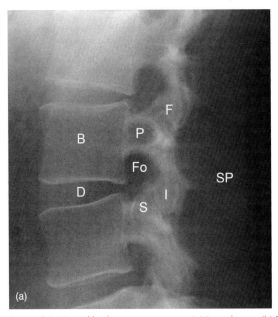

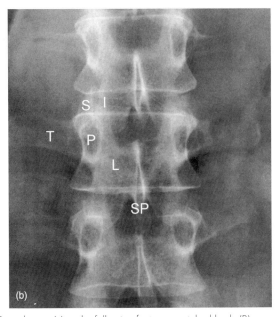

Figure 9.1 Normal lumbar spine anatomy. (a) Lateral view. (b) Frontal view. Note the following features: vertebral body (B), intervertebral disc (D), pedicle (P), facet joint (F), intervertebral foramen (Fo), inferior articular process (I), superior articular process (S), transverse process (T), lamina (L), spinous process (SP).

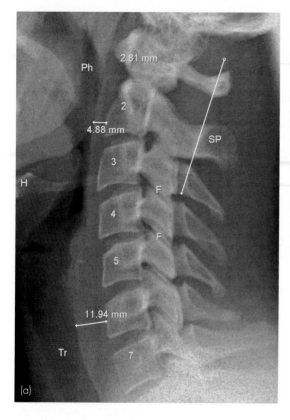

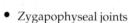

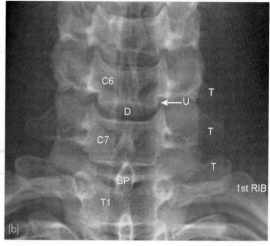

Figure 9.2 Normal cervical spine anatomy. (a) Lateral view. Note the following: facet joint (F), spinous process (SP), pharynx (Ph), hyoid bone (H), trachea (Tr) and posterior cervical line from C1 to C3. Note also measurements of predental space (between anterior arch of C1 and the odontoid peg), retropharyngeal space at C2 and retrotracheal space at C6. (b) Frontal view of lower cervical spine. Note the following: intervertebral disc (D), uncovertebral joint (U), transverse process (T), spinous process (SP).

- Zygapophyseal joints
  - Commonly known as facet joints
  - Formed by articular processes that project superiorly and inferiorly from the junction of pedicle and lamina
- Uncovertebral joints
  - Found in the cervical spine
  - Formed by a ridge or lip of bone that projects superiorly from the lateral edge of the vertebral body and articulates with the lateral edge of the vertebral body above.

The exception to the above pattern occurs at the first and second cervical vertebrae (C1 and C2). C1, also known as the 'atlas', consists of an anterior arch, two lateral masses and a posterior arch. Lateral masses of C1 articulate superiorly with the occiput (atlanto-occipital joints), and inferiorly with superior articular processes of C2 (atlanto-axial joints). The odontoid peg or dens is a vertical projection of bone that extends superiorly from the body of C2 and articulates with the anterior arch of C1.

9.2 SPINE TRAUMA

The roles of imaging in the assessment of spinal trauma are:
- Diagnosis of fractures/dislocation
- Assessment of stability/instability
- Diagnosis of damage to, or impingement on, neurological structures
- Follow-up
  - Assessment of treatment
  - Diagnosis of long-term complications, such as post-traumatic syrinx or cyst formation.

The principal imaging modalities used in the assessment of spine trauma are radiography, CT and MRI.

9.2.1 Cervical spine radiographs

Radiographic assessment of the cervical spine should be performed in all patients who have suffered major trauma as part of a trauma series that includes:
- Lateral radiograph cervical spine
- Frontal CXR
- Frontal radiograph of the pelvis.

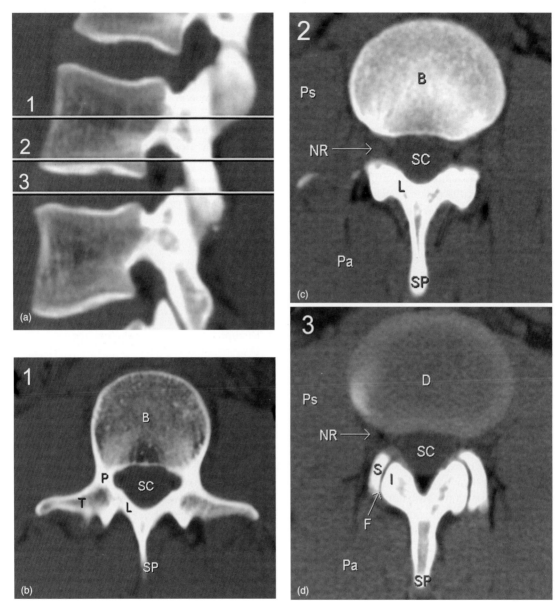

Figure 9.3 Normal lumbar spine anatomy: CT. (a) Reconstructed image in the sagittal plane showing the levels of the three following transverse sections. (b) Transverse section at level of pedicles. (c) Transverse section at level of intervertebral foramina. (d) Transverse section at level of intervertebral disc. In images (b), (c) and (d) note the following: vertebral body (B), pedicle (P), facet joint (F), inferior articular process (I), superior articular process (S), transverse process (T), lamina (L), spinous process (SP), nerve root (NR), spinal canal (SC), psoas muscle (Ps), paraspinal muscle (Pa).

Specific indications for cervical spine radiography in trauma patients include:

- Neck pain or tenderness
- Other signs of direct neck injury
- Abnormal findings on neurological examination
- Severe head or facial injury
- Near-drowning.

The following radiographs should be performed for suspected trauma of the cervical spine:

- Lateral view with patient supine showing all seven cervical vertebrae
  - Traction on the shoulders may be used to assist with visualization of the lower cervical spine

- Where the lower cervical vertebrae are obscured by the shoulders, a so-called 'swimmer's view' may be performed; this consists of a lateral view with one arm up and one down
  - Traction on the head must never be used
- AP view of the cervical spine
- AP open mouth view to show the odontoid peg.

Oblique views to show the facet joints and intervertebral foramina may also be performed where facet joint dislocation or locking is suspected. Functional views may be performed to diagnose posterior or anterior ligament damage where no fractures are seen on the neutral views. Functional views consist of lateral radiographs in flexion and extension with the patient erect. The patient must be conscious and cooperative and must actively flex and extend their neck; a doctor or radiographer must not move the patient's head passively.

Cervical spine radiographs should be checked in a logical fashion for radiographic features that may indicate trauma. These features include vertebral alignment, bone integrity, disc spaces and prevertebral swelling:

- Vertebral alignment
  - Disruption of anterior and posterior vertebral body lines: lines joining the anterior and posterior margins of the vertebral bodies on the lateral view
  - Disruption of the posterior cervical line: a line joining the anterior aspect of the spinous processes of C1, C2 and C3; disruption of this line may indicate upper cervical spine fractures, especially of C2 (Fig. 9.2)
  - Facet joint alignment at all levels; abrupt disruption at one level may indicate locked facets
  - Widening of the space between spinous processes on the lateral film
  - Rotation of spinous processes on the AP film
  - Widening of the predental space: >5 mm in children; >3 mm in adults
- Bone integrity
  - Vertebral body fractures
  - Fractures of posterior elements, i.e. pedicles, laminae, spinous processes
  - Integrity of odontoid peg: anterior/ posterior/lateral displacement

- Disc spaces
  - Narrowing or widening
- Prevertebral swelling
  - Widening of the retrotracheal space: posterior aspect of trachea to C6
    - >14 mm in children
    - >22 mm in adults
  - Widening of the retropharyngeal space: posterior aspect of pharynx to C2
    - >7 mm in adults and children.

9.2.2 Common patterns of cervical spine injury

9.2.2.1 Flexion: anterior compression with posterior distraction (Fig. 9.4)

- Vertebral body compression fracture
- 'Teardrop' fracture, i.e. small triangular fragment at lower anterior margin of vertebral body
- Disruption of posterior vertebral line
- Disc space narrowing
- Widening of facet joints
- Facet joint dislocation and locking
- Widening of space between spinous processes.

9.2.2.2 Extension: posterior compression with anterior distraction (Fig. 9.5)

- 'Teardrop' fracture of upper anterior margin of vertebral body: indicates severe anterior ligament damage
- Disc space widening
- Retrolisthesis (posterior shift of vertebral body) with disruption of anterior and posterior vertebral lines
- Fractures of posterior elements: pedicles, spinous processes, facets
- 'Hangman's' fracture: bilateral C2 pedicle fracture (Fig. 9.6).

9.2.2.3 Rotation (Fig. 9.7)

- Anterolisthesis (anterior shift of vertebral body) with disruption of posterior vertebral line
- Lateral displacement of upper vertebral body on AP view
- Abrupt disruption of alignment of facet joints: locked facets.

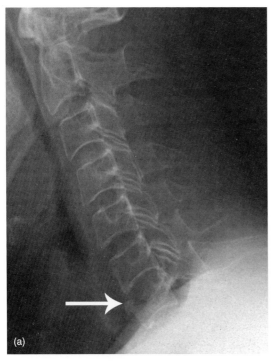

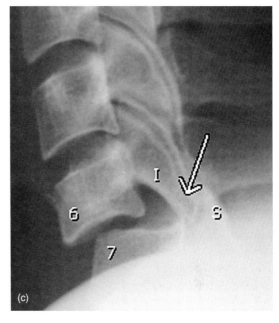

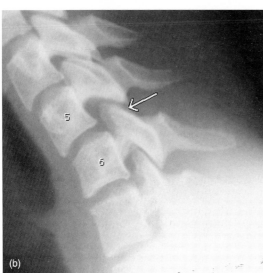

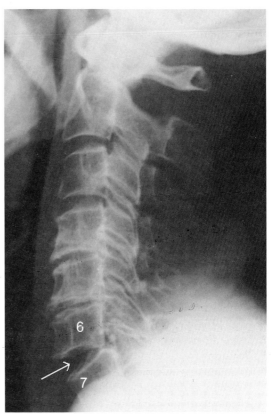

Figure 9.4 Flexion injuries of the cervical spine: three separate examples. (a) Crush fracture of C7 (arrow). (b) Facet joint subluxation. The space between the spinous processes of C5 and C6 is widened. The inferior articular processes of C5 are shifted forwards on the superior articular processes of C6 (arrow) indicating facet joint subluxation. (c) Bilateral locked facets. Both facet joints at C6/7 are dislocated. The posterior corners of the inferior articular processes (I) of C6 are locked anterior to the superior articular processes (S) of C7 (arrow).

Figure 9.5 Extension injury cervical spine. Note widening of the anterior disc space at C6/7 (arrow).

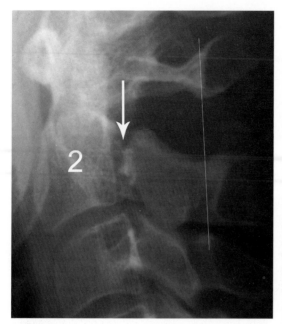

Figure 9.6 Hangman's fracture. Fracture of the pedicles of C2 (arrow) with loss of continuity of the posterior cervical line.

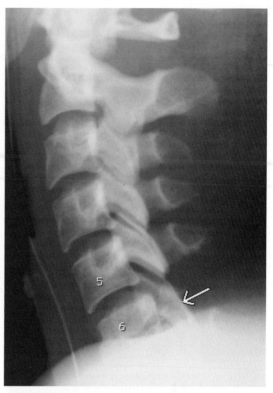

Figure 9.7 Flexion and rotation injury of the cervical spine: unilateral locked facet. There is widening of the space between the spinous processes of C5 and C6. Only one normally aligned facet joint is seen at C5/6. Compare this with the levels above where two normally aligned facet joints can be seen. Note the bare articular surface of one of the superior articular processes of C6 (arrow) due to dislocation of this facet joint.

9.2.3 Stability

As well as diagnosing and classifying cervical spine injuries, it is important to decide whether the injury is stable or not. Instability implies the possibility of increased spinal deformity or neurological damage occurring with mobilization or continued stress. Viewed laterally, the spine may be divided into three columns:

- Anterior: anterior two-thirds of the vertebral body
- Middle: posterior one-third of vertebral body and posterior longitudinal ligament
- Posterior: facet joints and bony arch of spinal canal (pedicles, laminae and spinous process).

It is generally accepted that two of these three columns must be intact for spinal stability to be maintained. Radiographic signs of instability include:

- Displacement of vertebral body
- 'Teardrop' fractures of vertebral body
- Odontoid peg fracture
- Widening or disruption of alignment of facet joints including locked facets
- Widening of space between spinous processes
- Fractures at multiple levels.

9.2.4 Thoracic and lumbar spine radiographs

Assessment of plain films of the thoracic and lumbar spine following trauma is similar to that outlined for the cervical spine, with particular attention to the following factors:

- Vertebral alignment
- Vertebral body height
- Disc space height
- Facet joint alignment
- Space between pedicles on AP film: widening at one level may indicate a burst fracture of the vertebral body.

9.2.5 Common patterns of thoracic and lumbar spine injury

9.2.5.1 Burst fracture

- Complex fractures of the vertebral body with a fragment pushed posteriorly (retropulsed) into the spinal canal
- Multiple fracture lines through vertebral end plates.

9.2.5.2 Compression (crush) fracture (Fig. 9.8)

- Common in osteoporosis
- Loss of height of vertebral body most marked anteriorly giving a wedge-like configuration.

9.2.5.3 Fracture/dislocation

- Vertebral body displacement
- Disc space narrowing or widening
- Fractures of neural arches, including facet joints
- Widening of facet joints or space between spinous processes.

9.2.5.4 Chance fracture (seatbelt fracture) (Fig. 9.9)

- Fracture of posterior vertebral body
- Horizontal fracture line through spinous process, laminae, pedicles and transverse processes
- Most occur at thoracolumbar junction

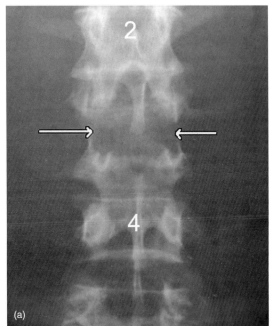

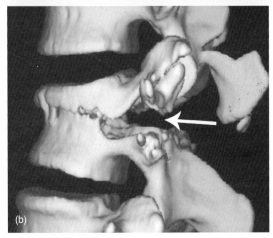

Figure 9.9 Chance fracture (seatbelt fracture) lumbar spine. (a) Frontal view showing a transverse fracture at L3 including horizontal splitting of the pedicles (arrows). (b) Three-dimensional CT reconstructed image showing the transverse fracture of the pedicles and posterior vertebral body (arrow).

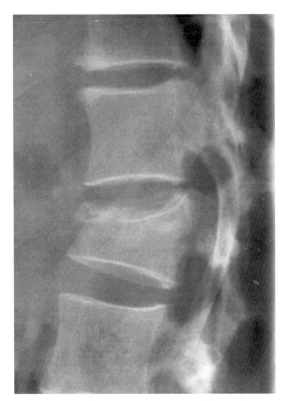

Figure 9.8 Crush fracture lumbar spine. Lateral view showing a crush fracture of the upper body of L1.

- High association with abdominal injury, i.e. solid organ damage, intestinal perforation, duodenal haematoma.

9.2.6 CT in spine trauma

CT is more sensitive than plain radiography in the diagnosis of bony spinal injuries. Particular advantages of CT in this clinical setting include:
- Accurate assessment of bony injuries, especially those of the neural arches and facet joints
- Retropulsed bone fragments projecting into the spinal canal and compressing neural structures are well seen (Fig. 9.10)
- Multiplanar and 3D images greatly assist in delineation of both subtle fractures and complex injuries.

CT examination of the cervical spine may be performed at the same time as a head CT in the setting of major trauma or an unconscious patient. Diagnostically adequate images of thoracic and lumbar spine may be reconstructed from multidetector CT of the chest and abdomen; this may obviate the need for radiographic assessment of these regions in patients with mid or lower back pain following trauma.

9.2.7 MRI in spine trauma

MRI is the investigation of choice for assessment of suspected spinal cord damage. Signs of spinal cord trauma that may be visualized on MRI include cord transection, cord oedema and haemorrhage, plus late sequelae such as arachnoid cyst, pseudomeningocele, myelomalacia and syrinx (Fig. 9.11). Other soft tissue changes, such as post-traumatic disc herniation, ligament tear and spinal canal haematoma are also seen on MRI.

Indications for MRI of the spine in the setting of trauma include:
- Where neurological symptoms or signs are present, regardless of radiographic findings
  - The phenomenon of spinal cord injury without radiographic abnormality

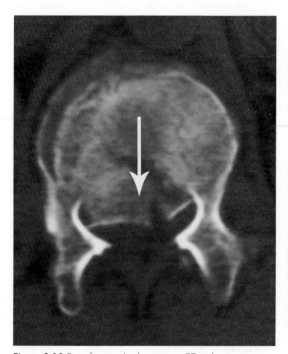

Figure 9.10 Burst fracture lumbar spine. CT in the transverse plane shows a fracture of the vertebral body with a retropulsed bone fragment (arrow) extending into the spinal canal.

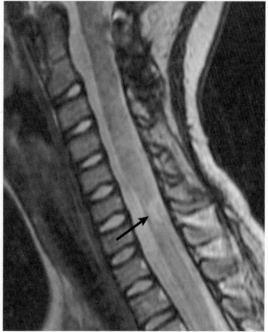

Figure 9.11 Spinal cord injury: MRI. Sagittal T2-weighted MRI of the cervical spine shows a high signal lesion associated with focal thinning of the spinal cord at C7 indicating myelomalacia (arrow).

(SCIWORA) is well described, particularly in children

- A normal radiograph should not preclude MRI where neurological injury is suspected on clinical grounds
- Suspected ligament injury and instability
- To differentiate acute crush fractures of the thoracic and lumbar spine from older healed injuries
  - This is an increasingly common indication in elderly patients with suspected osteoporotic crush fracture in whom MRI may assist with patient selection for percutaneous vertebroplasty (see Section 9.5.4).

9.3 NECK PAIN

Non-traumatic neck pain is an extremely common complaint. Most cases of neck pain are due to musculoligamentous strain or injury. Seventy per cent of episodes of neck pain resolve within one month. Most of the remaining 30 per cent resolve over the longer term with a small minority going on to have chronic neck problems. In the clinical assessment of neck pain, there are three major sources of diagnostic difficulty:

- Multiple structures including vertebral bodies, ligaments, muscles, intervertebral discs, vascular and neural structures are capable of producing pain
- Pain may be referred to the neck from other areas, such as shoulder, heart, diaphragm, mandible and temporomandibular joints
- Pain from the neck may be referred to the shoulders and arms.

9.3.1 Osteoarthritis of the cervical spine

Osteoarthritis (degenerative arthropathy) is a major cause of neck pain, with increasing incidence in old age. The primary phenomenon in osteoarthritis of the spine is degeneration of the intervertebral disc. Intervertebral disc degeneration in the cervical spine is most common at C5/6 and C6/7. Degenerate discs may herniate into the spinal canal or intervertebral foramina, with direct compression of the spinal cord or nerve roots. More commonly, disc degeneration

leads to abnormal stresses on the vertebral bodies and on the facet and uncovertebral joints. These abnormal stresses lead to formation of bone spurs or osteophytes. Osteophytes may project into the spinal canal causing compression of the cervical cord, or into the intervertebral foramina causing nerve root compression. Cervical cord compression presents clinically with neck pain associated with a stiff gait and brisk lower limb reflexes (myelopathy).

Causes of cervical myelopathy:

- Syrinx
- Spinal cord tumours: ependymoma, glioma, neurofibroma, meningioma
- Vertebral body tumours: metastases, giant cell tumour, chordoma.

Nerve root compression produces local neck pain plus pain in the distribution of the compressed nerve. Osteoarthritis uncomplicated by compression of neural structures may cause episodic neck pain with the following features:

- Tends to be increased by activity
- May be associated with shoulder pain or headache
- Usually resolves within 7–10 days.

9.3.2 Imaging of the patient with neck pain

The goals of imaging of the patient with neck pain should be to exclude conditions requiring urgent attention, to diagnose a treatable condition, and to direct management. With these goals in mind and given the fact that most neck pain resolves spontaneously, it follows that the majority of patients do not require imaging. Imaging should be reserved for those cases where symptoms are severe and persistent, or where there are other relevant factors on history or examination, such as trauma or a known primary tumour.

Initial imaging in the majority of cases consists of a plain film examination of the cervical spine. Radiographic signs of osteoarthritis of the cervical spine (Fig. 9.12) include:

- Disc space narrowing, most common at C5/6 and C6/7
- Osteophyte formation on the vertebral bodies and facet joints
- Osteophytes projecting into the intervertebral foramina.

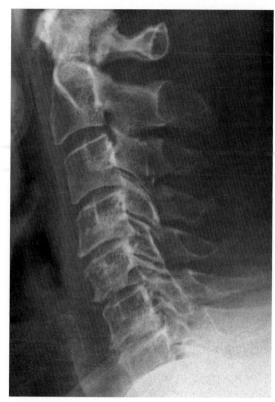

Figure 9.12 Osteoarthritis of the cervical spine. Note disc space narrowing at multiple levels.

MRI is the investigation of choice where further imaging is required for persistent nerve root pain, or for assessment of a possible spinal cord abnormality. CT is used in the investigation of neck pain where fine bone detail is required, such as in the assessment of vertebral body tumour.

9.4 LOW BACK PAIN

Low back pain refers to back pain that does not extend below the iliac crests. Pain extending to the buttocks or legs is referred to as sciatica; this is a separate clinical problem to back pain and is considered in Section 9.6. Low back pain may be classified into acute or chronic, with the term 'acute back pain' usually referring to pain of less than 12 weeks' duration. There are now well-developed evidence-based guidelines for the management and investigation of acute back pain from which

a number of consistent recommendations can be identified. Primary among these is the need for diagnostic triage of patients into three major groups:

- Non-specific low back pain, acute or chronic
- Specific low back pain
- Sciatica or radicular pain, with neurological findings such as positive straight leg raise test.

As discussed in Section 9.6, sciatica is best investigated with MRI or CT. Specific low back pain refers to back pain with associated clinical symptoms or signs, known as 'red flags', that may indicate an underlying problem. Examples of these 'red flags', some of which will be discussed below, include:

- Known primary tumour, such as prostate or breast
- Systemic symptoms: unexplained fever or weight loss
- Recent trauma
- Known osteoporosis or prolonged steroid use
- Age at onset of pain: <20 or >55 years
- Thoracic pain
- Neurological changes.

9.4.1 Acute non-specific low back pain

All of the evidence-based guidelines on acute back pain agree that imaging assessment, including radiography of the lumbar spine, is not indicated in patients with non-specific acute back pain. This reflects the fact that most cases of non-specific low back pain are due to musculoligamentous injury or exacerbation of degenerative arthropathy, and will usually resolve within a few weeks. Most guidelines emphasize the importance of reassurance, discouragement of bed rest, and the recognition of psychosocial risk factors that may predispose to chronic back pain.

9.4.2 Chronic non-specific low back pain

Most of the evidence in the medical literature dealing with the problem of chronic low back pain points to the exclusion of 'red flags' (see above). A multidisciplinary approach to therapy is often required, including exercise, education and counselling. A specific diagnosis as to the cause of pain is often not required. In some cases, however, particularly when pain is severe and debilitating, or due to other factors, such as loss of employment or depression, a specific diagnosis may be required as a guide to therapy.

Most cases of chronic back pain are due to facet joint pain, sacroiliac joint pain or internal disruption of intervertebral discs. Imaging techniques, such as radiography, CT and MRI, are able to show changes of degenerative arthropathy in a large percentage of patients examined (Fig. 9.13). A major problem with imaging in this context is that findings are very non-specific; imaging is often unable to pinpoint the cause of pain. For example, radiographs may show a narrowed disc space; this does not mean that this is definitely the cause of the patient's pain.

The only way to prove that a certain structure, such as a facet joint, is the cause of pain is to inject local anaesthetic into that structure and assess the response. Image-guided interventions are now commonplace in the management of chronic back pain and are performed under CT or fluoroscopic guidance (see below). It should be emphasized that in the absence of 'red flags', imaging is not indicated in the majority of patients with chronic non-specific low back pain.

9.4.3 Image-guided interventions in the diagnosis and management of back pain

Image-guided interventions are increasingly common in the management of back pain and sciatica. Most procedures outlined in this section have the following features in common:

- Performed under CT or fluoroscopic guidance
- Use of fine needles, 22–25 gauge
- Injection of local anaesthetic and corticosteroid (LACS).

Complications are very rare and may include haemorrhage or infection. Contraindications are few and include severe coagulopathy and unsuitable anatomy.

9.4.3.1 Facet joint injection

Facet joint injection of LACS (Fig. 9.14) has two roles:

- Diagnostic: confirm facet joint as pain generator
- Therapeutic.

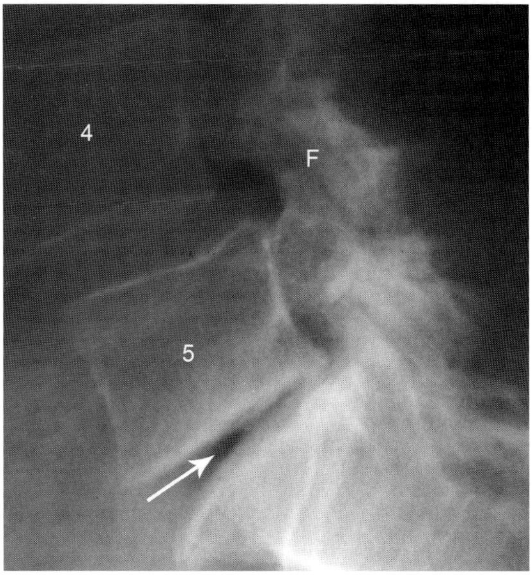

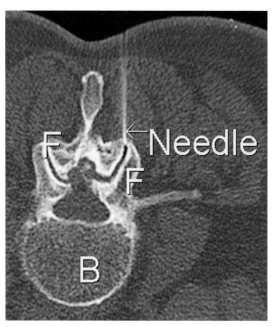

Figure 9.13 Osteoarthritis of the lumbar spine. Narrowing of the intervertebral disc space between L5 and S1 (arrow). Sclerosis of the facet joints at L4/5 (F) with degenerative spondylolisthesis at this level.

Figure 9.14 Facet joint block: computer tomography guidance. The patient is lying prone with the vertebral body (B) towards the bottom of the image. A fine needle is inserted into the facet joint (F) for injection of local anaesthetic and steroid.

9.4.3.2 Medial branch block

Each facet joint receives dual innervation from medial branches of two contiguous nerve roots:

- For example, each L4/5 facet joint receives innervation from medial branches of the L3 and L4 nerve roots
- These medial branches pass across the bases of the transverse processes of L4 and L5.

For medial branch block, fine needles are positioned under imaging guidance at the bases of the relevant transverse processes; LACS or local anaesthetic (LA) alone is injected to block the nerve supply to the facet joint.

Indications for medial branch block include:

- Recurrence of symptoms following successful facet joint block.
- Confirm facet joint as pain generator
- Prior to permanent medial branch ablation.

9.4.3.3 Medial branch ablation

The aim of medial branch ablation is long-term pain relief from facet joint denervation.

Facet joint denervation is usually achieved by radiofrequency (RF) ablation of the medial nerve branches supplying the joint. Following injection of LA, the RF probe is placed under imaging guidance with its tip at the known position of the medial nerve branch.

Medial branch ablation is often performed with mild intravenous conscious sedation. General anaesthetic is not used, as the patient must be able to respond to sensory and motor stimuli during the procedure.

9.4.3.4 Epidural injection

Injection of LACS into the epidural space (Fig. 9.15) may be performed for various indications including:

- Back pain and/or sciatica due to spinal stenosis
- 'Discogenic' back pain due to degenerative changes in intervertebral discs.

Although common, epidural injection is a controversial procedure for a number of reasons, including uncertainty over mechanism of action.

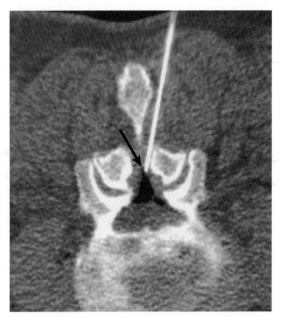

Figure 9.15 Epidural injection: CT guidance. Injection of a small amount of air confirms the needle tip position in the epidural space (arrow).

9.4.3.5 Discography

Discography is used to prove that pain is arising from one or more intervertebral discs. Under fluoroscopic guidance, a fine needle is positioned in the centre of the intervertebral disc. A small amount of dilute contrast material is injected to 'stress' the disc. The patient's pain response is recorded. Contrast material is used to assess the actual morphology of the disc and to diagnose annular tears.

9.5 SPECIFIC BACK PAIN SYNDROMES

Imaging may be required for assessment of back pain associated with 'red flags' as listed above. An initial radiographic examination of the lumbar spine is reasonable in these patients. This will help exclude obvious bony causes of pain, as well as delineate any other relevant factors such as scoliosis.

Limitations of radiographs of the lumbar spine:

- Soft tissue structures such as ligaments, muscles and nerve roots are not imaged
- Relatively insensitive for many painful bone conditions such as infection

- Cross-sectional dimensions of the spinal canal are not assessed.

In many conditions, such as suspected infection or suspected acute osteoporotic crush fracture, MRI is the investigation of choice.

CT is highly accurate for assessment of bony lesions such as suspected tumours or pars interarticularis defects.

Scintigraphy with ^{99}mTc-MDP may be indicated in certain instances:

- To exclude spinal metastases where there is a known primary tumour
- Suspected pars interarticularis fractures; these may be difficult to see on plain films, particularly in young patients with subtle stress fractures.

9.5.1 Pars interarticularis defects and spondylolisthesis

The pars interarticularis is a mass of bone between the superior and inferior articular processes of the vertebral body. Defect of the pars interarticularis, also known as spondylolysis, may be congenital or due to trauma:

- Congenital pars interarticularis defects are often associated with other developmental anomalies of the lumbar spine, especially failure of complete bony fusion of the laminae in the midline.
- Acute trauma may produce an acute fracture through the pars interarticularis, and stress fractures may occur associated with sports such as gymnastics and fast bowling (cricket).

Regardless of aetiology, pars interarticularis defects may be unilateral or bilateral, and are most common at L5. Bilateral pars defects may be associated with spondylolisthesis, i.e. anterior shift of L5 on S1. Back pain in spondylolysis and spondylolisthesis may be due to a number of factors including:

- The bony defects themselves
- Segmental instability
- Degenerative changes in the intervertebral disc.

Spondylolysis is suspected in otherwise healthy young adults presenting with back pain, particularly those participating in typical sporting activities. Spondylolisthesis also causes narrowing of the intervertebral foramina between L5 and S1 with compression of the exiting L5 nerve roots producing bilateral posterior leg pain and a sensation of hamstring tightness. Spondylolysis and spondylolisthesis may be investigated with radiographs, scintigraphy, CT and MRI.

Radiographically, pars interarticularis defects are best seen on oblique views of the lower lumbar spine. The complex of overlapping shadows from the superior and inferior articular processes, the pars interarticularis, and the transverse process forms an outline resembling that of a Scottish terrier dog. A pars defect is seen as a line across the neck of the 'dog' (Fig. 9.16).

Scintigraphy with ^{99}mTc-MDP and single photon emission CT–CT (SPECT–CT) may be used to diagnose subtle stress fractures not able to be visualized radiographically. Pars interarticularis defects are also well shown on CT, particularly with multidetector CT, which allows multiplanar reconstructions.

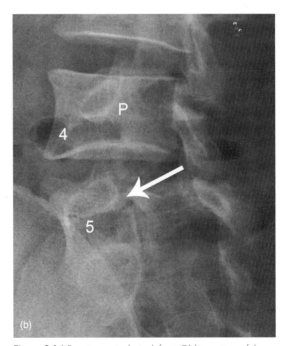

Figure 9.16 Pars interarticularis defect. Oblique view of the lower lumbar spine showing a pars interarticularis defect at L5 (arrow). Note also the intact pars interarticularis at L4 (P) and the facet joints.

When there is frank spondylolisthesis on the lumbar spine radiographs, MRI is often used. MRI provides more information on the state of the intervertebral disc and is also the best method for assessing the degree of narrowing of the intervertebral foramina and associated nerve root compression.

9.5.2 Vertebral infection

Most vertebral infection commences in the intervertebral disc (discitis). Discitis may spread to involve the vertebral body, causing vertebral osteomyelitis, or may invade the spinal canal to produce an epidural abscess. Discitis is usually due to blood-borne infection, may occur in children or adults, and is more common in the lower spine. Clinical features of discitis include rapid onset of back pain accompanied by fever and malaise. In young children, there may be less specific symptoms, such as limp or failure to weight bear.

Radiographic findings of discitis occur late in the disease process and include narrowing of the intervertebral disc with blurring of the vertebral endplates.

MRI is the investigation of choice for suspected vertebral infection. MRI is usually positive at the time of clinical presentation, before radiographic signs are evident (Fig. 9.17). MRI is also the best imaging method for showing the full extent of infection, including epidural abscess.

9.5.3 Vertebral metastases

Tumours with a high incidence of vertebral metastases include prostate, breast, lung, kidney and melanoma. Lymphoma and multiple myeloma may also involve the spine. Vertebral metastatic disease is suspected when back pain occurs in a patient with a known primary tumour. Other suspicious clinical factors include weight loss and raised PSA (prostate specific antigen).

Radiographs of the spine may show focal sclerotic (dense) lesions throughout the vertebral bodies in metastases from prostatic primary. Other primary tumours tend to produce lytic or destructive metastases that may be difficult to appreciate on radiographs (Fig. 9.18).

Scintigraphy with ^{99m}Tc-MDP is generally the investigation of choice in screening for skeletal metastases, including the spine.

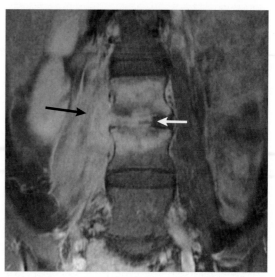

Figure 9.17 Discitis: MRI. Coronal T1-weighted, fat saturated contrast-enhanced MRI of the lumbar spine in a 14-year-old female with severe back pain and fever. Enhancement of L3/4 intervertebral disc (white arrow). Note also enhancement of adjacent vertebral bodies and spread of infection into the right psoas muscle (black arrow).

Occasionally, a vertebral metastasis may expand into the spinal canal and compress the spinal cord causing an acute myelopathy. Clinical features of myelopathy include:
- Motor problems in the legs leading to difficulty with walking
- Sensory disturbances; a band-like sensation around the abdomen
- Voiding difficulties.

Cord compression due to metastatic disease is most common in the thoracic region and may require acute surgical decompression or radiotherapy. MRI is the investigation of choice for suspected spinal cord compression (Fig. 9.19).

9.5.4 Acute osteoporotic crush fracture

Individuals with osteoporosis are at an increased risk for the development of a crush fracture of the spine. Osteoporotic crush fractures may occur at any level, though are most common in the lower thoracic and lumbar spine. The patient usually presents with acute back pain that is mechanical in type, i.e. worsened by movement or activity. There may be

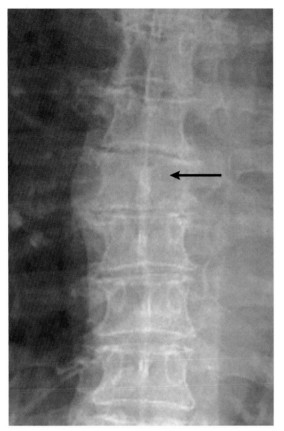

Figure 9.18 Vertebral metastasis. Sudden onset back pain and leg weakness in a 62-year-old female with a history of breast cancer. Frontal radiograph shows reduced height of the T6 vertebral body. Note loss of visualization of the left pedicle due to bone destruction (arrow).

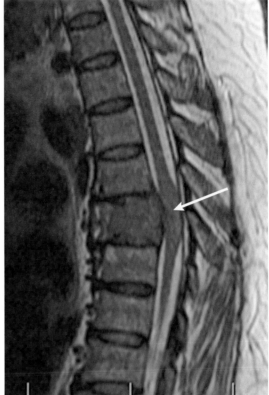

Figure 9.19 Vertebral metastasis: MRI. Same patient as Fig. 19.18. Sagittal T2-weighted MRI shows destruction and partial collapse of T6. Neoplastic tissue is invading the spinal canal and compressing the spinal cord (arrow).

an associated band-like distribution of pain around the chest wall or abdomen, depending on the level involved. The pain associated with osteoporotic crush fracture usually settles in a matter of weeks. In some patients, however, the pain may persist and produce numerous complications:

- Reduced mobility
- Inhibition of respiration
- Difficulty sleeping
- Significant mortality and morbidity in elderly patients.

Percutaneous vertebroplasty is now a well-accepted technique for the treatment of the pain associated with acute osteoporotic crush fractures. Radiographs of the spine will usually diagnose a crush fracture (Fig. 9.8). A major limitation of radiography is that there is no reliable way to distinguish an acute crush fracture from an older healed injury. This becomes particularly relevant where percutaneous vertebroplasty is being considered and multiple crush fractures are seen radiographically.

Prior to vertebroplasty, MRI is used to define the acute level(s), and therefore assists with patient selection and procedure planning. MRI is able to show bone marrow oedema in acutely crushed vertebral bodies (see Fig. 1.19). Older healed crush fractures show normal bone marrow signal with no evidence of oedema.

Vertebroplasty involves insertion of a large bore needle (11 or 13 gauge) into the vertebral body followed by injection of bone cement. The bone cement is mixed with barium powder so it can be visualized radiographically. Needle placement and cement injection are performed under direct fluoroscopic guidance to avoid injury to neurological structures (Fig. 9.20). Vertebroplasty is a highly effective technique for reducing pain, restoring mobility and reducing dependence on analgesics. Complications of vertebroplasty are uncommon and include:

- Haemorrhage
- Leakage of cement into the spinal canal or intervertebral foramina with impingement on spinal cord and nerve roots
- Embolization of tiny cement fragments into the lungs: usually not clinically significant.

9.5.5 Scoliosis

Scoliosis refers to abnormal curvature of the spine, with a lateral component of >10°. Recognized causes of scoliosis include:

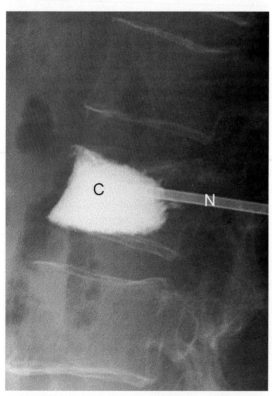

Figure 9.20 Vertebroplasty. Lateral view showing radio-opaque bone cement (C) being injected into the vertebral body via a large bone biopsy needle (N).

- Congenital due to abnormal vertebral segmentation (Fig. 9.21a)
- Underlying syndrome, such as neurofibromatosis
- Severe degenerative disease in elderly patients
- Acute painful scoliosis may indicate the presence of vertebral infection or a tumour such as osteoid osteoma.

Most commonly, scoliosis is idiopathic. Idiopathic scoliosis is classified according to the age of onset with three major groups described:

- Infantile: birth to four years
- Juvenile: four to ten years
- Adolescent: ten years or older.

Adolescent idiopathic scoliosis (AIS) accounts for 90 per cent of patients with scoliosis. The key clinical test for the diagnosis of AIS is the forward bend test. A positive forward bend test is indicated by convex bulging of the contour of the back on the side of the convexity of the spinal curve, due to rotation of the spine producing prominence of the posterior ribs on the convex side.

Patients with suspected scoliosis should be assessed radiographically with a single AP long film of the thoracic and lumbar spine taken with the patient standing erect. The key to radiographic diagnosis and follow-up is measurement of the Cobb angle:

- Identify the most tilted vertebral bodies above and below the apex of the curve
- Line drawn parallel to the superior vertebral end plate of the most tilted vertebral body at the upper end of the curve
- Similar line drawn parallel to the lower vertebral end plate of the lower most tilted vertebral body
- The angle between these lines is the Cobb angle (Fig. 9.21b).

A Cobb angle of 10° or greater is considered abnormal. Curves are described by their region, thoracic or lumbar, and by the direction of convexity, e.g. a 'right curve' is convex to the right. The largest curve is termed the 'major' or 'primary' curve. Compensatory or secondary curves occur above and/or below the primary curve; these usually have smaller Cobb angles than the primary curve. The most common pattern in AIS is a right thoracic primary curve with a left lumbar or thoracolumbar

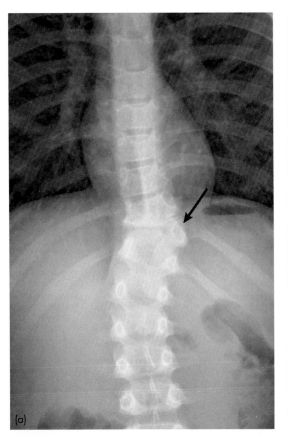 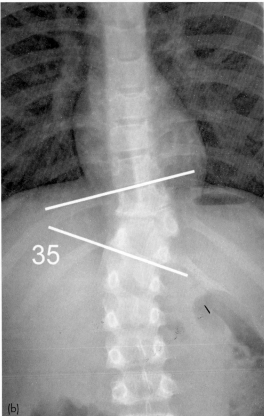

Figure 9.21 Vertebral anomaly causing scoliosis. (a) Frontal radiograph shows a left-sided hemivertebra on the left in the lower thoracic spine (arrow). Note that the hemivertebra articulates with an unpaired left rib. (b) Cobb angle measurement: note the method of Cobb angle measurement as outlined in text.

secondary curve. A single erect radiograph is usually sufficient for the imaging assessment of AIS.

Uncommonly, further imaging with MRI may be indicated for the following:

- Neurological signs
- Certain radiographic abnormalities, e.g. bone destruction such as may indicate the presence of a vertebral tumour
- Atypical curves
  - In particular, a left thoracic primary curve may be associated with a syrinx of the cord.

9.6 SCIATICA

Sciatica is usually caused by herniation of intervertebral disc, or by spinal stenosis due to degenerative disease. Each intervertebral disc is composed of a tough outer layer, the annulus fibrosis, and a softer semifluid centre, the nucleus pulposus. With degeneration of the disc, small microtears appear in the annulus fibrosis allowing generalized bulging of the nucleus pulposus. This causes the disc to bulge beyond the margins of the vertebral bodies causing narrowing of the spinal canal. Secondary effects of degenerative disc disease include abnormal stresses on the vertebral bodies leading to osteophyte formation, as well as facet joint sclerosis and hypertrophy. These changes may lead to further narrowing of the spinal canal producing spinal canal stenosis.

A common complication of disc degeneration is the occurrence of a localized tear in the annulus fibrosis through which the nucleus pulposus may herniate. Disc herniation may project into the spinal canal or posterolaterally into the intervertebral foramen, causing compression of nerve roots. 'Free fragment' and 'sequestration' are terms that refer to a fragment of disc that has broken off from the 'parent' disc; this fragment may migrate superiorly or inferiorly in the spinal canal.

9.6.1 Sciatica syndromes

Sciatica refers to pain confined to a nerve root distribution, with leg pain being more severe than back pain. Sciatica may be accompanied by other neurological symptoms such as paraesthesia, and by signs of nerve root irritation such as positive straight leg raise test. Sciatica or leg pain syndromes are classified based on whether the pain is acute or chronic, unilateral or bilateral:

- Unilateral acute nerve root compression: 'classical' sciatica
  - Usually caused by focal disc herniation
- Bilateral acute nerve root compression: cauda equina syndrome
  - Cauda equina syndrome refers to the sudden onset of bilateral leg pain accompanied by bladder and/or bowel dysfunction
  - Usually caused by a massive disc herniation or sequestration
- Unilateral chronic nerve root compression: sciatica lasting for months
  - Unilateral chronic sciatica may be caused by disc herniation or spinal stenosis
- Bilateral chronic nerve root compression
  - Bilateral chronic nerve root compression refers to vague bilateral leg pain aggravated by walking and slowly relieved by rest
  - Usually caused by spinal canal stenosis
  - A common clinical difficulty is differentiating neural compression from vascular claudication
    - Clinical pointers that indicate a vascular cause include absent peripheral pulses, pain is in the exercised muscles, and rapid pain relief with rest.

9.6.2 Imaging of sciatica

9.6.2.1 MRI and CT

MRI is the investigation of choice for most neurological disorders of the spine, including sciatica. Advantages of MRI in this context include:

- Better soft tissue contrast resolution than CT

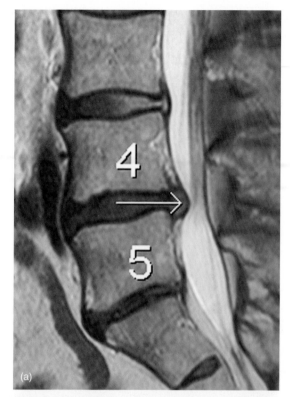

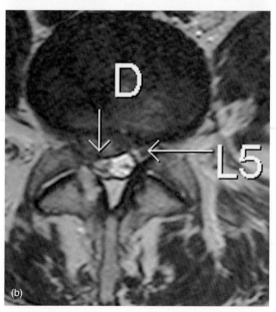

Figure 9.22 Intervertebral disc herniation: MRI. (a) Sagittal image showing posterior herniation of the L4/5 disc (arrow). (b) Transverse image through the intervertebral disc (D) showing herniation into the right side of the spinal canal (arrow). Note the normal left L5 nerve root. The right L5 nerve root is compressed and cannot be visualized.

- Nerve roots and the distal spinal cord and conus can be imaged without the use of contrast material
- Able to outline the anatomy of the spinal canal and the intervertebral discs
- Highly sensitive for the detection of spinal canal stenosis, disc herniation and narrowing of the intervertebral foramina (Fig. 9.22).

CT is a reasonable alternative for investigation of sciatica where MRI is not available.

9.6.2.2 Selective nerve root block

Selective nerve root block (SNRB) is used in patients with sciatica as both a diagnostic tool and a means for giving temporary pain relief. SNRB is a relatively simple procedure in which a fine needle is positioned adjacent to the nerve root under CT or fluoroscopic guidance, and a small volume of steroid and local anaesthetic injected. SNRB may be performed safely in the cervical, thoracic or lumbar spine.

Indications for SNRB include:
- To confirm the symptomatic level where imaging findings indicate nerve root compression at multiple levels
- Lack of imaging evidence of nerve root compression despite a convincing clinical presentation
- To provide temporary pain relief from sciatica while surgery is planned
- Surgery contraindicated due to anaesthetic risk or other factors.

Post-procedure care:
- Some patients experience transient lower limb numbness and a subjective feeling of weakness and may need to be assisted with standing and walking following the procedure
- Patients are advised not to drive a car for a few hours following the procedure.

SUMMARY BOX

Clinical presentation	Investigation of choice	Comment
Spine trauma	Radiography CT to define bony anatomy MRI to define soft tissue complications including spinal cord injury	
Neck pain	Imaging not indicated in most cases Radiography MRI/CT for radiculopathy/myelopathy	
Back pain	Imaging not indicated in most cases Radiography MRI/CT for radiculopathy/myelopathy	Imaging indicated in neck and back pain for chronic, relapsing or unremitting pain, or in the presence of clinical 'red flags' (see above)
Spondylolysis and spondylolisthesis	Radiography SPECT–CT	MRI if sciatica is the dominant symptom
Discitis	MRI	
Vertebral metastases	Bone scintigraphy	
Acute osteoporotic crush fracture(s)	Radiography	MRI where vertebroplasty is contemplated
Scoliosis	Radiography ('long films')	MRI in selected cases
Sciatica	MRI	CT where MRI is unavailable

SPECT–CT, single photon emission CT–CT.

Central nervous system

CT and MRI are the most common imaging investigations performed for assessment of brain disorders (Figs 10.1, 10.2 and 10.3). MRI is the investigation of choice for most indications. The two most common exceptions are acute trauma and suspected acute subarachnoid haemorrhage. Skull X-ray may occasionally be performed for a few uncommon skull vault disorders, such as craniosynostosis (premature fusion of cranial sutures in infants), or as part of a skeletal survey, e.g. multiple myeloma (see Fig. 8.65) or suspected non-accidental injury in children. Cranial US is a useful investigation in infants where the anterior fontanelle is open. The commonest indication for cranial US is the diagnosis and monitoring of cerebral haemorrhage in premature infants. Cranial US is also a useful screening test in older infants for assessment of increasing head circumference.

10.1 TRAUMATIC BRAIN INJURY

CT is the investigation of choice for the patient with head trauma and suspected traumatic brain injury. CT of the head provides rapid identification of cranial traumatic lesions that require urgent neurosurgical intervention, plus identification of non-surgical findings that may require treatment and follow-up. Indications for head CT in the setting of trauma vary from centre to centre and include:
- Confusion/drowsiness not improved at 4 hours
- New focal neurological signs
- Deterioration in level of consciousness
- Fully conscious with
  - Fitting
  - Nausea and vomiting
  - New and persisting headache
- Glasgow Coma Scale (GCS) <15
- Clinically obvious compound or depressed skull fracture
- Suspected fractured skull
  - Scalp laceration to bone; boggy scalp haematoma
- Signs of fractured base of skull
  - Discharge of blood or cerebrospinal fluid (CSF) from nose or ear
- Penetrating head injuries
- Suspected intracranial foreign body.

In all cases of major trauma and head injury, radiographs of the cervical spine should be obtained (see Chapter 9).

Owing to relatively poor visualization of acute haemorrhage, time taken for performance of examination and logistical problems with monitoring equipment, MRI has not been recommended for initial screening of acute head trauma. MRI is most useful in the assessment of an ongoing neurological or cognitive deficit. In particular, MRI is highly sensitive for the detection of diffuse axonal injury (DAI), a potentially serious injury that may be difficult to detect with CT.

10.1.1 Common CT findings of traumatic brain injury

Extradural haematoma (EDH) lies in the space between the dura and the inner table of the skull. EDH is usually associated with a skull fracture and

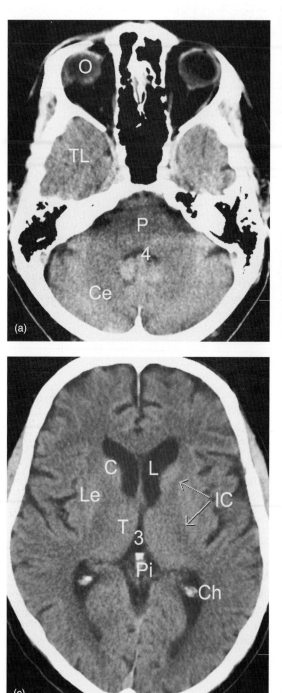

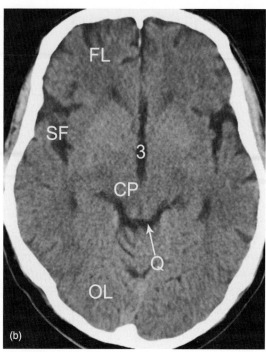

Figure 10.1 Normal brain anatomy: CT. (a) Transverse CT scan through the posterior fossa. (b) Transverse CT scan through the cerebral peduncles. Note the following: third ventricle (3), fourth ventricle (4), cerebellum (Ce), cerebral peduncles (CP), frontal lobe (FL), orbit (O), occipital lobe (OL), pons (P), quadrigeminal plate cistern (Q), sylvian fissure (SF), temporal lobe (TL). Normal brain anatomy: CT. (c) Transverse CT scan through the basal ganglia. Note the following: third ventricle (3), caudate nucleus (C), choroid plexus in lateral ventricle (Ch), internal capsule (IC), lateral ventricles (L), lentiform nucleus (Le), pineal gland (Pi), thalamus (T).

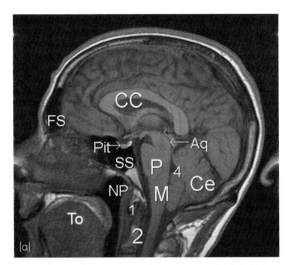

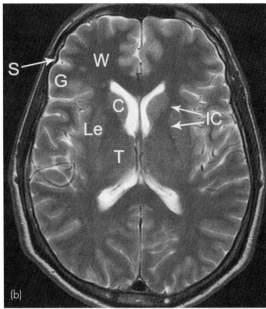

Figure 10.2 Normal brain anatomy: MRI. (a) Sagittal T1-weighted MRI in the midline. (b) Transverse T2-weighted MRI through the basal ganglia. Note the following: anterior arch of C1 (1), odontoid peg (2), fourth ventricle (4), aqueduct of Sylvius (Aq), caudate nucleus (C), corpus callosum (CC), cerebellum (Ce), frontal sinus (FS), gyrus (G), internal capsule (IC), lentiform nucleus (Le), nasopharynx (NP), pons (P), pituitary gland (Pit), sulcus (S), sphenoid sinus (SS), thalamus (T), tongue (To), white matter (W).

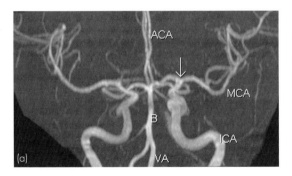

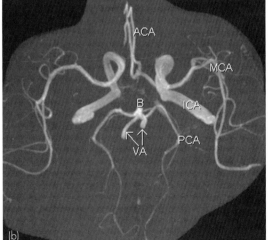

Figure 10.3 Normal brain anatomy: magnetic resonance angiogram. (a) Three-dimensional (3D) reconstruction of circle of Willis, viewed from the front. (b) 3D reconstruction of circle of Willis, viewed from above. Note the following: internal carotid arteries (ICA), bifurcation of ICA (arrow), vertebral arteries (VA), basilar artery (B), anterior cerebral artery (ACA), middle cerebral artery (MCA), posterior cerebral artery (PCA).

is the result of tearing of meningeal blood vessels. CT appearance of EDH:

- High-attenuation peripheral lesion with a convex inner margin (Fig. 10.4).

Subdural haematoma (SDH) lies in the space between the dura and the arachnoid. SDH is due to bleeding from bridging veins in the subdural space, and usually associated with cerebral oedema. CT appearance of SDH:

- High-attenuation peripheral lesion with a concave inner margin, often spreading over much of the cerebral hemisphere (Fig. 10.5)

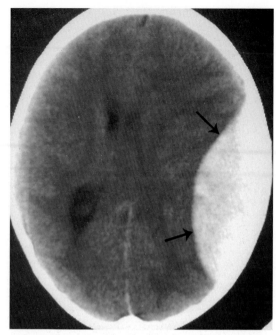

Figure 10.4 Extradural haematoma. Acute blood is of high attenuation on CT. Note the convex inner margin (arrows).

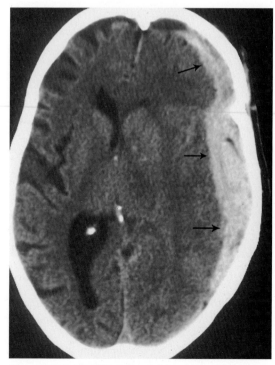

Figure 10.5 Subdural haematoma. Note the concave inner margin of the haematoma (arrows).

- Mass effect often severe due to combination of haematoma and swelling of the underlying brain
- Over 7–10 days, the attenuation of the haematoma gradually decreases to approximate that of adjacent brain tissue
- Over the ensuing couple of weeks, the attenuation decreases further to approximate that of CSF (black).

Subarachnoid haemorrhage (SAH) may occur with trauma, though more commonly is due to rupture of a cerebral aneurysm (see below).
CT appearance of SAH:
- High-attenuation material in the basal cisterns, sylvian fissures, cerebral sulci and ventricles.

Cerebral parenchymal injury may take several forms including intracerebral haematoma, cerebral oedema and contusion.
CT appearance of intracerebral haematoma:
- High-attenuation area in the brain tissue, usually surrounded by a low-attenuation rim of oedema.

CT appearance of cerebral oedema:
- Low-attenuation areas on CT that may be focal, multifocal or diffuse
- Associated mass effect with compression and distortion of cerebral ventricles and basal cisterns.

CT appearance of cerebral contusion:
- Areas of mixed high and low attenuation, which may be focal or multifocal
  - With time, the haemorrhagic component resolves leaving irregular areas of low attenuation.

Diffuse axonal injury occurs as a result of acute acceleration and deceleration of the brain. Cerebral cortex moves at a different speed to underlying white matter causing acute stretching of axons.
CT appearance of DAI:
- Small acute haemorrhages at the grey–white matter junctions, brainstem and corpus callosum.

CT tends to underestimate the degree of injury in DAI. DAI is suspected when the degree of neurological compromise following injury is out of proportion to CT findings. MRI is indicated

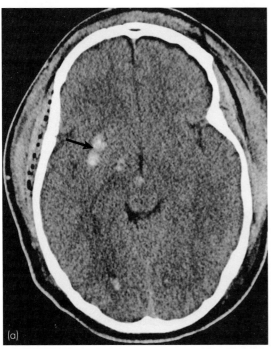 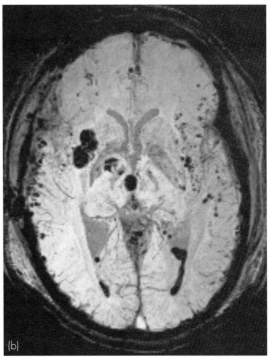

Figure 10.6 Diffuse axonal injury (DAI). Comatose 24-year-old male following head injury in high speed motor vehicle accident. (a) CT shows a small haemorrhage in the right basal ganglia (arrow). A couple of small haemorrhages are seen elsewhere plus a small amount of blood in the right lateral ventricle. (b) Transverse susceptibility-weighted MRI (SWI) shows the basal ganglia haemorrhage, blood in the lateral ventricles and extensive bilateral microhaemorrhages. These are seen as multiple foci of paramagnetic artefact producing small black spots. It can be seen that SWI is much more sensitive than CT for the detection of the microhaemorrhages associated with DAI.

in such cases, and is more accurate than CT at demonstrating typical features of DAI, such as focal microhaemorrhages and white matter oedema (Fig. 10.6).

Other CT signs that may be seen with cranial trauma:

- Fractures of skull base and skull vault
- Scalp swelling
- Intracranial air (pneumocephalus) due to penetrating injury or fractures through paranasal sinuses or temporal bones
- Fluid levels in paranasal sinuses
- Foreign bodies.

10.2 SUBARACHNOID HAEMORRHAGE

Patients with non-traumatic SAH present with sudden onset of severe headache, often accompanied by neck pain and stiffness, diminished consciousness and focal neurological signs. The most common causes of spontaneous SAH are ruptured cerebral artery aneurysm in 80–90 per cent and cranial arteriovenous malformation (AVM) in 5 per cent. Less common causes include spinal AVM, coagulopathy, tumour, and venous or capillary bleeding.

Most cerebral artery aneurysms are congenital 'berry' aneurysms. Berry aneurysms occur in 2 per cent of the population and are multiple in 10 per cent of cases. Increased incidence of berry aneurysms occurs in association with coarctation of the aorta and autosomal dominant polycystic kidney disease. Most berry aneurysms occur around the circle of Willis, the most common sites being:

- Anterior communicating artery
- Posterior communicating artery
- Middle cerebral artery

- Bifurcation of internal carotid artery
- Tip of basilar artery.

CT is the primary imaging investigation of choice in suspected SAH. CT that is positive for SAH is usually followed by CT angiography (CTA) to diagnose and define the cause. A negative CT does not exclude a small SAH; up to 5 per cent of patients with a proven SAH have a normal CT at initial presentation. In cases where there is strong clinical suspicion for SAH and CT is negative, CTA may be performed to try to demonstrate a berry aneurysm. Alternatively, in such cases, diagnostic lumbar puncture may be performed to look for blood in the CSF or xanthochromia. Potential problems with lumbar puncture include:

- False positive due to blood-stained ('traumatic') tap
- Problems with interpretation of xanthochromia
- Post-lumbar puncture headache.

10.2.1 CT

The roles of non-contrast-enhanced CT in SAH are:
- Confirm the diagnosis
- Suggest a possible site of bleeding and/or cause
- Diagnose complications.

Acute SAH shows on CT as high-attenuation material (fresh blood) in the basal cisterns, sylvian fissures, ventricles and cerebral sulci (Fig. 10.7). By localizing the greatest concentration of blood, a possible site of haemorrhage can be suggested, e.g. blood concentrated in a sylvian fissure indicates bleeding from the ipsilateral middle cerebral artery. Occasionally, the cause of SAH may be seen on non-contrast-enhanced CT, e.g. large aneurysm, AVM or tumour. Complications of SAH visible on CT include hydrocephalus and vasospasm. Hydrocephalus may occur within hours of the haemorrhage due to obstruction of CSF pathways with blood. Vasospasm may lead to ischaemia and infarction, seen on CT as areas of low attenuation.

10.2.2 CT angiography

Catheter angiography with selective catheterization of the carotid and vertebral arteries is the 'gold standard' for the diagnosis of cerebral aneurysms in the setting of SAH. In many centres, catheter

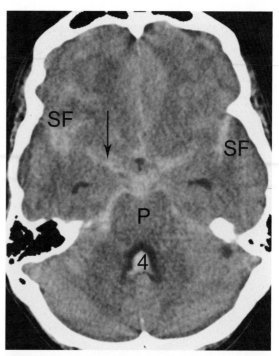

Figure 10.7 Subarachnoid haemorrhage. Acute blood is seen as high density material in the basal cisterns (arrow), anterior to the pons (P), in the Sylvian fissures (SF) and fourth ventricle (4).

angiography is reserved for use with interventional techniques (see below) and has been replaced by CTA (or MRA) for diagnosis. CTA is able to show the bleeding aneurysm (Fig. 10.8), demonstrate the relationship of the neck of the aneurysm to the vessel of origin, and to diagnose multiple aneurysms if present (10 per cent of cases). The sensitivity of CTA in the detection of cerebral artery aneurysms is similar to catheter angiography.

10.2.3 Screening for cerebral artery aneurysms

Indications for screening for cerebral artery aneurysms include:
- History of SAH or cerebral aneurysm in a first-degree relative
- Condition known to be associated with berry aneurysm including coarctation of the aorta and autosomal dominant polycystic kidney disease

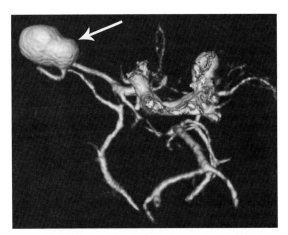

Figure 10.8 Cerebral aneurysm: CT angiogram. Three-dimensional reconstructed image from a CT angiogram shows an aneurysm of the right middle cerebral artery (arrow).

- Certain clinical presentations with a high probability of cerebral aneurysm, e.g. isolated third cranial nerve palsy, which may be caused by an aneurysm of the posterior communicating artery.

CT angiography and magnetic resonance angiography (MRA) may be used to image the cerebral vessels. Both techniques are of comparable sensitivity to catheter angiography for displaying aneurysms of 3 mm or greater. CTA and MRA each have relative advantages and disadvantages; choice of technique often depends on local expertise and availability.

Advantages of MRA:
- Non-invasive
- Contrast material injection is not required.

Disadvantages of MRA:
- Relatively long scan times that may be a problem in restless or claustrophobic patients
- Contraindicated in patients with pacemakers, ferromagnetic clips and implants, and ocular metal foreign bodies.

Advantages of CTA:
- Shorter scan times, therefore better tolerated in restless patients
- CTA performed with modern multidetector scanners has slightly higher sensitivity than MRA for detection of small aneurysms.

Disadvantages of CTA:
- Ionizing radiation
- Requires the use of iodinated contrast material.

10.3 STROKE

Transient ischaemic attack (TIA) is an acute neurological deficit that resolves completely within 24 hours. TIAs are thought to be caused by transient reduction of blood flow to the brain or eye due to emboli, and are associated with underlying stenosis of the internal carotid or cerebral arteries. Patients with TIA are usually investigated with CT of the brain and carotid Doppler US (see below).

The generic term 'stroke' refers to an acute event leading to a focal neurological deficit that lasts for more than 24 hours. Stroke may be caused by either decreased blood flow to the brain (ischaemia and infarction) or by intracranial haemorrhage.

Common causes of stroke:
- Cerebral ischaemia and infarction (acute ischaemic stroke): 80 per cent
- Parenchymal (primary intracerebral) haemorrhage: 15 per cent
  - Usually due to hypertension
  - Common sites: basal ganglia, brainstem, cerebellum and deep white matter of the cerebral hemispheres
- Spontaneous subarachnoid haemorrhage: 5 per cent (see above)
- Cerebral venous occlusion: <1 per cent.

Most acute ischaemic strokes are due to acute thromboembolic occlusion of cerebral arteries. Haemorrhagic infarction refers to haemorrhage into a region of infarcted brain. Haemorrhagic infarction may occur following clearing of an arterial occlusion with restoration of blood flow to damaged brain. Acute arterial occlusion produces a central region of infarcted brain tissue with a surrounding zone of hypoxic tissue. This hypoxic tissue is potentially salvageable and is termed the ischaemic penumbra. Intravenous infusion of thrombolytic agents such as tissue plasminogen activator (tPA) within the first 3 to 4.5 hours following stroke onset may salvage reversibly damaged brain tissue in the ischaemic penumbra. Thrombolysis with intravenous tPA is associated with improved neurological function in up to one in three patients. Risk of intracerebral haemorrhage producing an adverse outcome is about one in 30. tPA is contraindicated in the presence of haemorrhage.

10.3.1 Imaging of stroke

Based on the above principles, it can be seen that the primary goals of acute imaging in the investigation and management of stroke/TIA are:
- To diagnose the type of stroke, in particular to exclude haemorrhage in the acute situation
- Selection of patients suitable for treatment with tPA.

  Secondary goals of stroke imaging include:
- Identification of arterial stenosis and occlusion
- Identification of the source of emboli
- Identification of asymptomatic patients who may be at risk of stroke.

10.3.1.1 CT

CT is the investigation of choice in most centres for the initial assessment of the patient with symptoms of stroke or TIA. Early subtle CT changes of acute ischaemic stroke may be recognized within 3–6 hours of the onset of symptoms (Fig. 10.9):
- Mild cerebral swelling and mass effect
- Decreased attenuation of affected brain tissue
- Increased density of cerebral arteries due to thrombosis and vascular stasis.

  From 12 to 24 hours and over the next 3 days, there is increased oedema with more obvious flattening of cerebral gyri and mass effect. CT is sensitive to the presence of acute haemorrhage and is therefore highly accurate for the diagnosis of haemorrhagic causes of stroke, including haemorrhagic infarct, parenchymal haemorrhage and subarachnoid haemorrhage (Figs 10.10 and 10.11). The main limitation of CT is in the delineation of very subtle changes of early ischaemia.

10.3.1.2 CTA and perfusion CT

In specialist stroke centres, more sophisticated technologies based on interventional radiology may be used in the treatment of acute stroke, including:
- Intra-arterial infusion of tPA
  - Intra-arterial infusion of tPA has the theoretical advantage of achieving

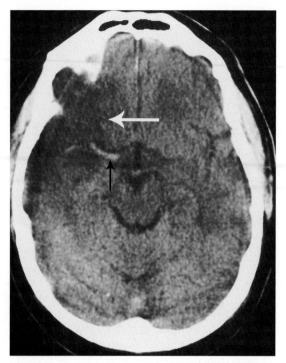

Figure 10.9 Early infarct seen on CT as an area of vague low attenuation (white arrow). Note also high attenuation in the right middle cerebral artery due to thrombosis (black arrow).

  recanalization of thrombosed arteries with use of a lower dose and therefore potentially fewer complications
- Various mechanical devices for removal of clot from occluded arteries.

  The main disadvantage of these interventional techniques is lack of availability. Where these techniques are available, the treatment window following acute stroke may be extended, in some cases up to 8 hours. In that time, more sophisticated imaging with CT or MRI may be performed to assist in patient and technique selection.

  CT angiography is able to provide visualization of the carotid arteries in the neck as well as the cerebral vessels; sites of arterial thrombosis and occlusion are clearly shown. For perfusion CT, CT scans of the brain are obtained during contrast infusion. Various parameters of cerebral perfusion are mapped, including:
- Cerebral blood flow
- Mean transit time
- Cerebral blood volume.

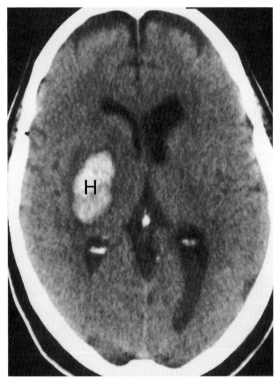

Figure 10.10 Primary hypertensive haemorrhage seen as an oval-shaped high attenuation lesion in the right basal ganglia (H).

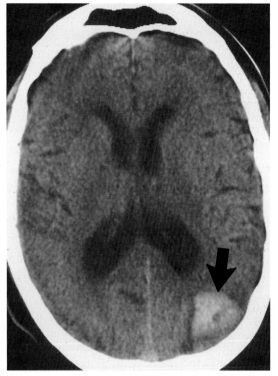

Figure 10.11 Haemorrhagic infarct seen as a peripheral wedge-shaped lesion in the left parieto-occipital region (arrow).

Areas of reduced perfusion demonstrated with perfusion CT may represent areas of 'salvageable' brain tissue. In some stroke centres CT now provides a detailed assessment of the patient with stroke as follows:

- Non-contrast-enhanced CT to exclude haemorrhage
- CTA to diagnose stenosis of internal carotid artery and occlusion of cerebral vessels
- Perfusion CT to map cerebral perfusion.

10.3.1.3 MRI

MRI with diffusion-weighted imaging (DWI) and perfusion-weighted imaging (PWI) is an alternative to CT in the identification of hyperacute infarction and ischaemia. DWI is sensitive to the random Brownian motion (diffusion) of water molecules within tissue.

Areas of reduced water molecule diffusion show on DWI as high signal. With the onset of acute ischaemia and cell death, there is increased intracellular water (cytotoxic oedema) with restricted diffusion of water molecules. An acute infarct therefore shows on DWI as an area of relatively high signal (Fig. 10.12). DWI is the most sensitive imaging test available for the diagnosis of hyperacute infarction.

Perfusion-weighted imaging can also be used to calculate the relative blood supply of a particular volume of brain. For PWI, the brain is rapidly scanned following injection of a bolus of contrast material (gadolinium). As for perfusion CT, the data obtained may be represented in a number of ways including maps of regional cerebral blood flow, cerebral blood volume and mean transit time. In general, the perfusion defects identified with PWI are larger than the diffusion abnormalities shown on DWI; the difference between these areas represents the ischaemic penumbra. MRI using DWI and PWI is therefore able to diagnose hyperacute infarction and identify the ischaemic penumbra.

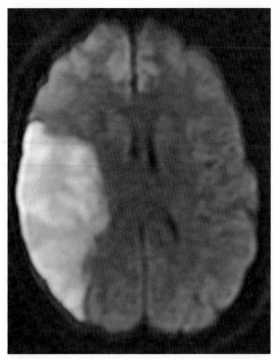

Figure 10.12 Acute cerebral infarct: MRI. Transverse diffusion-weighted MRI shows a large area of restricted diffusion in the right middle cerebral artery territory.

10.3.2 Identification of asymptomatic 'at risk' patients

Identification of patients at risk for developing stroke involves identification of risk factors plus the diagnosis of structural abnormalities.

Risk factors for stroke include:

- Hypertension
- Diabetes mellitus
- Hypercholesterolaemia
- TIA: approximately 30 per cent of patients with TIA will develop a subsequent infarct
- Coronary artery disease
- Severe peripheral artery disease.

Structural abnormalities include ischaemic changes in the brain and atheromatous disease of carotid, vertebral and basilar arteries.

10.3.2.1 Imaging of the brain

CT or MRI may be used to diagnose ischaemic changes in the brain including:

- Chronic deep white matter ischaemia
  - CT: low attenuation in the deep white matter (Fig. 10.13)
  - MRI: high signal in the deep white matter on T2-weighted and FLAIR images
- Old infarcts
- Lacunar infarcts
  - Small round infarcts in the basal ganglia and deep white matter.

10.3.2.2 Imaging of the carotid arteries

US examination of the carotid arteries is a useful screening test able to diagnose atheromatous disease causing stenosis and occlusion. Carotid US combines direct visualization of the arterial wall, colour Doppler examination of the arterial lumen, and measurement of blood flow velocity in the common carotid artery (CCA) and internal carotid artery (ICA). Blood flow velocity measurements include measurements of peak systolic velocity (PSV) and end diastolic velocity (EDV) given in cm/

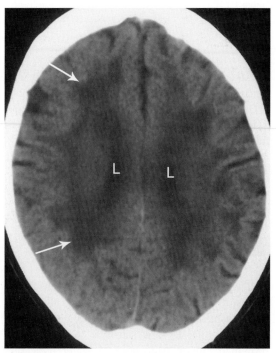

Figure 10.13 Chronic brain ischaemia: CT. A CT section at the level of the superior surfaces of the lateral ventricles (L) shows multiple bilateral areas of low attenuation in the white matter (arrows).

sec. Comparison of PSV for the CCA and ICA gives the ICA/CCA ratio. Stenosis is indicated by direct visualization of arterial narrowing plus increased measured flow velocity in the internal carotid artery (Fig. 10.14).

Based on the US appearance of the carotid arteries plus the measured blood flow velocities, the degree of ICA disease may be classified as follows:
- Normal: no plaque visualized; ICA PSV <125 cm/sec
- <50 per cent stenosis: plaque visualized; ICA PSV <125 cm/sec
- 50–69 per cent stenosis: plaque visualized; ICA PSV 125–230 cm/sec
- 70 per cent to near occlusion: plaque visualized; ICA PSV >230 cm/sec
- Near occlusion: markedly narrowed lumen visualized by colour Doppler
- Complete occlusion: no blood flow visualized by colour Doppler.

This classification is clinically relevant as carotid endarterectomy is beneficial in stenosis of 70 per cent to near occlusion, with no definite benefit shown for stenosis of <70 per cent. Complete ICA occlusion is considered to be inoperable. MRA or CTA may be performed where more definitive imaging of the carotid arteries is required.

10.4 BRAIN TUMOURS

Symptoms caused by brain tumours are quite variable as follows:
- Increased intracranial pressure caused by the tumour itself or hydrocephalus
  - Headache
  - Nausea and vomiting
  - Irritability
- Acute presentation (may be due to haemorrhage into the tumour)
  - Sudden severe headache
  - Stroke
  - Seizure
- Focal neurological disturbance
- Cranial nerve palsy
- Hormonal effects.

10.4.1 Classification and grading of brain tumours

Primary tumours of the central nervous system are classified and graded by the World Health Organization (WHO) (Table 10.1). WHO classifies primary tumours of the CNS into categories based on the cell or tissue of origin. WHO also grades primary brain tumours into four categories of increasing malignancy and aggressiveness: WHO grades I–IV. WHO grading does not always correlate with clinical outcome. A WHO I tumour may be in a location that makes it inoperable, e.g. pilocytic astrocytoma of the brainstem in children. Low grade astrocytomas have a tendency to progress to higher grade tumours.

Relative incidences of the various types of brain tumour vary between children and adults. In adults, metastases from non-CNS primary tumours account for 50 per cent of brain tumours. Of the primary brain tumours in adults, gliomas are the most common followed by meningioma, pituitary adenoma and vestibular schwannoma. Central nervous system (CNS) metastases are uncommon in children; most brain tumours in children are primary CNS lesions with the most common forms as follows:
- Astrocytoma of varying grade: 50 per cent

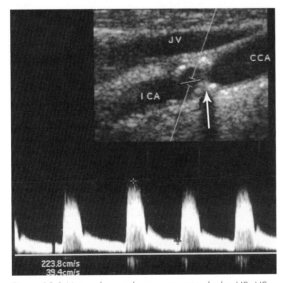

Figure 10.14 Internal carotid artery stenosis: duplex US. US shows a large calcified plaque (arrow) at the origin of the internal carotid artery (ICA). Velocity measurements indicate stenosis in the range of 50–69 per cent. Note also the common carotid artery (CCA) and internal jugular vein (JV).

Table 10.1 Brain tumours.

Tumour type	WHO grade	Age	Location
Pilocytic astrocytoma (Fig. 10.15)	I	Birth–9	Cerebellum, hypothalamus, optic nerves and chiasm
Diffusely infiltrating, low grade astrocytoma	II	20–40	Posterior fossa in children; supratentorial adults
Anaplastic astrocytoma	III	40–50	Frontal and temporal lobes
Glioblastoma multiforme	IV	45–70	Frontal and temporal lobes, pons, thalamus, corpus callosum
Ependymoma	II–III	Bimodal: 1–5; early 30s	Floor 4th ventricle (70%); supratentorial
Medulloblastoma (PNET-MB)	IV	<10	Cerebellar vermis, roof 4th ventricle
Supratentorial PNET	IV	<5	Frontal lobes
Meningioma	I	35–70	Supratentorial (90%): cerebral convexity, falx, sphenoid ridge Infratentorial (10%)
Schwannoma	I	35–60	8th cranial nerve (CN8) 90%; CN5, 7, 10, others rare
Pituitary adenoma	I	20–50	Pituitary gland

PNET, primitive neuroectodermal tumour; PNET-MB, PNET-medulloblastoma.

- Medulloblastoma: 15 per cent
- Ependymoma: 10 per cent
- Craniopharyngioma.

10.4.2 Imaging of brain tumours

The two imaging modalities used most commonly for the assessment of brain tumours are MRI and CT. MRI, including gadolinium enhancement, is generally regarded as the investigation of choice in most instances. MRI provides more detailed anatomical information and soft tissue characterization (Fig. 10.15). Use of specialized sequences including MR spectroscopy, DWI and PWI may occasionally be helpful. MRI of the entire neuroaxis (brain and spine) is often performed, particularly in the presence of tumours known to metastasize via CSF, e.g. medulloblastoma, germinoma.

CT may be used where MRI is unavailable, or for urgent clinical presentations such as sudden onset of severe headache or seizures. CT is more sensitive than MRI for the detection of calcification.

10.5 HEADACHE

Headache is a very common symptom. Common causes include stress or tension headache and migraine. Headache may also be a non-specific symptom of generalized malaise such as may occur in common viral or bacterial infections. Most patients with headache can be diagnosed and treated on clinical grounds, without any need for imaging assessment. There are, however, certain specific types of headache and associated clinical scenarios that do warrant imaging assessment and several examples of these are outlined below:

- Suspected subarachnoid haemorrhage (see above)
  - Sudden onset of severe headache
  - 'Worst headache of my life'
  - Associated neck pain and stiffness
  - Investigation of choice: CT
- Suspected space-occupying lesion: child
  - New onset headache, sleep related
  - No family history of migraine

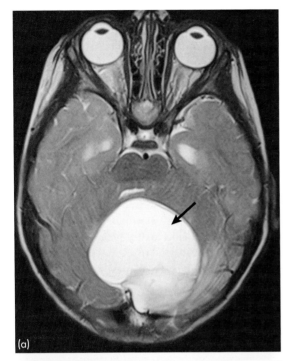

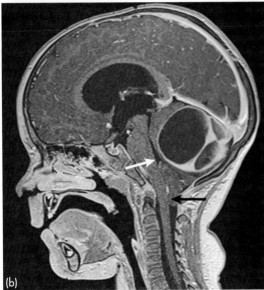

Figure 10.15 Juvenile pilocytic astrocytoma (WHO I): MRI. Four-year-old male with headaches and ataxia. (a) Transverse T2-weighted MRI shows a large space occupying lesion in the cerebellum. The lesion has a large cystic component (arrow). (b) Sagittal T1-weighted contrast-enhanced MRI shows enhancement of multiple septations plus the wall of the cystic component. Note that mass effect from the tumour is causing compression and distortion of the fouth ventricle (white arrow) and downward herniation of the cerebellar tonsils (black arrow).

- Papilloedema
- Investigation of choice: MRI (Fig. 10.15)
- Suspected space occupying lesion: adult
  - Signs of raised intracranial pressure
  - Headache, worse in the morning
  - Confusion; focal neurology: hemiparesis, focal seizures
  - Investigation of choice: MRI
  - CT if MRI contraindicated or difficult to obtain
- Suspected dissection of carotid or vertebral artery
  - Sudden onset of unilateral headache
  - Neck pain; ipsilateral Horner's syndrome
  - History of trauma or neck manipulation
  - Investigation of choice: MRI and MRA
- Suspected temporal arteritis
  - New headache in an elderly patient (>60)
  - Temporal tenderness
  - Increased ESR
  - Investigation of choice: MRI
- Suspected intracranial infection
  - New headache with fever
  - Neck stiffness with meningitis
  - Reduced consciousness with encephalitis
  - History of sinusitis or middle ear infection
  - History of immune compromise, including HIV
  - Investigation of choice: MRI with contrast material (gadolinium)
  - CT if MRI not available, although less sensitive than MRI for meningitis and encephalitis.

10.6 SEIZURE

Epilepsy is a common chronic condition that may be genetic or acquired, characterized by predisposition to recurrent seizures. Seizures are defined as abnormal electrical discharges in brain cells producing finite events of cerebral function. Classification of seizure type is important as this will help to guide the need for further investigation and subsequent management and counselling. The two broad categories of seizure type are primary generalized and partial. Primary generalized seizures originate simultaneously from both cerebral hemispheres and produce bilateral clinical symptoms.

Partial seizures originate from a localized area of the brain, based on clinical manifestations and EEG findings. Clinical manifestations of partial seizures may include focal motor or sensory disturbance, psychiatric symptoms, or autonomic signs or symptoms. Partial seizures are further classified as simple or complex: complex partial seizures are associated with loss of consciousness; simple partial seizures are not.

Most generalized seizure disorders are idiopathic. Most patients are referred for imaging for a first generalized seizure and in most cases this will not show an underlying abnormality. Partial seizures are more commonly associated with an underlying structural lesion:

- Vascular malformations
- Tumours
- Brain injury
- Developmental abnormalities.

In particular, developmental abnormalities of the temporal lobe and hippocampal formation are a common cause of partial complex seizures:

- Mesial temporal sclerosis: sclerosis and atrophy of the hippocampal formation
- Cortical dysplasia, characterized by abnormal areas of grey matter.

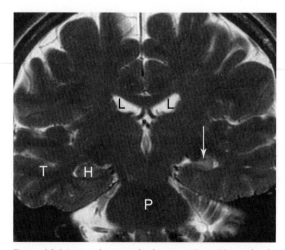

Figure 10.16 Mesial temporal sclerosis: MRI. A T2-weighted coronal scan through the temporal lobes (T) in a patient with complex partial seizures. Note the normal right hippocampus seen as an oval-shaped structure (H). The left hippocampus shows reduced size and increased signal indicating mesial temporal sclerosis (arrow). Note also the pons (P) and lateral ventricles (L).

MRI is the imaging investigation of choice for the assessment of seizure disorders. MRI of the brain is usually recommended in all patients presenting with a first seizure. MRI assessment should include high-resolution images of the temporal lobes in the coronal plane to search for developmental abnormalities, some of which may be extremely subtle (Fig. 10.16). Where MRI is unavailable, or in emergency situations, CT is able to detect surgical lesions such as haemorrhage or tumour.

10.7 DEMENTIA

The term dementia refers to deterioration of cognitive and intellectual functions not due to impaired consciousness or perception. Dementia should be differentiated clinically from delirium (acute transient confusion), psychiatric illness such as depression, and specific brain lesions leading to restricted function such as aphasia. Much research is currently directed at potential therapies for various types of dementia, making classification and accurate diagnosis increasingly important. Accurate diagnosis is also important for counselling of the patient and their family. The commonest causes of dementia are Alzheimer's disease (up to 80 per cent of cases) and multi-infarct dementia (10 per cent). Alzheimer's disease is suggested clinically by:

- Insidious onset of dementia after the age of 60 with progressive worsening
- Prominent loss of memory, especially of new material
- No focal neurological signs on examination.

Multi-infarct dementia occurs in patients with risk factors for atheromatous disease and stroke, such as tobacco smoking, hypertension and diabetes. Multi-infarct dementia is characterized clinically by:

- Sudden onset of cognitive decline with a step-wise deterioration in function
- Accompanying focal signs on neurological examination, such as weakness of an extremity or gait disturbance.

Less commonly, dementia may be due to communicating hydrocephalus or chronic subdural haematoma, with rare causes such as Pick's disease and Creutzfeldt–Jakob disease also described.

CT and MRI are the primary imaging investigations of the patient with dementia. MRI is more accurate than CT and is the investigation of choice. Signs of Alzheimer's disease on MRI include cortical atrophy in the parietal and temporal lobes with marked volume loss of the hippocampal formation. MRI and CT signs of multi-infarct dementia include multiple infarcts involving the basal ganglia, white matter and cortical grey matter (Fig. 10.13).

Scintigraphy may be useful in occasional cases where diagnostic difficulty is encountered with differentiating Alzheimer's disease from multi-infarct dementia on MRI. Scintigraphy may be performed to assess focal glucose metabolism with FDG-PET or regional cerebral blood flow with ^{99}mTc-HMPAO. FDG-PET shows reduced glucose metabolism in the temporal and parietal lobes in Alzheimer's disease; ^{99}mTc-HMPAO shows reduced blood flow in these regions. In multi-infarct dementia, FDG-PET shows focal areas of reduced cortical and white matter metabolism.

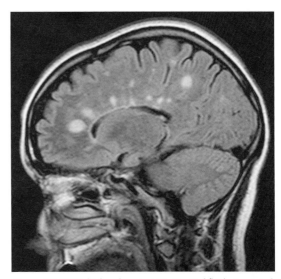

Figure 10.17 Multiple sclerosis: MRI. Sagittal fluid attenuated inversion recovery (FLAIR) MRI shows multiple high signal white matter lesions.

10.8 MULTIPLE SCLEROSIS

Multiple sclerosis (MS) is a chronic CNS disease of young adults characterized by the presence in the brain and spinal cord of focal lesions of demyelination, known as plaques. In the brain, MS has a fairly characteristic distribution, with plaques tending to occur along the walls of the cerebral ventricles, as well as the corpus callosum and posterior fossa. Plaques may also be seen in the spinal cord. Clinical presentation is extremely variable and may include double or impaired vision due to optic neuritis, weakness, numbness and tingling in the limbs, and gait disturbance. Clinical findings on neurological examination often reflect the multifocal nature of the disease. As well, the time course and nature of disease progression are quite variable.

Because of the importance of achieving a correct diagnosis in young adults, diagnostic criteria have been developed. Known as the 'McDonald criteria', these were released in 2001 and revised in 2005. The McDonald criteria incorporate a combination of clinical factors, CSF findings (oligoclonal IgG bands) and MRI appearances to diagnose MS.

MRI is the imaging investigation of choice for the diagnosis of MS. CT is not sensitive for the demonstration of MS plaques. Specific MRI sequences are required. FLAIR (fluid-attenuated

inversion recovery) sequence shows CSF as black and MS plaques as focal white lesions. FLAIR images provide accurate demonstration of subtle periventricular plaques (Fig. 10.17). Contrast material injection is also performed as so-called 'active' plaques may show enhancement. On follow-up MRI studies, the plaques may vary in appearance, with for example 'active' plaques becoming non-enhancing. This variation of appearances with time is an important feature of the McDonald criteria.

10.9 INTERVENTIONAL NEURORADIOLOGY

The basic tool of interventional neuroradiology is the microcatheter. Microcatheters can be advanced coaxially through larger catheters to access vascular pathology deep in the brain. Interventional neuroradiology encompasses a variety of endovascular techniques and indications, including:
- Coil embolization of aneurysms and occlusion of intracerebral AVMs, usually in the setting of SAH (Fig. 10.18)
- Intra-arterial infusion of vasodilator drugs for management of cerebral vasospasm, usually in the setting of subarachnoid haemorrhage
- Intra-arterial infusion of tPA in the treatment of stroke

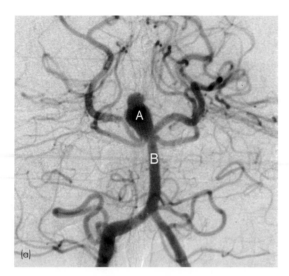

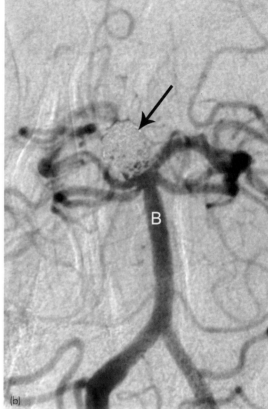

Figure 10.18 Treatment of cerebral aneurysm: interventional radiology. Aneurysm embolized with coils via superselective catheter. (a) Diagnostic angiogram showing an aneurysm (A) arising from the distal tip of the basilar artery (B). (b) Postprocedure subtracted angiogram image shows no blood flow into the aneurysm (arrow) indicating successful treatment.

- Intra-arterial infusion of tPA has the theoretical advantage of achieving recanalization of thrombosed arteries with use of a lower dose than with intravenous infusion, and therefore potentially fewer complications
- Mechanical devices for removal of thrombus from occluded arteries
- Angioplasty and arterial stenting in the management of atherosclerotic disease of the carotid and intracerebral arteries.

Patient preparation:
- Adequate informed consent
- Accurate imaging, including vascular supply and arterial anatomy
- Coagulation studies
- Pre-anaesthetic assessment.

Contraindications:
- Coagulopathy

- Lack of vascular access due to unsuitable arterial anatomy.

Disadvantages:
- Complications, though rare, are potentially devastating and include cerebral haemorrhage, stroke and death
- Imaging result often better than clinical outcome
  - For example, although intra-arterial tPA or mechanical thrombus retrieval may result in good rates of arterial recanalization, this may not always be accompanied by significant improvement in functional outcome
- Lack of evidence
  - Coiling of bleeding cerebral aneurysms is a well-established technique in the management of acute SAH
  - At the time of writing, large, multicentre randomized trials to assess the efficacy of most other neurointerventional techniques are yet to be published.

SUMMARY BOX

Clinical presentation	Investigation of choice	Comment
Traumatic brain injury	CT	MRI in selected cases
Subarachnoid haemorrhage	CT	
Screening for cerebral artery aneurysm	CTA/MRA	
TIA/stroke	CT head Carotid Doppler US	Increasing role in stroke centres for MRI and functional studies including DWI, PWI and perfusion CT
Brain tumour (suspected space-occupying lesion)	MRI	
Carotid or vertebral artery dissection	MRI/MRA	
Intracranial infection	MRI	
Seizure	MRI	
Dementia	MRI	Scintigraphy in selected cases: FDG-PET, ^{99m}Tc-HMPAO
Multiple sclerosis	MRI	

DWI, diffusion-weighted imaging; MRA, magnetic resonance angiography; PWI, perfusion-weighted imaging; TIA, transient ischaemic attack.

11 Head and neck

The topic of head and neck imaging covers a wide range of pathologies of the face and orbits, skull base and neck, and encompasses multiple specialties including ophthalmology, ENT, neurology, neurosurgery and endocrinology. The more common indications for head and neck imaging are outlined in this chapter.

11.1 FACIAL TRAUMA

For notes on head trauma, see Chapter 10.

11.1.1 Maxillary and zygomatic fractures

Radiographs using lateral, AP and angulated projections are usually performed in the initial assessment of facial trauma.

The zygomatic bone forms the 'cheekbone' at the inferolateral orbital margin. This outwardly convex part of the zygoma is composed of thick, tough bone. Zygomatic fractures occur in four points of relative weakness (Fig. 11.1):
- Inferior orbital margin
- Lateral wall of the maxillary sinus
- Zygomatic arch
- Lateral wall of orbit (usually diastasis of the zygomaticofrontal suture).

The Le Fort classification is used to describe fractures of the maxilla:
- Le Fort I: fracture line through the lower maxillary sinuses and nasal septum with separation of the lower maxilla
- Le Fort II: fracture lines extend from the nasal bones in the midline through the medial and inferior walls of the orbits and the lateral walls of the maxillary sinuses
- Le Fort III: fracture lines run horizontally

through the orbits and the zygomatic arches, causing complete separation of the facial bones from the cranium.

Other radiographic signs associated with facial fractures include:
- Soft tissue swelling
- Opacification or fluid levels in the maxillary sinuses
- Air in the orbit or other soft tissues.

CT is used commonly to define facial fractures and assist with planning of treatment (Fig. 11.2).

11.1.2 Orbital trauma

The most common type of orbital fracture is a blowout-type fracture of the orbital floor. Blowout orbital fracture is usually the result of a direct blow with sudden increase of intraorbital pressure producing a fracture of the orbital floor. This fracture may result in downward herniation of orbital contents into the maxillary sinus. Diplopia may occur due to entrapment of the inferior rectus muscle in the fracture. Radiographs may show a soft tissue mass in the shape of a 'teardrop' in the roof of the maxillary sinus (Fig. 11.3) due to downward herniation of orbital fat. The actual fracture is usually quite difficult to see radiographically. Coronal plane CT shows the fracture, as well as herniation of orbital structures into the maxillary sinus (Fig. 11.4).

Less commonly, due to blunt or penetrating trauma, there may be ocular injury. CT signs of ocular injury include:
- Deformity of the eyeball
- Intraocular haemorrhage seen on CT as an irregular area of increased attenuation in the vitreous.

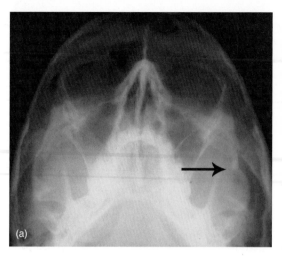

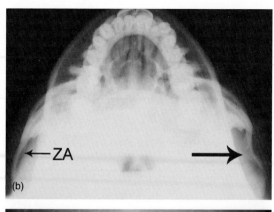

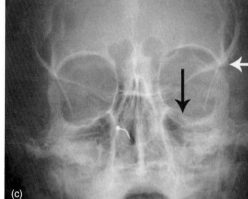

Figure 11.1 Zygomatic arch fracture: two examples. (a) Facial radiograph showing a depressed fracture of the left zygomatic arch (arrow). (b) Angulated view of (a) to show the zygomatic arches. Note the normal right zygomatic arch (ZA) and the fractured left arch (arrow). (c) Facial radiograph showing diastasis of the left zygomaticofrontal articulation (white arrow) plus a fracture of the orbital floor (black arrow). Note the fluid level in the left maxillary sinus due to blood. (The metal object is a nose stud.)

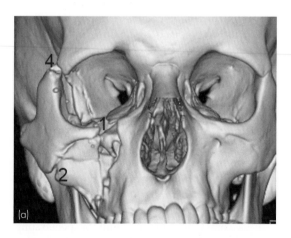

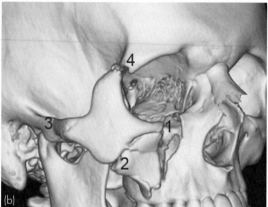

Figure 11.2 Zygomatic fracture: CT. Three-dimensional CT shows the four points of weakness at which zygomatic fractures occur: inferior orbital margin (1), lateral wall of the maxillary sinus (2), zygomatic arch (3) and zygomaticofrontal suture in lateral wall of orbit (4). (a) Frontal view. (b) Oblique view.

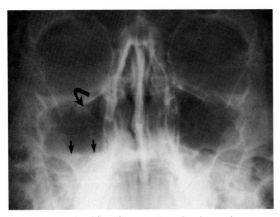

Figure 11.3 Orbital floor fracture. Frontal radiograph showing a fracture of the floor of the right orbit (curved arrow) with a round teardrop-shaped opacity in the roof of the maxillary sinus due to downward herniation of orbital fat. Note also the fluid level in the maxillary sinus due to blood (straight arrows).

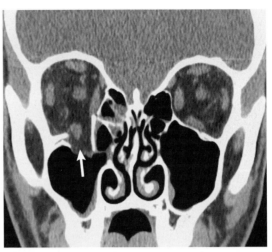

Figure 11.4 Orbital floor fracture: CT. Coronal CT images through the orbits showing a fracture of the right orbital floor with downward herniation of orbital fat and inferior rectus muscle (arrow) into the maxillary sinus.

Other extraocular injuries that may be seen on CT include optic nerve transection, retrobulbar haematoma and extraocular muscle damage.

11.1.3 Orbital foreign bodies

Radiographs may be used to diagnose radio-opaque foreign bodies and to localize these with respect to the bony margins of the orbit. Eye movement films give an idea of the position of a foreign body. US or CT may also be used for diagnosis and localization of orbital foreign bodies.

11.1.4 Mandibular fractures

Fractures of the mandible are usually the result of direct trauma. Being U-shaped, the mandible often fractures in two places. Due to the shape of the mandible plus the presence of complex, overlapping structures, radiography is often difficult. All parts of the mandible must be visualized in suspected mandibular fracture including midline, body, angle, ramus, condyle and coronoid process. Numerous radiographic views may be needed for full assessment of the mandible, including OPG (orthopantomogram). Used most commonly in dentistry, the OPG is a specialized radiographic technique, which gives a panoramic view of the tooth-bearing part of the mandible (Fig. 11.5).

11.2 IMAGING OF THE ORBIT

Imaging of orbital trauma is discussed above. Ophthalmologists and allied professionals diagnose most non-traumatic disorders of the eye and orbit without the need for imaging. Imaging is reserved for particular clinical indications including:
- Sudden loss of visual acuity
- Sudden onset of diplopia
- Exophthalmos (proptosis), especially when acute and progressive, painful or pulsatile
- Syndromes known to be associated with orbital pathology, such as neurofibromatosis
- To assess the extent of a known orbital tumour or vascular lesion.

Common orbital tumours include:
- Malignant tumours: retinoblastoma in children; ocular melanoma in adults; optic nerve glioma; lymphoma
- Optic nerve sheath meningioma
- Lacrimal gland tumours
- Vascular lesions: haemangioma; varix.

In many cases of suspected orbital pathology, imaging of the brain is also performed to diagnose lesions of the intracranial visual pathways or third, fourth and sixth cranial nerves. MRI and CT are the

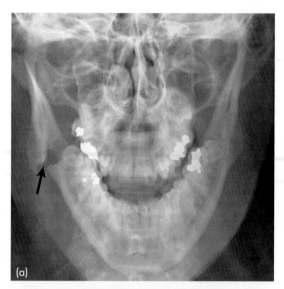

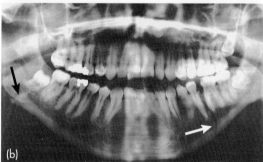

Figure 11.5 Mandible fractures: orthopantomogram (OPG). (a) Frontal radiograph shows a displaced fracture of the right angle of the mandible (arrow). (b) OPG shows a fracture of the left mandible (white arrow) as well as the right angle fracture (black arrow).

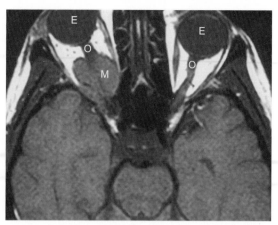

Figure 11.6 Orbital meningioma: MRI. Transverse T1-weighted transverse scan through the orbits shows the eyes (E) and optic nerves (O). A mass arising from the dural sheath of the right optic nerve has the typical appearance of a meningioma.

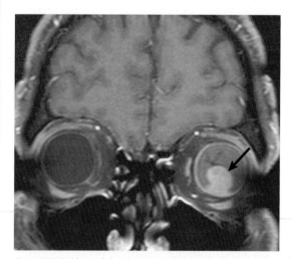

Figure 11.7 Choroidal melanoma: MRI. Coronal T1-weighted fat saturated contrast-enhanced MRI shows an enhancing mass in the posterior chamber of the left eye (arrow).

investigations of choice for orbital imaging. Both modalities have excellent natural contrast provided by the bony orbital margins and the orbital fat surrounding the optic nerve and extraocular muscles (Figs 11.6 and 11.7). MRI and CT often perform complementary roles in the imaging of orbital pathology. MRI has superior soft tissue contrast and is more accurate for delineating intracranial lesions of the visual pathways and cranial nerves. CT is more accurate for assessment of the bony margins of the orbit and for detecting calcification in vascular lesions and meningiomas.

11.3 IMAGING OF THE PARANASAL SINUSES

The paranasal sinuses are air-filled spaces in the medullary cavities of skull and facial bones. Named from the bones in which they occur, the paranasal sinuses consist of the frontal, ethmoid, maxillary and sphenoid sinuses. Paranasal sinuses drain by small ostia into the nasal cavities. Mucociliary action within the sinuses pushes debris towards the draining ostia. While a variety of congenital anomalies and tumours may affect the paranasal sinuses, the most common indication for imaging is inflammation. Paranasal sinus inflammation may be acute or chronic, and is commonly associated with disease in the nasal passages, in particular nasal polyposis in association with allergic sinusitis.

11.3.1 Acute sinusitis

Acute sinusitis is usually viral or bacterial and presents clinically with facial pain and headache, nasal discharge and fever. Diagnosis is usually made on clinical grounds and may be confirmed with nasal cultures or minimally invasive procedures such as endoscopic paranasal sinus aspiration. Imaging usually is not required for acute sinusitis. Indications for imaging in suspected acute paranasal sinusitis include:

- Lack of response to antibiotic therapy
- Immunocompromised patients
- Suspected complications, such as meningitis, subdural empyema or cerebral abscess.

Where imaging is required in acute sinusitis, CT is the investigation of choice. Radiographs may show fluid levels in the maxillary sinuses or sinus opacification, although are much less sensitive than CT.

11.3.2 Chronic sinusitis

Chronic sinusitis is defined as sinus inflammation of over 12 weeks' duration. Clinical presentation may include facial pain, nasal obstruction and reduced sense of smell. Chronic sinusitis may be bacterial, allergic or fungal. Functional endoscopic sinus surgery (FESS) is used to treat cases that do not respond to medical therapy. Imaging is performed to quantitate disease and to define relevant underlying anatomical anomalies that may restrict sinus drainage, as well as to assist in presurgical planning and postoperative follow-up. CT is the investigation of choice. The key images in assessing chronic sinusitis and planning FESS are coronal CT scans of the osteomeatal unit, i.e. the region of the drainage pathways of the maxillary, frontal and anterior ethmoid sinuses (Fig. 11.8).

11.4 IMAGING OF THE TEMPORAL BONE

The temporal bone is an extremely complex structure that contains the external auditory canal, middle and inner ear structures, and transmits the seventh cranial (facial) nerve (CN7). Middle ear structures include the tympanic membrane, aerated bony chambers, and three ossicles (malleus, incus,

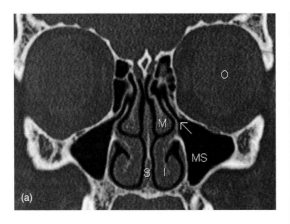
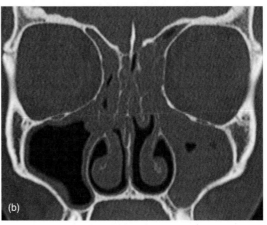

Figure 11.8 CT of the maxillary sinuses. (a) Normal sinuses: coronal CT through the osteomeatal unit. Note orbit (O), maxillary sinus (MS), sinus drainage pathway through maxillary ostium (arrow), middle turbinate (M), inferior turbinate (I), nasal septum (S). (b) Paranasal sinus disease: CT through the same level as (a). Note mucosal thickening on the right and almost complete opacification of the left maxillary sinus. Mucosal thickening is occluding both maxillary ostia. Compare this appearance with (a).

stapes) responsible for transmission of sound vibrations to the inner ear. Inner ear structures include the cochlea (responsible for hearing), vestibule and semicircular canals (responsible for balance), facial nerve canal and internal auditory canal (IAC). IAC transmits the facial nerve and the vestibular and cochlear components of the eighth cranial (vestibulocochlear) nerve (CN8). CN7 and CN8 exit the brainstem and pass laterally across a cerebrospinal fluid (CSF)-filled space known as the cerebellopontine angle (CPA) to enter the IAC.

11.4.1 Temporal bone fractures

Fractures of the temporal bone are usually discovered on CT performed for assessment of head injury. Less commonly, temporal bone fractures may present with hearing loss or CSF leak following recovery from acute head injury. Fractures are classified on CT as transverse or longitudinal depending on the relationship of the fracture line to the axis of the temporal bone.

Longitudinal temporal bone fractures run parallel to the long axis of the temporal bone, roughly in the coronal plane (Fig. 11.9). Longitudinal fractures may present with conductive hearing loss due to disruption of middle ear ossicles.

Transverse temporal bone fractures run in the

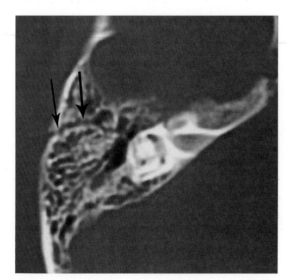

Figure 11.9 Temporal bone fracture (arrow): CT. Fracture runs in coronal plane parallel to long axis of temporal bone, i.e. longitudinal fracture.

sagittal plane, perpendicular to the long axis of the temporal bone. Transverse fractures often disrupt inner ear structures causing sensorineural hearing loss. Transverse fractures may also involve the facial nerve canal producing ipsilateral facial weakness.

11.4.2 Non-traumatic temporal bone pathology

Temporal bone pathology includes congenital anomalies, inflammatory conditions and tumours. Symptoms referable to the temporal bone and adjacent skull base include hearing loss, vertigo and tinnitus. These symptoms may occur in isolation or various combinations.

Hearing loss is assessed initially with audiometry. Hearing loss is classified as conductive, sensorineural or mixed, bilateral or unilateral. Conductive hearing loss results from lesions of the external or middle ear that prevent sound waves reaching the inner ear. Sensorineural hearing loss (SNHL) is due to pathologies of the cochlea or auditory nerve that prevent the transmission of neural impulses to the auditory cortex. Unilateral SNHL may be further classified clinically with brainstem electric response audiometry (BERA) into cochlear or retrocochlear pathology. Imaging is indicated if BERA indicates a retrocochlear cause for hearing loss.

Vertigo refers to an illusion of movement, such as rotation or tilt. Vertigo is classified as:
- Peripheral vertigo due to pathology of vestibule or semicircular canals
  - Suggested by features such as short duration, provocation with movement, pressure feeling in the ear
- Central vertigo due to pathology of the vestibular nerve or its connections in the brain.

Tinnitus refers to the subjective sensation of buzzing or ringing in the ear. Tinnitus may be classified as:
- Pulsatile: repetitive sound that accompanies the patient's pulse suggesting a vascular cause including glomus tumour, vascular malformation or acquired vasculopathy
- Non-pulsatile: constant sound that may be due to a lesion of the CPA, such as vestibular schwannoma.

Depending on clinical findings, imaging is commonly required for further assessment of hearing loss, vertigo and tinnitus. MRI with contrast enhancement is generally the imaging investigation of choice in cases of SNHL, tinnitus and central vertigo. MRI examination includes the brain, CPA and temporal bones. CT may be used as the first imaging investigation for conductive hearing loss. CT is also complementary to MRI in cases where fine bone detail is required.

11.4.3 Vestibular schwannoma ('acoustic neuroma')

One of the most common investigations in head and neck imaging is MRI to rule out acoustic neuroma. Acoustic neuroma refers to a nerve sheath tumour of CN8. These tumours are schwannomas, not neuromas, and usually involve the vestibular component of CN8, so 'vestibular schwannoma' is a more pathologically correct term. Vestibular schwannomas usually present in adults with slowly progressive unilateral SNHL, sometimes associated with tinnitus and vertigo. Vestibular schwannomas vary in size and are often quite small.

MRI is the imaging investigation of choice. High-definition MR scans are able to display the cranial nerves and inner ear structures in exquisite detail (Fig. 11.10). Where MRI is contraindicated, CT may be performed, though is less accurate for small tumours.

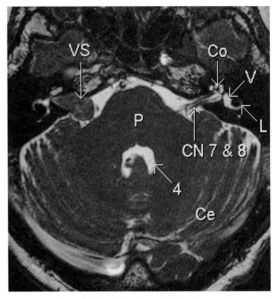

Figure 11.10 Vestibular schwannoma ('acoustic neuroma'): MRI. High resolution T2-weighted transverse scan through the posterior fossa shows the following: right vestibular schwannoma (VS), pons (P), fourth ventricle (4), cerebellum (Ce), normal left seventh and eighth cranial nerves (CN7 & 8), cochlea (Co), vestibule (V), lateral semicircular canal (L). (See also Fig. 1.36.)

11.5 NECK MASS

The anatomy of the neck is extremely complex and includes:
- Multiple compartments or spaces, separated by fat planes
- Multiple muscles, blood vessels and nerves
- Airway in the midline
- Cervical spine posterior
- Salivary glands and thyroid gland
- Lymph glands.

To make sense of this anatomy and to narrow the differential diagnosis for pathologies, the neck is divided by the hyoid bone into the suprahyoid and infrahyoid neck. Suprahyoid neck is further subdivided into various anatomical compartments including the parapharyngeal, masticator, parotid, carotid, retropharyngeal and perivertebral spaces. Spaces of the infrahyoid neck include visceral, anterior cervical, posterior cervical, carotid, retropharyngeal and perivertebral spaces. These anatomical spaces are all definable on CT and MRI, and to a lesser extent on US.

The roles of imaging in the investigation of neck masses include:
- Localization
- Characterization
  - Cystic or solid
  - Calcification or fat
  - Enhancement with intravenous contrast material
- Anatomical relations: position relative to the great vessels, thyroid gland, laryngeal cartilages
- Evidence of malignancy
  - Invasion of surrounding structures
  - Lymphadenopathy.

US is an accurate and non-invasive screening test for initial localization and characterization of a neck mass (Fig. 11.11). A specific diagnosis may often be made with US, particularly for cystic lesions such as branchial cleft cyst and thyroglossal cyst. US provides an excellent modality for guidance of fine needle aspiration (FNA), biopsy or cyst aspiration.

Depending on local availability and expertise, CT or MRI may be used to further delineate neck masses, particularly deep masses or complex and multifocal pathologies such as extensive lymphadenopathy. Both CT and MRI provide good localization of the plane of origin of a mass, plus definition of anatomical relations (Figs 11.12 and 11.13). Complications, such as invasion of surrounding structures and lymphadenopathy, are well seen. Some of the more commonly encountered neck masses include:

- Lymph node enlargement (lymphadenopathy)
  - Infection
  - Head and neck malignancy, such as squamous cell carcinoma (SCC) of the larynx or oral cavity
  - Systemic malignancy, including lymphoma
- Abscess: usually occurs in close relation to the airway in the parapharyngeal or retropharyngeal spaces
- Second branchial cleft cyst: presents in young adults with a mass of the upper neck anterior to the sternomastoid muscle

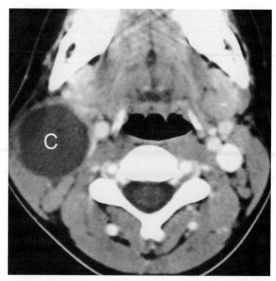

Figure 11.12 Second branchial cleft cyst (C): CT.

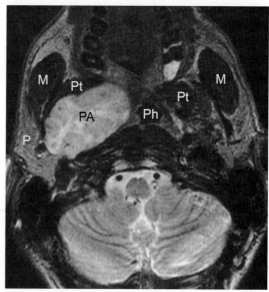

Figure 11.13 Mixed benign tumour: MRI. T2-weighted transverse scan through the oropharynx shows a mass (PA) arising from the deep lobe of the right parotid gland. Note also the superficial lobe of the right parotid gland (P), masseter muscles (M), oropharynx (Ph) and pterygoid muscles (Pt), compressed on the right by the mass.

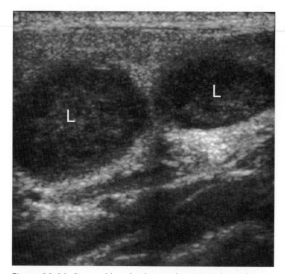

Figure 11.11 Cervical lymphadenopathy: US. Enlarged neoplastic lymph nodes seen on US as round hypoechoic masses (L).

- Thyroglossal duct cyst: cyst of remnants of the thyroglossal duct occurring anteriorly in the midline
- Lymphatic malformation (previously referred to as cystic hygroma)
  - Occurs in infants and young children

- Complex cystic mass of the lower lateral neck
  - Associated with Turner syndrome
- Dermoid cyst: midline cyst containing fat in the floor of the mouth
- Carotid body tumour: paraganglioma located in the bifurcation of the common carotid artery
- Masses and diffuse diseases of the thyroid gland are considered in Chapter 12.

11.6 SALIVARY GLAND SWELLING

Focal or diffuse salivary gland swelling may be due to inflammation, systemic disease or tumour. Causes of salivary gland inflammation:
- Bacterial: usually unilateral
- Viral: commonly bilateral
- Due to obstruction of salivary duct by a calculus.

Bilateral parotid gland swelling may be caused by various systemic diseases, including Sjogren syndrome and sarcoidosis.

Salivary gland tumours may be classified as follows:
- Benign
  - Benign mixed tumour (pleomorphic adenoma)
  - Adenolymphoma (Warthin's tumour)
- Malignant
  - Adenoid cystic carcinoma (cylindroma)
  - Mucoepidermoid carcinoma.

Other soft tissue tumours that may occur in the parotid gland include lipoma, neuroma and melanoma. Ratio of incidences of benign and malignant tumours varies according to which particular salivary gland is involved:
- Parotid: 80 per cent benign, 20 per cent malignant
- Submandibular: 50 per cent benign, 50 per cent malignant
- Sublingual: 20 per cent benign, 80 per cent malignant.

US is the initial imaging investigation of choice for salivary gland swelling:
- Differentiates intraparotid from extraparotid masses
- Able to diagnose most parotid and submandibular calculi (Fig. 11.14)

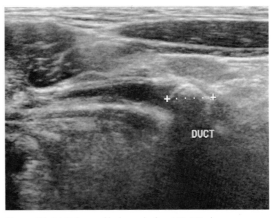

Figure 11.14 Submandibular calculus: US. US shows a dilated submandibular duct (arrows) with a calculus at its distal end (+).

- Visualization of dilated ducts
- Guidance of FNA.

MRI may be required for assessment of deep or large masses, particularly masses of the deep lobe of the parotid gland (Fig. 11.13).

Radiographs may be used where salivary gland calculus is suspected clinically:
- Most salivary calculi are visible on plain radiographs
- Specific views may be used for the gland of interest, such as intraoral films to show the submandibular ducts.

Sialography provides the most detailed visualization of salivary ducts:
- Salivary duct cannulated with a fine catheter
- Contrast medium injected
- Radiographs performed
- A salivary calculus appears as a filling defect within a localized expansion of the salivary duct.

Sialography is contraindicated in the presence of acute salivary gland infection. With increased expertise in the performance of US, sialography is no longer commonly performed in modern practice.

11.7 STAGING OF HEAD AND NECK CANCER

For principles of cancer staging, please see Chapter 14.

Head and neck cancer refers to cancers arising from the surface mucosa of four basic regions of the upper aerodigestive tract:

- Nasal cavity and paranasal sinuses
- Oral cavity: anterior two-thirds of tongue, hard palate, floor of mouth, buccal mucosa
- Pharynx
  - Nasopharynx: posterior to nasal passages
  - Oropharynx: posterior one-third of tongue, soft palate, tonsils, posterior pharyngeal wall
  - Hypopharynx: piriform sinuses, postcricoid posterior surface of larynx
- Larynx
  - Supraglottis: epiglottis, aryepiglottic folds, arytenoids, false vocal cords
  - Glottis: true vocal cords
  - Subglottis: from 1 cm below true cords to trachea.

Histologically, most head and neck cancers are SCC. Other less commonly encountered tumour types include adenocarcinoma, sarcoma and lymphoma. Major risk factors for the development of SCC of the head and neck include tobacco use and heavy alcohol intake. These tumours are most common in male adults, although the relative incidence of head and neck SCC in females is rising. There is also an increasing incidence of SCC of the hypopharynx in younger adults, associated with human papilloma virus (HPV). These HPV-positive tumours tend to have a better prognosis than HPV-negative SCC.

Clinical presentation of head and neck cancer may include sore throat, hoarse voice or stridor. Another common presentation is with a painless neck lump due to lymph node metastasis (Fig. 11.11). SCC of the head and neck spreads by local invasion through the mucosal surface to deep structures. Lymph node metastases are common. Distant metastases may also occur, most commonly in the lungs. Relevant factors for staging of head and neck cancer include size of primary tumour, extent of local invasion and presence of cervical lymphadenopathy.

Squamous cell carcinoma of the head and neck is assessed initially with direct clinical examination. Laryngoscopy is used for assessment of the laryngeal mucosal surface. CT is the traditional imaging investigation of choice for further staging of head and neck cancer. SCC of the head and neck appears on CT as a high attenuation mass causing asymmetry and anatomical distortion of the airway. Invasive tumours cause obliteration of surrounding fat planes. MRI may be used in a problem-solving role, e.g. for confirmation of laryngeal cartilage invasion. Increasingly, MRI is used as the initial staging modality for head and neck cancer. US-guided FNA of cervical lymph nodes is useful for assessment of nodes that are considered equivocal on CT or MRI. US-guided FNA also has an increasing role in primary diagnosis for tumours that present clinically with an enlarged lymph node and no obvious mucosal lesion. Positron emission tomography (PET)–CT may be useful to assess response to therapy, and in postoperative patients to diagnose recurrent SCC.

SUMMARY BOX

Clinical presentation	Investigation of choice	Comment
Facial trauma	Radiography	CT to define anatomy
Symptoms of orbital pathology, e.g. visual symptoms, proptosis	MRI/CT	MRI and CT often complementary in orbital pathology
Chronic sinusitis	CT	
Symptoms of temporal bone pathology, e.g. hearing loss, tinnitus, vertigo	MRI/CT	MRI and CT often complementary in skull base pathology
Neck mass	US: initial assessment CT/MRI: further definition	
Salivary gland swelling	US: initial assessment MRI: complex or deep lesions	
Staging of head and neck cancer	CT/MRI	US-guided FNA for enlarged or equivocal lymph nodes

FNA, fine needle aspiration.

12 Endocrine system

12.1 IMAGING OF THE PITUITARY

The pituitary gland consists of two functionally separate components:
- Adenohypophysis (anterior lobe): secretes hormones including adrenocorticotropic hormone (ACTH), thyroid stimulating hormone (TSH), luteinizing hormone (LH), follicle stimulating hormone (FSH) and growth hormone
- Neurohypophysis (posterior lobe): stores hormones secreted by hypothalamus (vasopressin and oxytocin).

The pituitary stalk connects the pituitary gland to the hypothalamus and contains axons that transport releasing hormones. Tumours of the pituitary region include:
- Pituitary adenomas, classified on hormonal status (Table 12.1) and on size criteria
  - Macroadenoma: >10 mm (Fig. 12.1)
  - Microadenoma: <10 mm (Fig. 12.2)
- Pituitary carcinoma (rare)
- Meningioma
- Craniopharyngioma
- Metastasis
- Optic chiasm glioma
  - Commonly associated with neurofibromatosis, type 1.

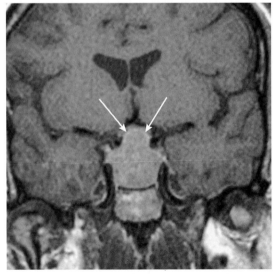

Figure 12.1 Pituitary macroadenoma: MRI. Coronal T1-weighted contrast-enhanced MRI of the pituitary gland shows an enhancing mass projecting superiorly from the pituitary fossa and compressing the optic chiasm (arrows).

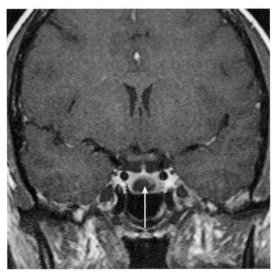

Figure 12.2 Pituitary microadenoma: MRI. Coronal T1-weighted contrast-enhanced MRI of the pituitary gland shows a small non-enhancing mass (arrow) surrounded by normally enhancing pituitary tissue.

Table 12.1 Clinical syndromes associated with pituitary adenomas.

Adenoma type	Relative incidence (%)	Hormone produced	Clinical presentation
Prolactinoma	30	Prolactin	Amenorrhoea, galactorrhoea, infertility
Corticotrophic adenoma	14	ACTH	Cushing syndrome
Somatotrophic adenoma	14	Growth hormone	Gigantism; acromegaly
Gonadotroph cell adenoma	7	FSH, LH	Menstrual irregularity; headache
Thyrotroph cell adenoma	1	TSH	Thyrotoxicosis
Plurihormonal adenoma	5	Multiple	Variable
Non-functioning adenoma	27	None	Pressure effects

ACTH, adrenocorticotropic hormone; FSH, follicle stimulating hormone; LH, luteinizing hormone; TSH, thyroid stimulating hormone.

Pituitary region tumours may present clinically in multiple ways depending on the size, location and hormonal status of the tumour:
- Compression of structures
  - Pituitary: hypopituitarism
  - Optic chiasm: bitemporal hemianopia
- Raised intracranial pressure due to a large tumour or obstructive hydrocephalus
  - Headache, nausea, vomiting
- Endocrine syndromes.

Endocrine syndromes associated with pathology of the pituitary gland and hypothalamus include:
- Pituitary dwarfism
  - Hypoplasia of adenohypophysis
  - Ectopic neurohypophysis
  - Absent pituitary stalk
- Central diabetes insipidus
  - Dysfunction of neurohypophysis or hypothalamus due to tumour, Langerhans cell histiocytosis, infection or trauma
- Precocious puberty
  - Hamartoma or other neoplasm of hypothalamus
- Hypersecretion syndromes
  - Pituitary adenomas (see Table 12.1).

MRI is the investigation of choice for imaging of the pituitary gland and adjacent structures. Sagittal T1-weighted images demonstrate the lobar anatomy of the pituitary (see Fig. 10.2a):
- Adenohypophysis of similar signal intensity to brain tissue

- Neurohypophysis seen as a posterior 'bright spot'.

Coronal T1-weighted scans with contrast enhancement are particularly useful for the diagnosis of microadenomas. Where MRI is unavailable or contraindicated CT may be used, however it is much less sensitive.

12.2 THYROID IMAGING

Common clinical indications for imaging of the thyroid gland include hyperthyroidism (thyrotoxicosis), diffuse thyroid enlargement, and focal thyroid mass or nodule. The most commonly used imaging techniques for the investigation of thyroid diseases are US, US-guided fine needle aspiration (FNA), and scintigraphy with ^{99}mTc or radioiodine. CT or MRI may be used to outline the anatomy of large goitres prior to surgical removal, particularly where there is retrosternal extension into the upper mediastinum.

12.2.1 Hyperthyroidism (thyrotoxicosis)

Thyrotoxicosis refers to a spectrum of clinical and biochemical findings that occur due to excess thyroid hormone:
- Heat intolerance, inability to sleep, weight loss and palpitations
- Elevated serum triiodothyronine (T3) and/or thyroxine (T4)

- Rarely, elevated TSH levels may indicate a TSH-secreting pituitary adenoma
- More commonly, TSH levels are low indicating a thyroid problem.

In cases with a typical presentation for Grave's disease, treatment may be instituted without further investigation.

Where imaging is required scintigraphy with ^{99m}Tc or radioiodine is the investigation of choice. ^{99m}Tc is more widely available than radioiodine and has a lower radiation dose. In the context of thyrotoxicosis, scintigraphy with ^{99m}Tc is useful for differentiating Grave's disease from other causes of thyrotoxicosis, including subacute thyroiditis, multinodular goitre and toxic adenoma.

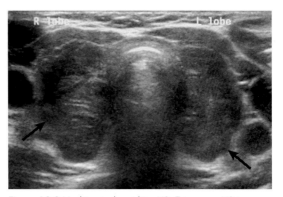

Figure 12.3 Hashimoto thyroiditis: US. Transverse US image of the lower neck shows symmetrical enlargement and reduced echogenicity of the thyroid gland (arrows).

12.2.2 Diffuse thyroid enlargement

Causes of diffuse thyroid enlargement include Grave's disease, Hashimoto thyroiditis, subacute thyroiditis and multinodular goitre. Diagnosis is often achieved by clinical history and examination, plus laboratory tests for thyroid function and antibodies. These may be complemented by thyroid scintigraphy with ^{99m}Tc, and US with colour Doppler (Table 12.2 and Fig. 12.3).

12.2.3 Thyroid nodules and masses

A thyroid nodule is defined as a discrete mass lesion in the thyroid gland, distinguishable from thyroid parenchyma on US. Thyroid nodules most commonly are benign colloid nodules. Follicular adenoma is a true benign neoplasm of the thyroid gland. Thyroid carcinoma is usually of epithelial origin and is classified into papillary, follicular, medullary and anaplastic. Papillary carcinoma is the most common type (75–80 per cent); it has an excellent prognosis with a 30-year survival rate of 95 per cent.

Thyroid nodules are extremely common, found in up to 40 per cent of adults on US examination. Thyroid cancer, on the other hand, is quite uncommon. It follows that the majority of thyroid nodules are benign. Thyroid nodules may be assessed clinically and with imaging, the aim being to decide which nodules may be malignant.

Clinical factors associated with an increased likelihood of a nodule being malignant include:

- Family history of thyroid cancer
- History of irradiation to the neck
- Patient age <20 or >60
- Rapid growth of the nodule
- Fixation to adjacent structures
- Vocal cord paralysis
- Adjacent lymphadenopathy.

US is the imaging investigation of choice for characterization of thyroid nodules. Features of thyroid nodules assessed with US include:

Table 12.2 Imaging appearances of common diffuse thyroid diseases.

Disease	^{99m}Tc scintigraphy	US
Grave's disease	Intensely increased uptake	Enlarged, hypoechoic and hypervascular thyroid
Hashimoto thyroiditis (chronic lymphocytic thyroiditis)	Reduced uptake	Hypoechoic and hypervascular thyroid
Subacute (De Quervain) thyroiditis	Reduced uptake	Mildly enlarged and hypervascular thyroid
Multinodular goitre	Patchy uptake	Enlarged thyroid with multiple solid nodules

- Size: the incidence of cancer in nodules smaller than 1 cm is extremely low
- Composition: cystic, solid or mixed
- Margins: well-defined margin or 'halo'; irregular margins
- Calcification: coarse or fine
- Vascularity.

US-guided FNA is usually definitive (Fig. 12.4). FNA is indicated for solitary nodules with the following features:

- >1.0 cm with fine calcifications
- >1.5 cm if predominantly solid or with coarse calcifications
- >2.0 cm if mixed solid and cystic components.

Where multiple nodules are present, each nodule is judged on its merits using the criteria above. Nodules not meeting the above criteria may still be referred for FNA if there is suspicion of malignancy on clinical grounds.

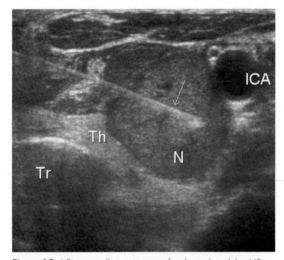

Figure 12.4 Fine needle aspiration of a thyroid nodule: US guidance. A transverse US image shows a fine needle (arrow) entering a nodule (N) in the left lobe of the thyroid (Th). Note also the trachea (Tr) in the midline and the internal carotid artery (ICA) lateral to the nodule.

12.3 PRIMARY HYPERPARATHYROIDISM

Primary hyperparathyroidism is the most common indication for imaging of the parathyroid glands. Causes of primary hyperparathyroidism:

- Solitary parathyroid adenoma: 80 per cent
- Multiple parathyroid adenomas: 7 per cent
- Parathyroid hyperplasia: 10 per cent
- Parathyroid carcinoma: 3 per cent.

Imaging is indicated in hyperparathyroidism to localize the causative lesion prior to surgery; this is relevant where minimally invasive surgery is intended. In centres where bilateral neck exploration is the standard procedure, preoperative imaging for localization of parathyroid adenoma is not always performed. Where preoperative localization is required, US is the investigation of first choice. US with high-resolution equipment has a high sensitivity (80–90 per cent) for the detection of parathyroid adenoma. US appearance of parathyroid adenoma is a well-defined hypoechoic mass usually of around 1.0–1.5 cm in diameter (Fig. 12.5). Most parathyroid adenomas lie behind or immediately below the thyroid gland. The principal cause of a false-negative US is ectopic adenoma, which may be present in up to 10 per cent of cases; ectopic sites include mediastinum and carotid sheath.

Where US is negative further imaging may be performed, i.e. scintigraphy, CT or MRI. The imaging technique chosen usually reflects local expertise and availability. Scintigraphy with ^{99}mTc-sestamibi shows a high rate of uptake in parathyroid adenoma and is especially useful for ectopic or multiple adenomas (Fig. 12.6). Postoperative imaging for recurrent or persistent hyperparathyroidism is best performed with US complemented by sestamibi scintigraphy.

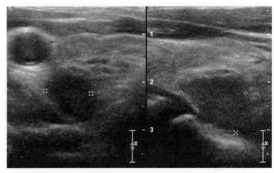

Figure 12.5 Parathyroid adenoma: US. Two US images, transverse on the left and longitudinal on the right, show a small hypoechoic nodule posterior to the right lobe of the thyroid gland.

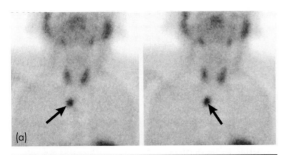

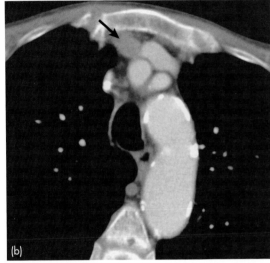

Figure 12.6 Ectopic parathyroid adenoma: scintigraphy and CT. (a) Sestamibi scan shows a small focus of increased activity in the right mediastinum (arrow) in a patient with hypercalcaemia. Note normal physiological uptake of sestamibi by the salivary and thyroid glands. (b) Transverse contrast-enhanced CT confirms a small mass in the upper right mediastinum (arrow).

12.4 ADRENAL IMAGING

The adrenal gland is essentially made up of two separate organs, the adrenal cortex and the adrenal medulla:

- Adrenal cortex: endocrine gland composed of fat-rich cells
  - Secretes cortisol, aldosterone and androgenic steroids
- Adrenal medulla: develops from the neural crest
  - Secretes adrenaline and noradrenaline.

Indications for imaging of the adrenal glands include:

- Endocrine syndromes
  - Cushing syndrome
  - Hyperaldosteronism
- Suspected phaeochromocytoma
- Incidentally discovered adrenal mass.

CT is the investigation of choice for imaging of the adrenal glands. MRI and scintigraphy may occasionally be useful for specific indications. More specialized techniques, such as adrenal vein sampling and percutaneous biopsy, rarely may be required.

12.4.1 Adrenal endocrine syndromes

12.4.1.1 Cushing syndrome

Causes of Cushing syndrome:

- Excessive ACTH production (70 per cent) (Cushing disease)
  - Usually due to pituitary adenoma
- Ectopic ACTH production by tumours (10 per cent)
  - Bronchial carcinoid, thymoma, islet cell tumour
- Adrenal disease 20 per cent

Adrenal causes of Cushing syndrome may be further classified as follows:

- Bilateral adrenal hyperplasia (70 per cent)
- Unilateral adrenocortical adenoma (20 per cent)
- Adrenal carcinoma (10 per cent).

Biochemical assessment of the patient with Cushing syndrome includes measurement of serum ACTH levels. Elevated ACTH indicates pituitary or ectopic production; low or undetectable levels of ACTH indicate adrenal disease. Patients with elevated ACTH may then undergo a high-dose dexamethasone suppression test. Cortisol suppression indicates a pituitary source of ACTH; lack of cortisol suppression suggests an ectopic source.

Imaging investigation of Cushing syndrome guided by biochemical testing is therefore as follows:

- Suspected pituitary source of ACTH: MRI of the pituitary gland
- Suspected ectopic source of ACTH: CT of chest and abdomen
- Suspected adrenal disease: CT of the adrenal glands.

12.4.1.2 Primary hyperaldosteronism (Conn syndrome)

Primary hyperaldosteronism is thought to be responsible for up to 10 per cent of cases of hypertension. The diagnosis of primary hyperaldosteronism is established biochemically with measurement of plasma aldosterone concentration to plasma renin activity ratio (PAC/PRA). Causes of primary hyperaldosteronism (Conn syndrome):

- Solitary unilateral adrenal adenoma (70 per cent)
- Multiple adrenal adenomas (20 per cent)
- Bilateral adrenal hyperplasia (10 per cent)
- Adrenal carcinoma (rare).

CT of the adrenal glands is the initial investigation of choice. When bilateral adrenal disease is seen on CT, or when CT is normal, bilateral selective adrenal vein sampling for aldosterone levels may be helpful to localize a small abnormality and therefore guide management.

12.4.1.3 Primary adrenal insufficiency (Addison disease)

Causes of primary adrenal insufficiency (Addison disease):

- Usual cause: idiopathic (probably autoimmune) adrenal atrophy
- TB
- Sarcoidosis
- Bilateral adrenal haemorrhage
  - Birth trauma, hypoxia, and sepsis in neonates
  - Anticoagulation therapy or sepsis in adults.

CT of the adrenal glands is the investigation of choice.

12.4.2 Phaeochromocytoma

Phaeochromocytoma is a tumour arising from chromaffin cells of the adrenal medulla. Ninety per cent occur in the adrenal gland and 10 per cent in ectopic extra-adrenal locations. Phaeochromocytoma usually presents with symptomatology related to excess catecholamine production:

- Paroxysmal or sustained hypertension
- Headaches, sweating, flushing
- Nausea and vomiting
- Abdominal pain.

Urine analysis reveals elevated levels of vanillylmandelic acid (VMA).

Phaeochromocytoma may also be discovered due to a hypertensive crisis brought on by surgery or some other stress. Ten per cent arise as part of a syndrome, e.g. multiple endocrine neoplasia, familial phaeochromocytoma, tuberous sclerosis, and Von Hippel–Lindau disease, neurofibromatosis. Ten per cent are malignant. Phaeochromocytomas are usually large tumours, measuring up to 12 cm with an average around 5 cm.

CT of the abdomen, with particular attention to the adrenal glands is the initial imaging investigation of choice in the diagnosis of phaeochromocytoma. When the adrenal glands are normal on CT and no obvious mass is seen elsewhere, whole body scintigraphy with iodine-labelled metaiodobenzylguanidine (^{131}I-/^{123}I-MIBG) may be useful. MRI of the abdomen may be used where MIBG is not available.

12.4.3 The incidentally discovered adrenal mass

Benign adrenal adenomas occur in 1–2 per cent of the population. Incidental adrenal masses are a common finding on CT of the abdomen. Patients with an incidentally discovered adrenal mass should be assessed for clinical evidence of Cushing syndrome and hypertension; depending on the clinical findings, biochemical screening for Cushing syndrome, hyperaldosteronism or phaeochromocytoma may be indicated.

Adrenal mass is a particularly significant finding where there is a history of malignancy. Tumours with a high incidence of metastasizing to the adrenal glands include melanoma, lung, breast, renal, gastrointestinal tract and lymphoma. Fifty per cent of adrenal masses seen in patients with primary carcinoma elsewhere are benign adenomas, not metastases. It is important to differentiate benign from malignant masses, specifically adrenal adenoma from adrenal metastasis or carcinoma.

CT features of a benign adrenal adenoma (Fig. 12.7):

- Small size (<3 cm)
- Smooth contour

- Low density on unenhanced scans due to the high fat content of normal adrenal cells (Fig. 9.10).

CT features of adrenal carcinoma include:
- Relatively large size (>5 cm)
- Higher density on unenhanced scans with low density centrally due to necrosis
- Other evidence of malignancy, such as liver metastases, lymphadenopathy, venous invasion.

Adrenal metastases also tend to be larger in size (>3 cm) and of higher density on unenhanced scans.

Equivocal lesions may be further assessed with multiphase contrast-enhanced CT. Attenuation value of the adrenal mass is measured pre-contrast injection and then at 60 seconds and 15 minutes after injection. Adrenal adenomas show rapid enhancement and subsequent washout with intravenous contrast material. Adrenal adenoma will show low attenuation pre-contrast, high attenuation at 60 seconds, and significantly reduced attenuation at 15 minutes.

MRI, including chemical shift imaging may also be useful in differentiating adrenal adenoma from malignancy. Chemical shift imaging exploits the slightly different precession frequency of hydrogen atoms in water from those in fat. At certain time intervals, the hydrogen atoms in water and fat will be perfectly in phase and at other times, out of

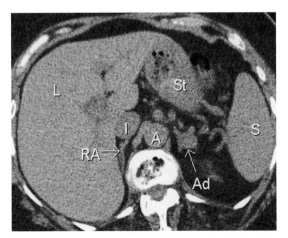

Figure 12.7 Adrenal adenoma: CT. A low attenuation mass (Ad) is seen arising on the left adrenal gland. Note also right adrenal gland (RA), liver (L), inferior vena cava (I), aorta (A), stomach (St), spleen (S).

phase. A good analogy is to think of two children on swings in a playground, one swinging slightly faster than the other. At certain times, both children will be at the top of their arcs at the same time; at other intervals, the swings will be at opposite ends of their arcs. Where fat and water molecules are in close contact, such as in fat-rich adrenal cells, scans timed to detect the molecules in phase will show high signal, while scans timed to be out of phase will show reduced signal. So it is that with chemical shift MRI, normal adrenal tissue and adrenal adenomas show reduced signal on out of phase scans (Fig. 12.8). Adrenal metastases show relatively increased signal on the out of phase scans allowing differentiation from benign adrenal adenoma.

Occasionally, when imaging is unable to confidently classify an adrenal mass as either benign or malignant, and where that adrenal mass is the only evidence of metastasis in a patient with a primary tumour, percutaneous biopsy under CT guidance may be required for definitive diagnosis.

12.5 OSTEOPOROSIS

Osteoporosis may be defined as a condition in which the quantity of bone per unit volume or bone mineral density (BMD) is decreased. Osteoporosis is an enormous public health issue, increasing in incidence with the gradual ageing of the population. It leads to fragility of bone with an increased incidence of fracture, particularly crush fractures of the vertebral bodies, and hip and wrist fractures. Treatment of osteoporosis can help to prevent further bone loss and reduce the incidence of fragility fractures. The three most important factors in the decision to treat osteoporosis are the age of the patient, the presence of a previous fragility fracture and the BMD.

Accurate measurement of BMD is the key to the diagnosis of osteoporosis and the decision to institute treatment. Dual X-ray absorptiometry (DEXA) is widely accepted as a highly accurate, low radiation dose technique for measuring BMD. DEXA uses an X-ray source, which produces X-rays of two different energies. The lower of these energies is absorbed almost exclusively by soft tissue. The higher energy is absorbed by bone and soft tissue. Calculation of the two absorption patterns gives

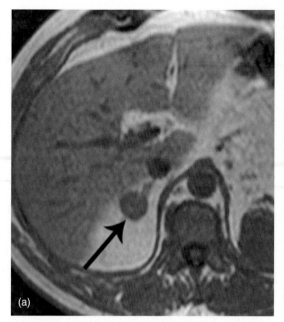
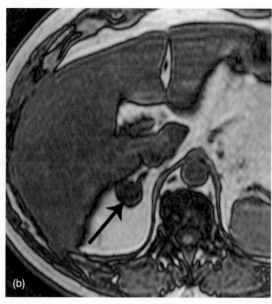

Figure 12.8 Adrenal adenoma: chemical shift MRI. (a) In-phase gradient echo scan shows a small round mass on the right adrenal gland (arrow). (b) Out-of-phase gradient echo scan shows reduced signal intensity in the mass (arrow) typical of an adrenal adenoma.

an attenuation profile of the bone component from which BMD may be estimated. Measurements are usually taken from the lumbar spine (L2–L4) and the femoral neck. The DEXA report gives an absolute measurement of BMD expressed as grams per square centimetre (g/cm^2). This value is compared with a normal young adult population to give a 'T score', expressed as the number of standard deviations from the mean.

Osteoporosis is defined as a BMD of 2.5 standard deviations below the young normal adult mean, i.e. a T score of equal to or less than −2.5. A T score of −1 to −2.5 is defined as osteopaenia, with normal being a T score of more than −1.

Treatment of osteoporosis includes drug regimes including biphosphonates, hormone replacement therapy, and weight-bearing exercise. There is good evidence for the following treatment guidelines based on BMD as calculated with DEXA:

- T score more than −1: no treatment
- T score −1 to −2.5: treatment if there is a previous fragility fracture
- T score less than −2.5: treatment recommended whether there is a previous fracture or not.

SUMMARY BOX

Clinical presentation	Investigation of choice	Comment
Suspected pituitary pathology: endocrine syndromes, optic chiasm compression, raised intracranial pressure	MRI	
Hyperthroidism	Scintigraphy with ^{99m}Tc	
Diffuse thyroid enlargement	US Scintigraphy with ^{99m}Tc	
Thyroid nodule/mass	US ± FNA	
Primary hyperparathyroidism	US	^{99m}Tc-sestamibi, CT or MRI where US negative
Cushing syndrome	MRI pituitary CT adrenals CT chest and abdomen	Imaging directed by results of biochemical tests
Conn syndrome	CT adrenals	
Phaechromocytoma	CT abdomen/adrenals	Scintigraphy with MIBG or MRI where CT negative
Incidental adrenal mass	Multiphase contrast-enhanced CT MRI	
Osteoporosis	DEXA	

DEXA, Dual X-ray absorptiometry; FNA, fine needle aspiration; MIBG, metaiodobenzylguanidine.

13 Paediatrics

Paediatric radiology is an extremely diverse subject encompassing many subspecialty areas. Many of the topics covered in other chapters of this book, such as musculoskeletal trauma and oncology, are relevant to paediatrics. Other topics in paediatrics are considered to be beyond the scope of a student text. These include congenital heart disease, which is imaged with echocardiography and MRI, and congenital brain disorders, imaged with MRI. For further information on these topics, the reader is referred to more specialized texts. This chapter discusses some of the more common clinical problems unique to paediatric practice that require imaging.

13.1 NEONATAL RESPIRATORY DISTRESS: THE NEONATAL CHEST

An approach to interpretation of CXR is outlined in Chapter 2. Specific features that may be seen on a normal neonatal CXR include (see Fig. 2.3b):

- Thymus may be prominent
- Heart shadow is often prominent and globular in outline; normal cardiothoracic ratio up to 65 per cent
- Air bronchograms may be seen in the medial third of the lung fields
- Diaphragms normally lie at the level of the sixth rib anteriorly.

The more common causes of neonatal respiratory distress tend to produce quite typical radiographic patterns as described below. When assessing a neonatal CXR, the clinical setting should always be borne in mind, for example:

- Premature infant with respiratory distress: hyaline membrane disease will be the most likely diagnosis
- Distressed term infant following Caesarean delivery: retained lung fluid will be most likely
- Term delivery with meconium-stained liquor: consider meconium aspiration syndrome.

Finally, it should be remembered that acutely ill neonates may have various tubes and vascular catheters visible on CXR, and it is important to check that these are correctly positioned (Fig. 13.1):

- Endotracheal tube: tip above carina
- Nasogastric tube: tip in stomach
- Umbilical artery catheter: tip in lower thoracic aorta, projected over lower thoracic vertebral bodies (T6–T10)
- Umbilical vein catheter: tip just above diaphragm in lower right atrium.

13.1.1 Surfactant deficiency disease

Formerly known as hyaline membrane disease or respiratory distress syndrome, surfactant deficiency disease (SDD) is a generalized lung condition of premature infants caused by insufficient surfactant production. Clinical presentation is usually respiratory distress and cyanosis soon after birth.

CXR changes of SDD (Figs 13.1 and 13.2):

- Reduced lung volume
- Granular pattern throughout the lungs
- Air bronchograms.

Surfactant therapy for SDD usually produces rapid improvement of respiratory distress

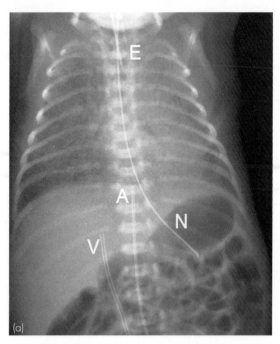
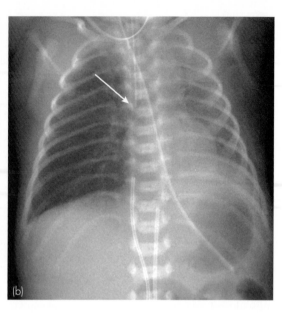

Figure 13.1 Surfactant deficiency disease (SDD) and tube placement: two separate examples. (a) Fine granular opacification throughout both lungs indicating SDD. Note placement of various tubes: endotracheal tube (E) in mid to upper trachea; nasogastric tube (N) in stomach; umbilical venous catheter tip in liver (V); umbilical artery catheter tip at T9 (A). (b) Subtle granular opacification throughout both lungs indicating mild SDD. Note placement of various tubes: nasogastric tube in stomach; umbilical venous catheter tip in right atrium; umbilical artery catheter tip at T11. Tip of endotracheal tube inappropriately positioned in right main bronchus (arrow): partial collapse of left lung due to lack of ventilation.

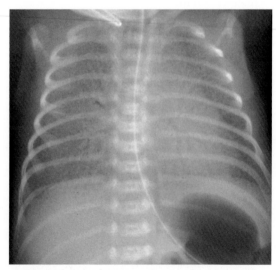

Figure 13.2 Surfactant deficiency disease. Note a fine granular pattern throughout both lungs with air bronchograms.

accompanied by resolution of the radiographic abnormalities. Failure of resolution of the radiographic changes of SDD after a couple of days may imply an added abnormality such as persistent ductus arteriosus (PDA) or infection. New or worsening airspace consolidation may indicate a pulmonary haemorrhage; this is a recognized complication of surfactant therapy. Other complications of SDD that may be seen on CXR relate to air leaks and include:

- Pulmonary interstitial emphysema (PIE) (Fig. 13.3)
- Pneumothorax (Fig. 13.4)
- Pneumomediastinum.

13.1.2 Transient tachypnoea of the newborn

Also known as retained fetal lung fluid or wet lung syndrome, transient tachypnoea of the newborn (TTN) is a self-limiting condition due to persistence

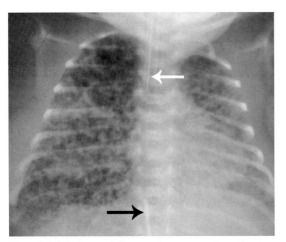

Figure 13.3 Surfactant deficiency disease complicated by pulmonary interstitial emphysema. Note the presence of multiple small air bubbles throughout both lungs, more obvious on the right. Note also an endotracheal tube (white arrow) and umbilical artery catheter (black arrow).

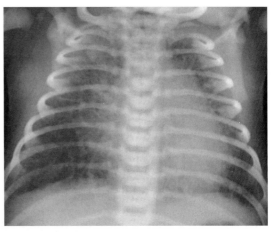

Figure 13.5 Transient tachypnoea of the newborn (TTN). CXR in a term infant born by Caesarian section shows widespread linear opacities throughout both lungs, plus small pleural effusions, better seen on the right.

- Prominent linear pattern with thickening of lung fissures, small pleural effusions
- Resolution of changes within 24 hours.

13.1.3 Meconium aspiration syndrome

Passage of meconium *in utero* may occur in response to fetal distress. Meconium aspiration may be seen in distressed neonates, in association with meconium-stained liquor.

CXR signs of meconium aspiration (Fig. 13.6):

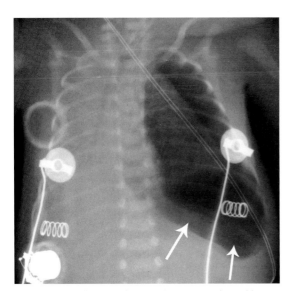

Figure 13.4 Surfactant deficiency disease complicated by a left tension pneumothorax. Note increased volume of the left hemithorax with shift of the mediastinum to the right. Also as the infant is supine most of the pneumothorax lies anteriorly and inferiorly producing lucency of the inferior left chest and upper abdomen (arrows).

of fetal lung fluid at birth. TTN usually presents with respiratory distress in a term infant following a prolonged labour or Caesarean section.

CXR signs of TTN (Fig. 13.5):
- Increased lung volume

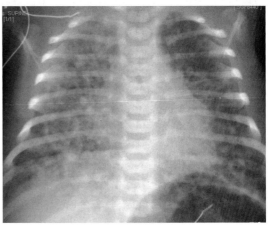

Figure 13.6 Meconium aspiration. Term infant, prolonged labour, heavy meconium staining of liquor, severe respiratory distress. CXR shows extensive coarse opacity throughout both lungs.

- Increased lung volume
- Dense, patchy opacities in central lungs
- Complications such as pneumonia or pneumothorax.

13.1.4 Cardiac failure

Specific patterns of cardiac enlargement and alterations of the cardiac outline may be seen with congenital heart disease. Suspected congenital heart disease is assessed with echocardiography and MRI. Cardiomegaly on CXR is a feature of cardiac failure, though is not a reliable sign in neonates. More commonly, signs of cardiac failure on neonatal CXR include alveolar and interstitial opacification bilaterally, and pleural effusions (Fig. 13.7). Pleural fluid in neonates commonly extends up the chest wall lateral to the lung, rather than forming a fluid level and meniscus.

13.1.5 Neonatal pneumonia

Neonatal pneumonia may produce a variety of CXR appearances including lobar consolidation or patchy widespread consolidation. Dense bilateral consolidation may mimic the appearances of HMD. Correlation of CXR abnormality with clinical findings, particularly the presence of a fever, is important for the diagnosis of neonatal pneumonia.

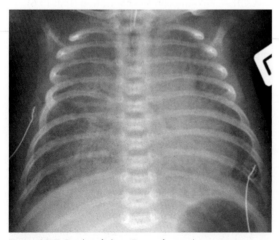

Figure 13.7 Cardiac failure. Term infant with respiratory distress. CXR shows cardiac enlargement, bilateral alveolar and interstitial opacity, and right pleural effusion. Note that in neonates, pleural fluid tracks lateral to the lung. Subsequent investigations including echocardiography revealed total anomalous pulmonary venous drainage.

13.1.6 Chronic neonatal lung disease

Previously known as bronchopulmonary dysplasia, chronic neonatal lung disease (CNLD) occurs in premature infants. Incidence of CNLD increases with low birthweight, early gestational age and duration of pulmonary ventilation.

Radiological changes of CNLD evolve over time:
- First 3 days: CXR signs are those of HMD
- Next week: increased opacification of both lungs
- Next couple of weeks: development of a 'bubbly' pattern through the lungs, i.e. air-filled 'bubbles' separated by irregular lines
- First month: 'bubbles' expand producing increased lung volumes.

Most infants with CNLD will survive, though with a high incidence of poor neurological development. CXR changes generally resolve over time, though often with some minor residual pulmonary overexpansion and linear stranding.

13.2 PATTERNS OF PULMONARY INFECTION IN CHILDREN

Most pulmonary infections in children are due to viruses such as respiratory syncytial virus (RSV), influenza, parainfluenza and adenovirus, or *Mycoplasma pneumoniae*. Viral infections tend to be seasonal and occur in epidemics. Bacterial infections are less common, and tend to be sporadic and less seasonal. Bacteria that commonly cause pulmonary infections in children include *Streptococcus pneumonia*, *Staphylococcus aureus* and *Haemophilus influenzae*.

Although there is some overlap in CXR appearances, viruses tend to produce an interstitial pattern while bacteria tend to produce alveolar consolidation. Community-acquired pneumonia caused by *Mycoplasma pneumoniae* may produce an interstitial or alveolar pattern, or a combination of the two. The most important question on the CXR of a child with a lower respiratory infection is: 'Is alveolar consolidation present?' If the answer is 'No', treatment will usually consist of supportive measures without the use of antibiotics. If the answer is 'Yes', bacterial aetiology is suspected and antibiotics may be required.

13.2.1 Viral infection

Children with viral lower respiratory tract infection usually present with a history of a couple of days of malaise, tachypnoea and cough. The most common CXR pattern seen with viral pulmonary infection is bilateral parahilar 'infiltration' (Fig. 13.8). This consists of irregular linear opacity extending into each lung from the hilar complexes, with bronchial wall thickening a prominent feature. Hilar lymphadenopathy may increase the amount of hilar opacification. Atelectasis due to mucous plugs and bronchial inflammation may complicate this pattern. Atelectasis may involve whole lobes, or may be seen as linear opacities that are transient and migratory on serial radiographs.

Large areas of atelectasis may mimic consolidation; it is important to recognize the lung volume loss associated with atelectasis, as this will help to differentiate it from consolidation. Consolidation may rarely complicate viral infection, and is often due to haemorrhagic bronchiolitis rather than a genuine exudate.

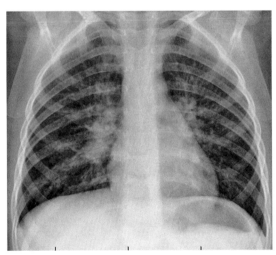

Figure 13.8 Viral lower respiratory tract infection. CXR in a three-year-old female shows bronchial wall thickening in the parahilar regions with no focal areas of airspace consolidation.

13.2.2 Bronchiolitis

Bronchiolitis is usually caused by the respiratory syncitial virus, with a peak incidence at around six months of age. Affected children present with tachypnoea, dyspnoea, cough and cyanosis.

The usual CXR pattern seen with bronchiolitis is overexpansion of the lungs due to bilateral air trapping. Severe cases may be complicated by atelectasis (Fig. 13.9). Where bronchiolitis is recurrent or prolonged, underlying asthma or cystic fibrosis should be considered.

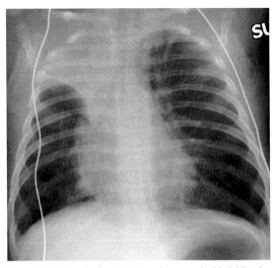

Figure 13.9 Bronchiolitis. CXR in a three-month-old child with fever and respiratory distress shows overexpansion of left lung with flattening of the left diaphragm. There is complete collapse of the right upper lobe.

13.2.3 Bacterial infection

Children with a bacterial pulmonary infection usually present with abrupt onset of malaise, fever and cough. The typical CXR pattern of bacterial infection is alveolar consolidation, i.e. fluffy opacity with air bronchograms, which may be lobar or patchy in distribution (see Chapter 2).

Round pneumonia is a common pattern of early bacterial infection in children. Round pneumonia appears on CXR as a dense round opacity, which may be mistaken for a mass (Fig. 13.10). The clinical setting of suspected infection (fever, cough, chest pain) should suggest the diagnosis. Follow-up CXR in 6–24 hours will usually show evolution of the round opacity to a more lobar pattern. Round pneumonia is much less common in adults.

Established cases of bacterial infection are usually easily diagnosed on CXR. Difficulties may arise with early infections where the consolidation may be extremely subtle.

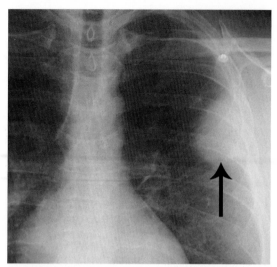

Figure 13.10 Round pneumonia. Round opacity with slightly blurred margins in the left upper lobe (arrow). This resolved rapidly with antibiotic therapy.

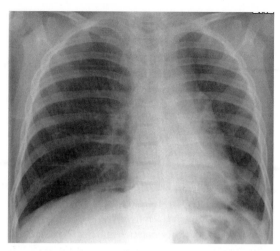

Figure 13.11 Asthma complicated by left lower lobe collapse. Note reduced volume left lung, triangular opacity behind heart, and loss of definition of left diaphragm.

Overlying structures may obscure certain parts of the lung and consolidation in these areas may be very difficult to see; in a febrile child with suspected chest infection, particular attention should be given to the following review areas:

- Apical segments of the lower lobes, obscured by the hilar complexes
- Lung bases, obscured by the diaphragms
- Left lower lobe, which lies behind the heart
- Apical segments of the upper lobes, obscured by overlying ribs and clavicles.

13.2.4 Asthma

Between acute attacks, the CXR of an asthma sufferer is often normal. 'Baseline changes' that may be seen include overexpanded lungs, thickening of bronchial walls most marked in the parahilar regions, and focal scarring from previous infections. During acute asthma attacks, the lungs are overinflated due to air trapping. Lobar or segmental collapse due to mucous plugging is common (Fig. 13.11). It is important to differentiate collapse from consolidation to avoid unnecessary use of antibiotics. Other complications of asthma that may be diagnosed on CXR include pneumonia, pneumomediastinum and pneumothorax, and secondary aspergillosis.

13.2.5 Cystic fibrosis (mucoviscidosis)

Cystic fibrosis is an autosomal recessive condition with dysfunction of exocrine glands and reduced mucociliary function. Pancreatic insufficiency leads to steatorrhoea and malabsorption. Meconium ileus may be seen in infants (see Section 13.5.5). Complications in older children include recurrent pancreatitis, biliary cirrhosis and meconium ileus equivalent, also known as distal intestinal obstruction syndrome (DIOS). Pulmonary symptoms include recurrent infections and chronic cough.

CXR changes associated with cystic fibrosis (Fig. 13.12):

- Overinflated lungs with thickening of bronchial walls and dilated bronchi
- Localized finger-like opacities due to mucoid impaction in dilated bronchi
- High incidence of pneumonia producing focal areas of consolidation
- Large pulmonary arteries due to pulmonary arterial hypertension.

13.3 INVESTIGATION OF AN ABDOMINAL MASS

A child with an abdominal mass may present in a number of ways:

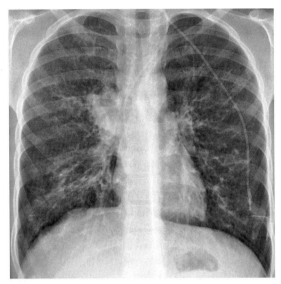

Figure 13.12 Cystic fibrosis. CXR in a 14-year-old female shows overexpanded lungs with extensive linear densities due to bronchial wall thickening and mucous plugs. Prominence of right hilum due to lymphadenopathy. Tunnelled central venous catheter inserted via left internal jugular vein.

- Hydronephrosis and other congenital masses are frequently diagnosed on obstetric US
- Detection by attending paediatrician of a congenital mass at birth
- In older children, an abdominal mass may produce a visible bulge or may be felt by a parent
- Depending on location, there may be specific signs or symptoms, such as jaundice or intestinal obstruction.

Common causes of abdominal masses in children are as follows:
- Benign renal conditions (see below)
  - Hydronephrosis
  - Multicystic dysplastic kidney
  - Polycystic syndromes
- Nephroblastoma (Wilms' tumour)
- Neuroblastoma
- Hepatic
  - Hepatoblastoma
  - Hepatocellular carcinoma
  - Haemangioendothelioma.

The roles of imaging for an abdominal mass are:
- Diagnosis of a mass

- Define organ of origin
- Characterize margins: well defined or infiltrative
- Characterize contents: calcification, necrosis, cyst formation, fat
- Diagnose complications and evidence of malignancy
  - Metastases
  - Lymphadenopathy
  - Invasion of surrounding structures
  - Vascular invasion
- Treatment planning
- Guidance of percutaneous biopsy or other interventional procedures, such as nephrostomy
- Follow-up: response to therapy, diagnosis of recurrent tumour.

13.3.1 US

US is the first investigation of choice in children for assessing the site of origin of a mass and as guidance for further investigations. Following confirmation of an abdominal mass and development of a differential diagnosis on US, further imaging with MRI, CT or scintigraphy is usually required for more accurate definition, and for staging in the case of malignancy.

13.3.2 MRI and CT

MRI has several advantages in children and in many centres is performed in preference to CT for the assessment of an abdominal mass:
- MRI uses no ionizing radiation
- In most cases, due to superior soft tissue definition and multiplanar capabilities, MRI is able to provide better definition of relevant structures than CT.

Disadvantages of MRI compared with CT include:
- Relatively long scanning time requiring general anaesthetic in young children
- Inability to accurately image the lungs; CT of the chest is required for accurate staging of those tumours known to metastasize to lung.

In centres where MRI has limited availability, multidetector CT (MDCT) is used for imaging of abdominal masses in children. MDCT provides accurate characterization of an abdominal mass and its organ of origin, and is highly sensitive for the presence of calcification and fat. Disadvantages of CT include use of ionizing radiation and iodinated contrast material.

A common protocol for investigation and staging of malignancy in children is a non-contrast-enhanced CT of the chest for accurate assessment of the lungs followed by MRI of the abdomen. Depending on the layout of the medical imaging department this may be done under a single general anaesthetic in young children.

13.3.3 Scintigraphy

Renal scintigraphy complements US in the assessment of benign renal conditions that may present as an abdominal mass. ^{99}mTc-DTPA or ^{99}mTc-MAG3 may be used. MAG3 (mercaptoacetyltriglycine) has more efficient renal extraction than DTPA and is more widely used in paediatric patients. Renal scanning with DTPA or MAG3 provides physiological information such as differential renal function and diuretic 'wash-out', as well as anatomical information such as level of obstruction (see Fig. 5.1).

Other scintigraphic studies that may be used in the context of an abdominal mass include bone scintigraphy with ^{99}mTc-MDP for suspected skeletal metastases, and ^{123}I-MIBG in the staging of neuroblastoma.

13.3.4 Nephroblastoma (Wilms' tumour)

Nephroblastoma is the most commonly occurring solid intra-abdominal tumour in childhood. Most cases present between the ages of one and five years with an asymptomatic renal mass, although there may be associated haematuria or abdominal pain. Fifteen per cent of nephroblastomas are associated with congenital anomalies including non-familial aniridia, congenital hemihypertrophy and Beckwith–Weidemann syndrome.

On US, nephroblastoma appears as a hyperechoic mass with hypoechoic areas due to necrosis. The mass tends to replace renal parenchyma with progressive enlargement and distortion of the kidney. MRI (or CT) of the abdomen shows a renal mass and distortion of kidney. The mass shows less intense contrast enhancement than functioning renal tissue (Fig. 13.13). Complications

of nephroblastoma that may be seen on CT or MRI include lymphadenopathy, invasion of renal vein and inferior vena cava (IVC), liver metastases, and invasion of surrounding structures. Chest CT is more accurate than CXR for the initial diagnosis of pulmonary metastases. Although less accurate than CT for initial diagnosis, CXR may be performed to establish a baseline for follow-up examinations.

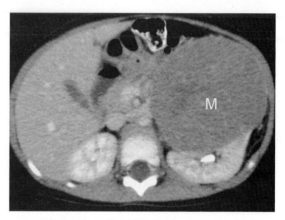

Figure 13.13 Wilms' tumour (nephroblastoma): CT. Transverse CT scan shows a large mass (M) arising from and distorting the left kidney.

13.3.5 Neuroblastoma

Neuroblastoma is a malignant childhood tumour arising from primitive sympathetic neuroblasts of the embryonic neural crest. Sixty per cent occur in the abdomen; of these, two-thirds arise in the adrenal gland. Other common abdominal sites of origin of neuroblastoma are the periaortic sympathetic ganglia in the chest and abdomen, and ganglia at the aortic bifurcation. The peak age of incidence is two years with most neuroblastomas occurring below five years of age. A less common subgroup is congenital neuroblastoma in infants. Congenital neuroblastoma has a better prognosis due to its tendency to spontaneous regression.

US shows a mass with a heterogeneous texture due to areas of necrosis, haemorrhage and calcification. MRI (or CT) shows a heterogeneous mass with displacement or invasion of the kidney. Calcification is seen on CT in most cases. Neuroblastoma tends to spread across the midline, encasing or displacing the aorta (Fig. 13.14). Other

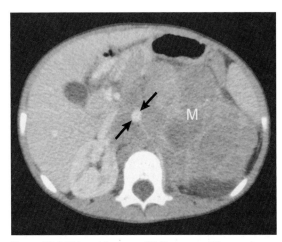

Figure 13.14 Neuroblastoma: CT. Transverse CT scan shows a large left-sided mass (M) with extension across the midline and encasement of the aorta (arrows).

complications seen on MRI or CT include invasion of surrounding structures, extension into the spine, lymphadenopathy and liver metastases (Fig. 13.15). Further staging is performed with chest CT for pulmonary metastases and bone scintigraphy with ^{99}mTc-MDP. Scintigraphy with ^{123}I-MIBG (metaiodobenzylguanidine) may also be used for staging, and to assess response to therapy in advanced cases.

13.3.6 Hepatoblastoma

Hepatoblastoma is the most common hepatic tumour in children. Hepatoblastoma has an

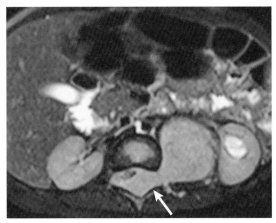

Figure 13.15 Neuroblastoma: MRI. Transverse T2-weighted, fat saturated MRI shows a tumour medial to the left kidney. Tumour can be seen invading the spinal canal (arrow).

increased incidence in Beckwith–Weidemann syndrome, hemihypertrophy and biliary atresia; it is not associated with cirrhosis. Most hepatoblastomas occur under the age of three.

US of hepatoblastoma shows a well-circumscribed mass of higher echogenicity than surrounding liver. MRI or CT shows a hepatic mass in which areas of necrosis, calcification and, occasionally, fat may be seen. Hepatoblastoma may be complicated by vascular invasion, seen on MRI or CT as a filling defect within an enlarged portal vein or IVC.

13.3.7 Hepatocellular carcinoma

Hepatocellular carcinoma is uncommon in children, with an increased incidence in chronic liver diseases, such as cirrhosis, biliary atresia or tyrosinaemia. US shows an ill-defined hypoechoic mass in the liver. MRI or CT may show a solitary hepatic mass or multiple confluent masses.

13.3.8 Haemangioendothelioma

Haemangioendothelioma is a highly vascular benign multicentric liver tumour, which may be associated with cutaneous haemangiomas. Haemangioendothelioma usually presents in infancy with hepatomegaly, cardiac failure or acute haemorrhage. US shows multiple discrete hyperechoic masses in the liver. MRI or CT shows multiple hepatic masses with occasional calcification.

13.4 URINARY TRACT DISORDERS IN CHILDREN

13.4.1 Urinary tract infection

Urinary tract infection (UTI) is one of the most common indications for imaging in paediatrics. UTI is more common in young children. UTI in infants occurs with equal incidence in males and females and usually presents with signs of generalized sepsis including fever, vomiting and anorexia. In children older than six months, UTI is more common in females. Clinical presentation in these children is usually more specific for UTI with fever, frequency and dysuria. Flank pain may indicate pyelonephritis.

Roles of imaging in the investigation of a child with UTI:

- Diagnose underlying urinary tract abnormalities
- Diagnose and grade vesicoureteric reflux (VUR)
- Differentiate cystitis (UTI confined to the bladder) from pyelonephritis (UTI involving one or both kidneys)
- Document renal damage
- Establish a baseline for subsequent evaluation of renal growth
- Establish prognosis and guide management.

13.4.1.1 US

US of the renal tract is the initial investigation of choice for the child with urinary tract infection. US is performed to detect abnormalities of the urinary tract that may predispose the child to the development of recurrent UTI. Most children with uncomplicated UTI have a normal US examination, and in the majority of these cases no further imaging is required. In the minority of cases in which US is abnormal, the more common findings include hydronephrosis, neurogenic bladder (usually associated with congenital neurological abnormalities such as spina bifida) and renal duplex. Depending on the results of US as well as the clinical situation, further imaging may be performed to diagnose VUR, document renal function and diagnose renal scars.

13.4.1.2 Micturating cystourethrogram

Micturating cystourethrogram (MCU), also known as voiding cystourethrogram (VCU), is performed primarily to diagnose VUR and grade its severity as follows (Fig. 13.16):

- Grade 1: Reflux into non-dilated ureter
- Grade 2: Reflux into non-dilated collecting system
- Grade 3: Reflux into mildly dilated collecting system
- Grade 4: Reflux into moderately dilated collecting system
- Grade 5: Reflux into grossly dilated collecting system with dilated, tortuous ureter.

Micturating cystourethrogram may be performed radiographically or with scintigraphy; both methods involve catheterization of the child. Radiographic MCU provides more precise anatomical imaging of the urinary tract including the urethra (Fig. 13.17). Radiographic MCU may therefore be helpful in documenting the site of insertion of the ureter, as well as diagnosing underlying anomalies, such as posterior urethral valves in males. Once the diagnosis of VUR is established, scintigraphic reflux studies may be performed for follow-up. When moderate to severe VUR is diagnosed, or in the presence of underlying urinary tract anomalies, further imaging with scintigraphy may be required.

13.4.1.3 Scintigraphy

Scintigraphy with ^{99}mTc-MAG3 or ^{99}mTc-DTPA may be performed to differentiate obstructive from non-obstructive hydronephrosis and to quantitate differential renal function. Differential renal

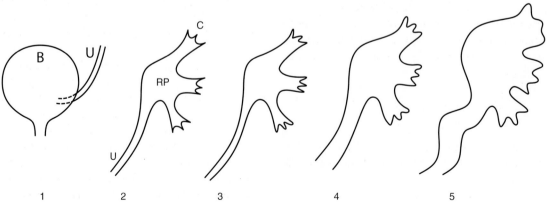

Figure 13.16 Schematic diagram illustrating the five grades of vesicoureteric reflux. For orientation note the following labels: bladder (B), ureter (U), renal pelvis (RP) and calyces (C).

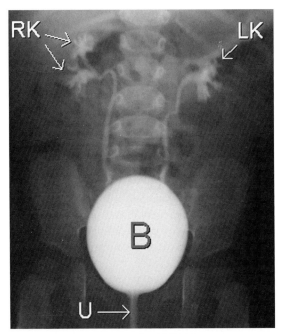

Figure 13.17 Vesicoureteric reflux (VUR). Micturating cystourethrogram in a female infant shows contrast material filling the bladder (B) and outlining the urethra (U). There is bilateral grade 3 VUR. Note the reduced number of calyces on the left (LK) compared with the right (RK) indicating reflux into the lower moiety of a duplex collecting system.

function is expressed as the percentage of overall renal function contributed by each kidney.

Scintigraphy with ^{99m}Tc-DMSA is much more sensitive than US for the documentation of renal scars (see Fig. 1.13). DMSA is taken up by cells of the proximal convoluted tubule and retained in the renal cortex. Cortical scars show on DMSA scans as focal areas of reduced tracer uptake, with irregularity of the outline of the kidney. DMSA scans are also used to diagnose pyelonephritis, seen as focal areas of reduced tracer uptake in an acutely febrile child.

13.4.1.4 Guidelines for imaging children with urinary tract infection

Recommendations may be made as to which children with UTI should be investigated with imaging:
- Males of any age with a first UTI
- Females under three years of age with a first UTI

- Females older than three years with UTI and complicating factors such as
  - Atypical organism
  - Recurrent UTI
  - Family history of UTI and VUR
  - Abnormal voiding
  - Poor growth
  - Hypertension.

Recommendations may also be made as to the use of the various imaging modalities:
- US as the first-line investigation in all
  - MAG3 scan if obstruction suspected on US
- MCU for children younger than 12 months
- DMSA for young males and recurrent UTI in others
  - May also be used to make the specific diagnosis of pyelonephritis if this will alter management
- More aggressive investigation for recurrent or complicated cases.

13.4.2 Renal duplex

Renal duplex is a single kidney with two separate collecting systems. (The term 'renal duplication' should be reserved for cases where there are two separate kidneys on one side.) The part of the kidney drained by each collecting system of a duplex kidney is referred to as a moiety. The term 'duplex kidney' refers to a range of anomalies including bifid renal pelvis, two separate ureters that join above the bladder, or two ureters that drain separately into the bladder (complete ureteric duplication).

With complete ureteric duplication, the ureter draining the upper moiety usually inserts inferior and medial to the ureter from the lower moiety (Weigert-Meyer rule) (Fig. 13.18). The upper moiety ureter may enter the inferior bladder or may have an ectopic insertion. Possible sites of ectopic ureteric insertion include bladder neck, urethra, vagina or perineum in females and prostatic urethra and ejaculatory system in males. Regardless of the site of insertion the upper moiety ureter is prone to obstruction. Ureterocele may also complicate the bladder or ectopic insertion of the upper moiety ureter (Fig. 13.19). Ureterocele is a cyst-like expansion of the distal end of the ureter projecting into the bladder. The ureter draining the lower moiety of a duplex kidney is prone to VUR.

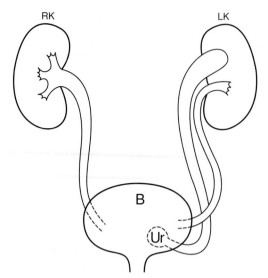

Figure 13.18 Schematic diagram illustrating the potential problems of a duplex renal collecting system. For orientation note the right kidney (RK), left kidney (LK) and bladder (B). The ureter from the upper moiety implants lower than that from the lower moiety and is sometimes complicated by ureterocele (Ur) and obstruction. The ureter from the lower moiety implants higher and is prone to reflux.

13.4.3 Hydronephrosis

Hydronephrosis is the most common cause of a neonatal abdominal mass. Hydronephrosis may also present with UTI, or may be detected on prenatal (obstetric) screening US. Widespread use of obstetric US screening has led to a significantly increased incidence of prenatal diagnosis of hydronephrosis.

Common causes of hydronephrosis in children include:

- Pelviureteric junction (PUJ) obstruction
- Vesicoureteric junction (VUJ) obstruction
- VUR
- Primary megaloureter
- Duplex kidney with obstruction of upper pole moiety ureter.

US and scintigraphy are the primary imaging modalities for assessment of hydronephrosis.

The roles of imaging of hydronephrosis are:
- Document severity of urinary tract dilatation
- Differentiate obstructive from non-obstructive causes
- Define level of obstruction
- Diagnose underlying anatomical anomalies.

13.4.3.1 US

US is the initial imaging modality of choice in the investigation of hydronephrosis.

Signs of hydronephrosis on US include:
- Dilated renal pelvis and calyces
- Underlying anomalies, such as ureterocele or duplex collecting system
- PUJ obstruction: round, dilated renal pelvis (Fig. 13.20)
- VUJ obstruction: dilated ureter can be followed down to the bladder

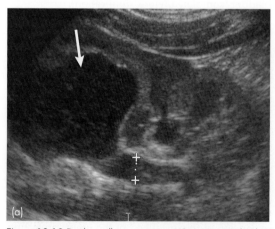
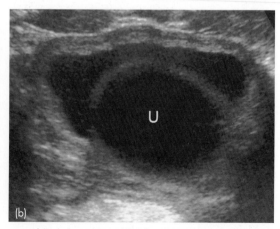

Figure 13.19 Duplex collecting system: US. (a) Longitudinal US image of the kidney shows dilated upper moiety collecting system (arrow), dilated upper moiety ureter (+) and normal lower moiety. (b) Transverse US image of the bladder shows a ureterocele (U) at the insertion of the upper pole ureter.

- Chronic hydronephrosis may cause thinning of the renal cortex.

13.4.3.2 Scintigraphy

Diuretic scintigraphy with ^{99}mTc-MAG3 or ^{99}mTc-DTPA is used to differentiate mechanical urinary tract obstruction from non-obstructive causes of hydronephrosis. Furosemide is injected after the renal collecting system is filled with isotope. Rate of washout of isotope is then assessed. With mechanical obstruction, such as PUJ obstruction, isotope continues to accumulate in the collecting system following diuretic injection (see Fig. 5.1). Isotope is rapidly washed out of the dilated collecting system in cases of non-obstructive hydronephrosis, such as VUR. Scintigraphy is also used to quantitate differential renal function and to show the level of obstruction at either PUJ or VUJ. Vesicoureteric reflux is suspected when scintigraphy shows a non-obstructive hydronephrosis. In such cases, MCU may be indicated to confirm and grade vesicoureteric reflux.

13.4.4 Multicystic dysplastic kidney

Multicystic dysplastic kidney (MCDK) is the second most common cause of an abdominal mass in a neonate, after hydronephrosis. Pathological features of MCDK include:

- Multiple cysts of varying size replace the kidney
- Absence of the ipsilateral ureter
- Ipsilateral renal artery is hypoplastic
- Congenital abnormality of the contralateral kidney in 30 per cent of cases, usually PUJ obstruction
- The natural history of MCDK is involution: many adults diagnosed with a solitary kidney were probably born with MCDK
- Bilateral MCDK is incompatible with life.

US is the investigation of choice for suspected MCDK. US of MCDK shows the kidney replaced by a lobulated collection of variably sized non-communicating cysts (Fig. 13.21). MCDK is often diagnosed prenatally on obstetric US (see Fig. 6.7). Scintigraphy with ^{99}mTc-MAG3 or ^{99}mTc-DTPA may be used to confirm MCDK by showing absence of renal function on the affected side.

13.4.5 Polycystic renal conditions

Polycystic renal conditions are classified according to genetic inheritance, pathological findings and clinical presentation.

Autosomal recessive polycystic kidney disease (ARPKD) refers to a spectrum of disorders with associated liver disease, with infantile and juvenile forms described. In the infantile form, renal disease tends to be more severe with less hepatic involvement; in older children, liver disease is the dominant

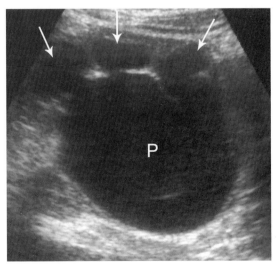

Figure 13.20 Hydronephrosis due to pelviureteric junction obstruction: US. US shows a markedly dilated renal pelvis (P) communicating with dilated calyces (arrows).

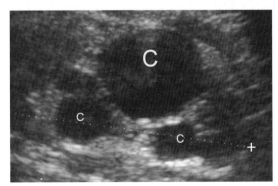

Figure 13.21 Multicystic dysplastic kidney: US. The left kidney is replaced by a collection of non-communicating cysts (C).

feature. US in ARPKD shows symmetrically enlarged hyperechoic kidneys (Fig. 13.22).

Autosomal dominant polycystic kidney disease (ADPKD) usually presents in middle age with enlarged kidneys and hypertension. US in adults with ADPKD shows enlarged kidneys containing multiple cysts of varying size. ADPKD may occasionally present in childhood with bilateral enlarged kidneys, which may be asymmetrical. On US examination, the kidneys are of increased echogenicity due to multiple cysts that are too tiny to be seen individually. Occasionally, separate small anechoic cysts are seen.

Various hereditary syndromes, including tuberous sclerosis and von Hippel–Lindau disease, may be associated with renal cysts.

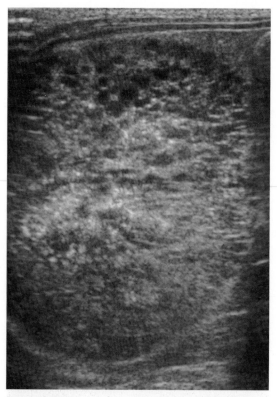

Figure 13.22 Autosomal recessive polycystic kidney disease. US in a 3-day-old female infant shows marked enlargement of the kidneys. Transverse view of the kidney shows loss of normal parenchymal pattern and innumerable tiny cysts.

13.5 GUT OBSTRUCTION AND/OR BILE-STAINED VOMITING IN THE NEONATE

Neonatal gut obstruction with or without bile-stained vomiting is a common clinical problem with a wide differential diagnosis. AXR is the investigation of choice for most neonates with suspected gut obstruction. For some causes, such as duodenal obstruction, AXR is often sufficient for diagnosis. In other conditions, such as malrotation, the AXR may be normal. Contrast studies, such as upper GI series and contrast enema, are often required for diagnosis of neonatal gut obstruction, particularly malrotation and large bowel disorders.

13.5.1 Duodenal obstruction

Causes of congenital duodenal obstruction:
- Duodenal atresia: most common
- Duodenal stenosis or web
- Annular pancreas: rare congenital anomaly whereby pancreatic tissue encircles and constricts the second part of the duodenum.

Thirty per cent of patients with duodenal atresia have Down syndrome. Anomalies that may be associated with duodenal atresia include oesophageal atresia, imperforate anus, renal anomalies and congenital heart disease. Duodenal atresia may be diagnosed on prenatal US with visualization of a fluid-filled 'double bubble' in the fetal abdomen due to dilated stomach and duodenal cap (Fig. 13.23).

Signs of duodenal atresia on AXR (Fig. 13.24):
- Classic 'double bubble' sign due to gas in distended stomach and duodenal cap
- Absence of gas in distal bowel
- Occasionally, gas in the gallbladder may produce a third bubble.

13.5.2 Small bowel atresia

Atresia of the small bowel most commonly occurs in the proximal jejunum. AXR shows a few dilated small bowel loops in the left upper quadrant. Occasionally, as a result of small bowel perforation, widespread abdominal calcification due to meconium peritonitis may be seen.

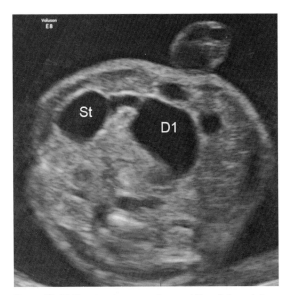

Figure 13.23 Duodenal atresia: obstetric US at 34 weeks' gestation for assessment of polyhydramnios. Transverse view shows a 'double bubble' due to stomach (St) and dilated first part of duodenum (D1).

13.5.3 Anorectal atresia

Absence of an anus indicates anorectal atresia. Anorectal atresia is classified as either a low or high anomaly. The key anatomical feature in classification of anorectal atresia is the levator sling:

- Low anomaly: bowel ends below the levator sling
- High anomaly: bowel ends above the levator sling, usually associated with fistula into vagina or posterior urethra.

Lateral and frontal abdominal radiographs are performed to classify anorectal atresia by assessing the relationship of the most distal part of the bowel to the pelvic floor (Fig. 13.25). Gas in the bladder or vagina indicates the presence of a fistula. Associated sacral anomalies may also be seen, including failure of sacral segmentation or sacral agenesis. US of the perineum may be used to determine the distance between the anal dimple on the perineal surface and the distal bowel end and thus aid in surgical planning.

13.5.4 Hirschsprung disease

Hirschsprung disease refers to an aganglionic segment of distal large bowel. Distal colonic

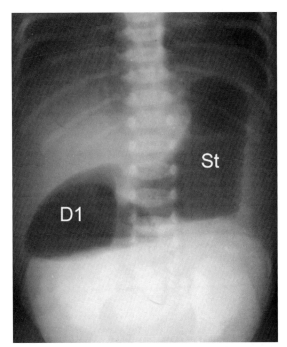

Figure 13.24 Duodenal atresia. AXR shows the characteristic 'double bubble' due to gas filling the stomach (St) and first part of the duodenum (D1). Gas is unable to pass more distally due to atresia of the second part of the duodenum.

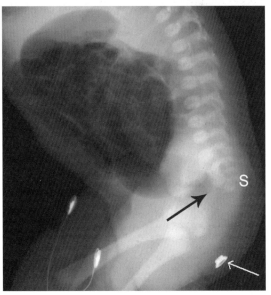

Figure 13.25 Anorectal atresia. Lateral radiograph showing the high termination of the distal large bowel (black arrow), marker placed on perineum (white arrow), and failure of formation of distal sacral segments (S).

aganglionosis occurs during embryological development due to arrest of normal craniocaudal migration of neuroblasts. The most common form of Hirschsprung disease is a short distal aganglionic segment, which causes distal large bowel obstruction. Normally innervated bowel proximal to the aganglionic segment is dilated. Hirschsprung disease usually presents in neonates with abdominal distension and constipation. Less commonly, it may be a cause of chronic constipation in an older child.

AXR in Hirschsprung disease may show dilated bowel loops (Fig. 13.26). Contrast enema is definitive when it shows an abrupt transition from narrow distal aganglionic segment to dilated normally innervated bowel. Total colonic aganglionosis occurs in 5 per cent of cases; this may be very difficult to diagnose with imaging due to lack of a transition point. Diagnosis of Hirschsprung disease is confirmed with biopsy.

13.5.5 Meconium ileus

Meconium ileus occurs in association with cystic fibrosis (mucoviscidosis) and is due to viscous meconium impacted in the distal ileum. Obstetric US may show polyhydramnios and hyperechoic contents in fetal small bowel.

Signs of meconium ileus on AXR (Fig. 13.27):
- 'Soap bubble' appearance in right lower quadrant due to complex retained meconium in the distal small bowel
- Dilated small bowel loops of variable calibre with no fluid levels on the erect view.

Contrast enema shows a small colon (microcolon), plus a large distal ileum with filling defects due to meconium. Contrast enema may be therapeutic in that it may disimpact the viscous meconium.

13.5.6 Meconium plug syndrome

Meconium plug syndrome refers to inspissated meconium causing distal large bowel obstruction.

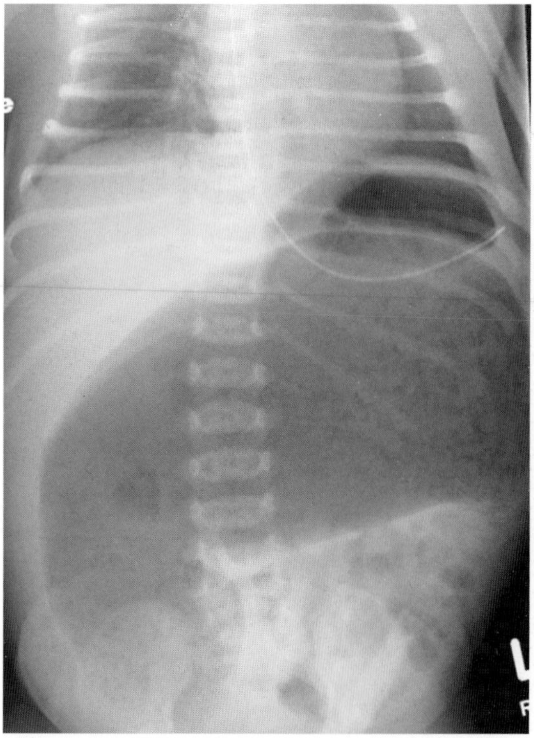

Figure 13.26 Hirschsprung disease. AXR in an infant with abdominal distension shows marked dilatation of transverse colon. Stomach can be seen pushed upwards with nasogastric tube *in situ*.

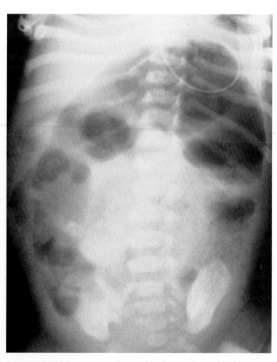

Figure 13.27 Meconium ileus. AXR shows distended large bowel with a characteristic 'soap-bubble' appearance on both sides of the abdomen.

It is not related pathologically to meconium ileus. AXR usually shows non-specific dilated small bowel loops. Contrast enema shows a dilated rectum with large filling defects in the colon, and is often therapeutic.

13.5.7 Malrotation and midgut volvulus

Small and large bowel from the second part of duodenum to the distal transverse colon are formed from the embryological midgut in several stages:

- Up to the 6th week of gestation: midgut lies within the abdominal cavity
- 6th to 10th weeks of gestation: midgut develops outside the abdominal cavity (physiological herniation)
- 10th week: midgut returns to the abdominal cavity.

During these various stages of embryological development, the midgut rotates through 270°. This rotation produces the final normal orientation of the small bowel mesentery and bowel loops:

- Junction of fourth part of duodenum with jejunum (duodeojejunal flexure) lies to the left of midline
- Proximal small bowel loops lie to the left
- Caecum lies in the right lower abdomen.

Malrotation refers to a wide spectrum of anatomical variants, the common feature being abnormal rotation of the midgut. Anatomical variations seen with malrotation include:

- Duodenojejunal flexure in abnormal position, usually to the right of midline (key feature)
- Colon to the left of midline
- Caecum in the left upper abdomen
- Transverse colon lying posterior to the superior mesenteric artery
- Peritoneal (Ladd) bands: fibrous bands that cross the duodenum and may cause compression
- Internal paraduodenal hernia
- Shortened small bowel mesenteric attachment.

The anatomical variations seen in malrotation may produce clinically significant complications, including volvulus of the small bowel and duodenum, and intestinal obstruction due to Ladd bands or paraduodenal hernia. These complications lead to two common types of clinical presentation:

- Severe bile-stained vomiting in neonates
- Intermittent vomiting, nausea and abdominal pain in older children.

Imaging investigation of suspected malrotation consists of AXR plus a contrast study of the upper gastrointestinal tract (GIT). AXR in a child with malrotation is often normal, particularly if performed when the child is asymptomatic. In the symptomatic child, AXR may show non-specific signs, such as dilatation of the duodenum. Upper GIT contrast study is usually definitive in the diagnosis or exclusion of malrotation. The key finding in malrotation is malposition of the duodenojejunal junction to the right or in the midline. As well as examining the upper GIT, contrast material may be followed through the small bowel to the caecum and colon. Other signs of malrotation that may be seen on the contrast study include (Fig. 13.28):

- Duodenal obstruction
- Proximal jejunum lying in the right abdomen

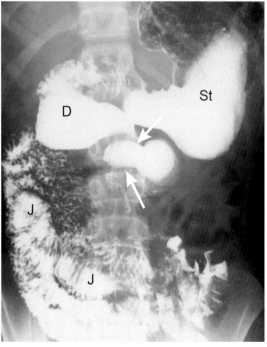

Figure 13.28 Malrotation: barium study. Note normally located stomach (St), duodenum (D) does not pass across the midline to the left, 'corkscrew' configuration of proximal small bowel (arrows), jejunum (J) located abnormally on the right.

- 'Corkscrew' appearance of small bowel loops
- Abnormally high caecum on follow-through films.

13.6 OTHER GASTROINTESTINAL TRACT DISORDERS IN CHILDREN

13.6.1 Oesophageal atresia and tracheo-oesophageal fistula

During early embryological development, the foregut develops into a ventral respiratory component (lungs and trachea) and a dorsal digestive component (oesophagus and stomach). Congenital foregut malformations due to failure of complete separation of dorsal and ventral foregut components occur in 1:3000 live births. Congenital foregut malformations are classified as shown in Fig. 13.29.

With the widespread use of obstetric US, oesophageal atresia and tracheo-oesophageal fistula (TOF) may be suspected prenatally. Findings on obstetric US may include polyhydramnios and absence of a normal fluid-filled fetal stomach.

Most cases of oesophageal atresia and TOF may be diagnosed with radiographs (CXR and AXR) of the neonate. Radiographic findings depend on the type of malformation (Fig. 13.30):

- Air in a blind-ending upper oesophageal pouch posterior to trachea, best seen on a lateral view

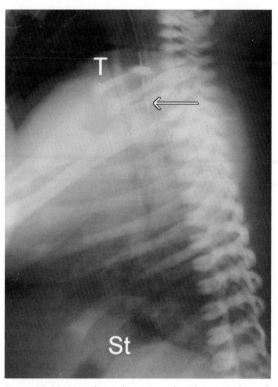

Figure 13.30 Oesophageal atresia and tracheo-oesophageal fistula. Lateral view shows a nasogastric tube in the blind-ending upper oesophageal segment (arrow). Gas in the stomach (St) indicates the presence of a fistula from trachea to the distal oesophagus. Note also that the trachea (T) is narrowed due to tracheomalacia, which is commonly associated with oesophageal atresia.

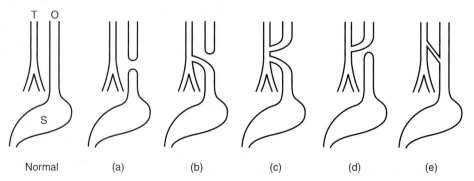

Figure 13.29 Schematic diagram illustrating the classification and relative incidences of oesophageal atresia and tracheo-oesophageal fistula. Note the normal orientation of trachea (T), oesophagus (O) and stomach (St). (a) Oesophageal atresia with no fistula: 9 per cent. (b) Oesophageal atresia with distal fistula: 82 per cent. (c) Oesophageal atresia with proximal and distal fistulas: 2 per cent. (d) Oesophageal atresia with proximal fistula: 1 per cent. (e) Fistula without oesophageal atresia ('H' type fistula): 6 per cent.

- Nasogastric tube curled in pouch
- Air in GIT implies a distal fistula
- Gasless abdomen is seen with no TOF or a proximal TOF
- Signs of aspiration pneumonia on CXR.

Contrast studies are usually not needed except for the diagnosis of 'H-type' TOF.

In this uncommon variant, the oesophagus is formed normally with no oesophageal atresia; upper oesophagus is joined to the trachea by a thin fistula. Plain films are often normal, apart from possible signs of aspiration pneumonia. Contrast studies are usually required for demonstration of the fistula, with water-soluble contrast material injected through a feeding tube placed in the upper oesophagus.

Associated anomalies occur in approximately 25 per cent of cases of oesophageal atresia and TOF including:

- Vertebral anomalies
- Anorectal atresia
- Duodenal atresia
- Renal anomalies, such as MCDK and renal agenesis
- Cardiac anomalies, such as ventricular septal defect, atrial septal defect, PDA
- Radial dysplasia and other limb anomalies.

Due to these associations, all patients with a TOF should have a renal US and an echocardiogram. Radiographs of the chest and abdomen should be closely perused for vertebral anomalies. Right-sided aortic arch is seen in 5 per cent of cases. It is important to diagnose right-sided aortic arch preoperatively, as the surgical approach may have to be amended.

13.6.2 Hypertrophic pyloric stenosis

Hypertrophic pyloric stenosis refers to progressive gastric outlet obstruction due to idiopathic hypertrophy of the circular muscle fibres of the pylorus. Clinical presentation is usually at around 6 weeks of age, with forceful non-bile stained vomiting leading to dehydration and hypokalaemic alkalosis. Palpation of a pyloric muscular mass in the right upper quadrant of an infant with a typical clinical history is diagnostic of hypertrophic pyloric stenosis and imaging is not required in such cases.

US is the investigation of choice, and is useful in infants with equivocal symptomatology, or with typical symptoms where a mass cannot be palpated.

US signs of pyloric stenosis (Fig. 13.31):

- Thickened pylorus seen as a rim of hypoechoic thickened muscle with a hyperechoic centre producing a target appearance
- US measurements indicating hypertrophic pyloric stenosis
  - Total pyloric diameter >13 mm
  - Pyloric muscle thickness >3 mm
  - Pyloric length >16 mm
- Distended stomach
- Lack of passage of gastric contents through the thickened pylorus on real-time scanning.

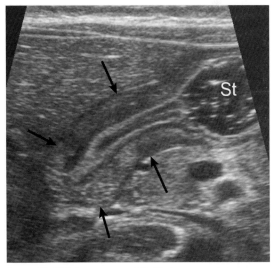

Figure 13.31 Pyloric stenosis: US. Thickening and elongation of the pylorus (arrows), with failure of passage of fluid from the stomach (St).

13.6.3 Intussusception

Intussusception refers to prolapse or telescoping of a segment of bowel (referred to as the intussusceptum) into the lumen of more distal bowel (the intussuscepiens). The most common form of intussusception is ileocolic, i.e. prolapse of distal small bowel into the colon. Intussusception occurs most commonly in young children, usually from six months to two years of age, with a peak incidence at around nine months. At this age, intussusception is usually regarded as idiopathic, although enlarged lymph nodes secondary to viral infection are thought to be responsible in most cases. In older children, a lead point should be suspected. Causes of a lead point include Meckel diverticulum, mesenteric cyst and lymphoma. (Intussusception may also occur in adults with underlying causes including benign small bowel tumours such as lipoma, Meckel diverticulum and foreign body.) Signs and symptoms of intussusception include vomiting, blood-stained stool, colicky abdominal pain, listlessness and palpable abdominal mass. Imaging in suspected intussusception consists of an AXR followed by US.

13.6.3.1 AXR

Signs of intussusception on AXR (Fig. 13.32):
- 'Target' lesion in right upper quadrant due to swollen hepatic flexure seen end-on with layers

of peritoneal fat within and surrounding the intussusception
- Meniscus sign due to air outlining intussusceptum
- Relatively gasless right side of abdomen
- Small bowel obstruction
- Free air indicates intestinal perforation.

13.6.3.2 US

US of intussusception shows a multilayered mass that consists of hypoechoic and hyperechoic concentric rings due to layers of oedematous bowel wall and mesentery (Fig. 13.33). In older children or adults, US may occasionally show a lead point such as lymphoma or duplication cyst.

13.6.3.3 Reduction

Intussusception is a surgical emergency and early involvement of radiological and surgical teams is mandatory. Non-surgical treatment of intussusception, known as 'reduction', consists of pushing the intussusceptum back into its normal position. Reduction is most commonly performed under fluoroscopic screening using barium or gas introduced via an enema tube. Some centres use US-guided liquid reduction.

Gas reduction is now widely used and has several advantages:

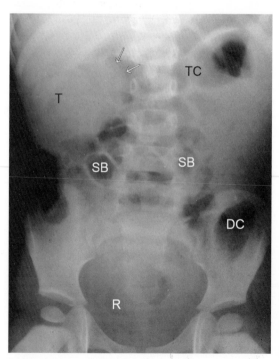

Figure 13.32 Intussusception. AXR shows normal rectum (R) and descending colon (DC) with a few moderately distended loops of small bowel (SB). A round soft tissue opacity (arrows) is seen projecting into the transverse colon (TC). This is the leading edge of the intussusception. Note also a target-shaped 'mass' (T) in the right upper abdomen due to multiple thickened layers of bowel seen 'end-on'.

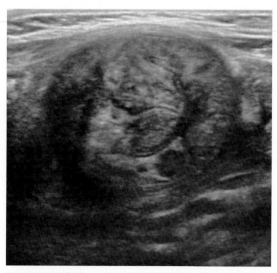

Figure 13.33 Intussusception: US. US shows a complex, target-like lesion.

- Relatively quick and clean
- Highly effective
- Low complication rate.

Contraindications to radiological reduction:

- Shock: the child must be adequately hydrated prior to attempting reduction
- Intestinal perforation, as indicated by clinical signs of peritonism and/or visualization of free air on AXR
- Duration of symptoms greater than 12 hours or small bowel obstruction make radiological reduction more difficult and decrease the likelihood of success, but are not of themselves absolute contraindications.

Recurrent intussusception occurs in 5–10 per cent of cases and should lead to repeat enema reduction. Surgery is indicated for multiple recurrences or suspected pathological lead point.

13.7 SKELETAL DISORDERS IN CHILDREN

13.7.1 Non-accidental injury

Non-accidental injury (NAI) refers to injury of a child due to the violent actions of another person. NAI is encountered most commonly in young children aged less than one year of age. Clinical presentation may include symptoms and signs of a specific skeletal injury or non-specific symptoms, such as apnoea, seizures or lethargy. Diagnosis relies on recognition of suspicious features including:

- Nature of injury not consistent with clinical history
  - May include brain injury, subdural haematoma, rib fractures and metaphyseal corner fractures
- Bruises or other evidence of injury to multiple body parts
- Burns
- Multiple fractures at different stages of healing
- Fractures at unusual sites, such as sternum or scapula.

Imaging findings are often crucial to the diagnosis of NAI. Radiographs of affected areas, plus skeletal survey (radiographs of the ribs, skull and long bones) are important in the diagnostic workup.

Patterns of skeletal injury suggestive of NAI (Fig. 13.34):

- Long bones
  - Periosteal new bone formation related to prior fractures
  - Metaphyseal or epiphyseal plate fractures
  - Spiral diaphyseal fractures
- Ribs
  - Posterior rib fractures
  - Up to 80 per cent of rib fractures are occult and may only become visible with healing
- Skull
  - Multiple/complex fractures
  - Depressed fractures, especially in the occipital bone
  - Wide fractures, i.e. >5 mm.

Soft tissue injuries may also occur in NAI, including hepatic, splenic and renal damage.

Brain injuries are common. Subdural haematomas in infants, unusual in accidental injury, are commonly associated with severe shaking of the child. Differential diagnosis of NAI includes accidental injury, birth-related trauma and conditions causing abnormally fragile bones, such as osteogenesis imperfecta.

13.7.2 Developmental dysplasia of the hip

Developmental dysplasia of the hip (DDH) occurs in 1–2 per 1000 births. Females are more commonly affected than males with a ratio of 8:1. Left hip is more commonly involved than the right. Previously known as congenital hip dislocation, the term DDH more accurately reflects the underlying disorder, which is dysplasia of the acetabulum. Dysplasia of the acetabulum may lead to varying degrees of hip joint subluxation, dislocation and dysfunction. Risk factors for the development of DDH include family history, breech presentation, neuromuscular disorders and foot deformities. Early diagnosis is essential to the prevention of long-term complications including worsening dysplasia, abnormal gait and premature osteoarthritis. Conservative measures, such as splinting for a few weeks, are usually successful in all but the most severe cases.

US is the investigation of choice for suspected DDH in infants (Fig. 13.35). US has a number of advantages including:

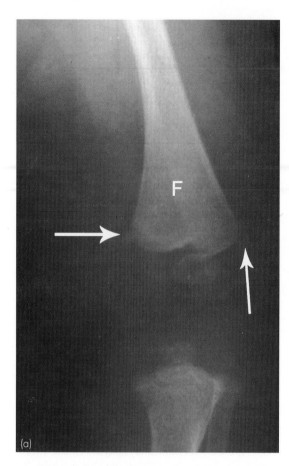

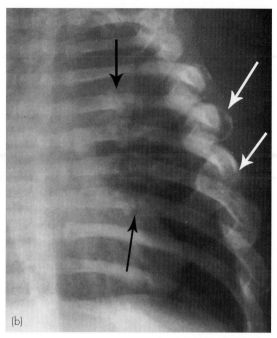

Figure 13.34 Non-accidental injury. (a) Radiograph of the femur (F) shows typical metaphyseal corner fractures (arrows). (b) CXR shows multiple posterior (black arrows) and lateral (white arrows) rib fractures.

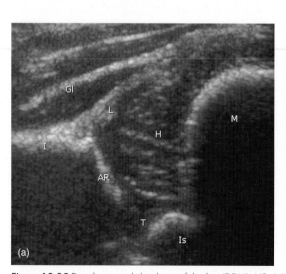

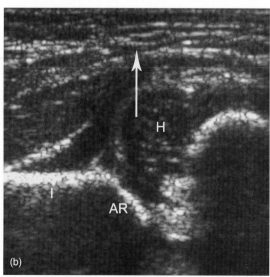

Figure 13.35 Developmental dysplasia of the hip (DDH): US. (a) Coronal US of a normal infant hip showing the following: lateral wall of the ileum (I), acetabular roof (AR), femoral head (H), femoral metaphysis (M), triradiate cartilage (T), ischium (Is), gluteal muscles (Gl). (b) Coronal US of DDH showing a shallow angle between the acetabular roof and ileum plus displacement of the femoral head out of the acetabulum (arrow).

- Lack of ionizing radiation
- Cartilage structures are well seen including femoral head, hyaline acetabular cartilage and fibrocartilagenous labrum
- Reproducible measurements of the angle of the acetabular roof and the position of the femoral head may be taken and used in follow-up examinations
- Dynamic real-time US is used to assess hip stability
- Position of the hip in a splint may be confirmed.

Radiography has limited accuracy in infants as most of the essential structures, such as the femoral head and acetabular rim, are composed of cartilage and cannot be seen. Radiographic assessment is used in children over nine months of age.

In severe cases, including those that do not respond to splinting, MRI or arthrogram may be indicated for further assessment of the internal structures of the hip joint, including the fibrocartilagenous labrum. Choice of modality usually reflects local availability and expertise.

The child with missed DDH usually presents with late walking or a limp. In cases of missed DDH, permanent acetabular dysplasia and delayed femoral head ossification may occur with long-term complications including limp, early and severe osteoarthritis, and tearing of the acetabular labrum.

13.7.3 Osteomyelitis

Osteomyelitis refers to infectious inflammation of bone. Osteomyelitis may occur at any age, though is more common in young children with over 50 per cent of cases occurring before the age of five. Common sites of involvement are the metaphyses of long bones, growth centres (metaphyseal equivalents) in the pelvis, mandible and spine. Osteomyelitis is usually due to haematogenous spread from respiratory or urinary tract infection. Less commonly, osteomyelitis may be due to direct penetration, especially of the calcaneus or distal toes. The most common organisms causing childhood osteomyelitis are *Staphylococcus aureus*, *β-haemolytic streptococcus* and *Streptococcus pneumoniae*. (In adults, osteomyelitis may occur from a number of causes including compound fractures, adjacent soft tissue infection, diabetes and intravenous drug use.) Clinical presentation of osteomyelitis in children

is variable, although usually consists of pain, local tenderness and fever. In younger children, symptoms may be less specific, e.g. development of a limp, unwillingness to use affected limb, lethargy and poor feeding in neonates.

13.7.3.1 Radiography

Radiographs are usually the first investigation performed, though are often normal at the time of initial presentation. Radiographic signs of osteomyelitis usually develop over a few days and include:
- Soft tissue swelling
- Bony lucency that progresses to frank destruction
- Subperiosteal new bone formation, usually visible after symptoms present for 7–10 days.

Brodie abscess is a type of chronic circumscribed osteomyelitis, most common in the lower extremity, and seen radiographically as a focal lucency with marginal sclerosis.

13.7.3.2 MRI

MRI is the investigation of choice where osteomyelitis is suspected clinically and radiographs are normal or equivocal (Fig. 13.36). Advantages of MRI for the investigation of suspected osteomyelitis in children:
- MRI is usually positive at the time of presentation
- Whole body STIR images are often included for two reasons:
  - Localization of symptoms is often difficult in children
  - Osteomyelitis may occasionally be multifocal
- MRI is usually able to differentiate conditions such as Ewing sarcoma or Langerhans cell histiocytosis, which may mimic osteomyelitis clinically or radiographically.

Bone scintigraphy with ^{99}mTc-MDP will be positive within 24–72 hours of infection and is used where MRI is unavailable. Depending on local expertise, US may also be used.

13.7.4 Septic arthritis of the hip

Septic arthritis of the hip most commonly presents before the age of three, and is usually due to

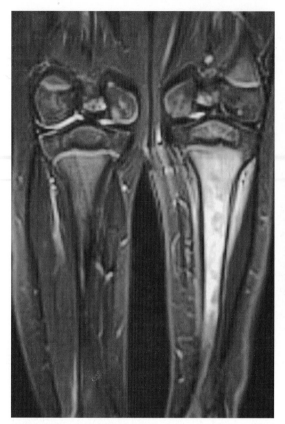

Figure 13.36 Osteomyelitis: MRI. Limp and fever in a two-year-old male. Coronal STIR image of the legs shows extensive high signal in the marrow cavity of the left tibia. Oedema is also seen in adjacent soft tissue with no evidence of a soft tissue mass.

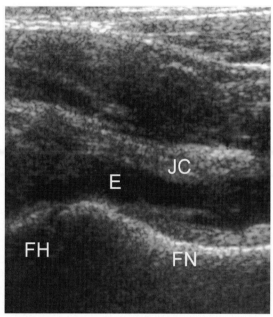

Figure 13.37 Hip joint effusion: US. US image obtained with the probe parallel to the femoral neck (FN) with the round surface of the femoral head (FH) seen medially. The effusion is seen as anechoic fluid (E) elevating the joint capsule (JC).

Transient synovitis usually settles with bed rest, and imaging usually is not required. Radiographs, if performed, are usually normal. If imaging is required, US is the investigation of choice to diagnose a joint effusion.

haematogenous spread from respiratory or urinary tract infection. Radiographs are insensitive and early scintigraphy may be negative.

US is the investigation of choice to diagnose the presence of a hip joint effusion (Fig. 13.37). Diagnostic aspiration of the hip joint may be performed safely under US control.

13.7.5 Transient synovitis (irritable hip)

Transient synovitis is a benign, self-limiting hip disorder. Peak age of incidence is four to ten years, with males more commonly affected than females. Clinical presentation usually suggests the diagnosis of transient synovitis and consists of a limp that develops rapidly over 1–2 days, often following a history of a recent viral illness and mild fever.

13.7.6 Perthes disease

Perthes disease refers to avascular necrosis of the proximal femoral epiphysis. Perthes disease has a peak age of incidence of four to seven years; 10 per cent of cases are bilateral. Radiography of the hips is the initial investigation of choice.

Early radiographic signs of Perthes disease:
- Reduced size and sclerosis of the femoral epiphysis with joint space widening
- Subchondral fracture producing a linear lucency deep to the articular surface of the femoral head.

Radiographs may be normal at the time of initial presentation. In such cases, bone scintigraphy with ^{99}mTc-MDP or contrast-enhanced MRI may show signs of ischaemia of the femoral head prior to development of visible irregularity or collapse.

Radiographic signs later in the course of Perthes disease (Fig. 13.38):

- Delayed maturation and fragmentation of the femoral head with cyst formation in the femoral neck
- Flattening of the femoral head (coxa plana)
- Widening of the femoral neck (coxa magna).

13.7.7 Slipped capital femoral epiphysis

Slipped capital femoral epiphysis (SCFE) refers to posteromedial slip of the capital femoral epiphysis, producing acute onset of hip or groin pain and a limp. SCFE occurs most commonly in adolescent males; 20 per cent of cases are bilateral. Associations of SCFE include obesity and avascular necrosis of the femoral head. Radiographic signs of SCFE are best appreciated on a lateral projection, where the slip of the femoral head is well seen.

Signs on the AP film may be more difficult to appreciate and include:

- Widening and irregularity of the femoral growth plate
- Reduced height of the epiphysis (Fig. 13.39).

13.7.8 Langerhans cell histiocytosis

Langerhans cell histiocytosis (LCH) describes a spectrum of disorders, the common feature being

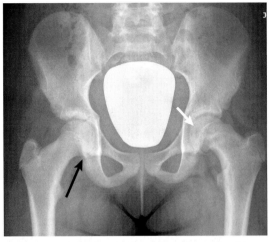

Figure 13.39 Slipped capital femoral epiphysis. Slip of the left capital femoral epiphysis (white arrow). Note the normal metaphyseal overlay sign on the right side producing a white triangle where the lower corner of the femoral metaphysis overlays the acetabulum (black arrow). This appearance is lost on the left due to the metaphysis being pushed laterally.

histiocytic infiltration of tissues and aggressive bone lesions. LCH may be subclassified as restricted or extensive LDH. Extensive LDH refers to visceral organ involvement with or without bone lesions. Visceral involvement may produce organ dysfunction and failure. Skin rash and diabetes insipidus are common. Restricted LCH refers to monostotic bone

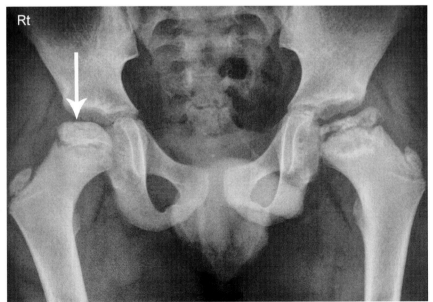

Figure 13.38 Perthes disease. Advanced changes of Perthes disease on the left with flattening, irregularity and sclerosis of the femoral epiphysis, widening of the metaphysis, and widening of the hip joint. There are much more subtle early changes on the right with slight irregularity and flattening of the femoral head (arrow).

or polyostotic bone lesions, or isolated skin lesions. The monostotic bone lesion of LCH occurs in children with a peak age of incidence of five to ten years, though may also be seen in older patients. Clinical presentation may be with local pain or pathological fracture (see Fig. 8.9). Radiographically, LCH produces focal well-defined lytic skeletal lesions in the skull, spine and long bones.

SUMMARY BOX

Clinical presentation	Investigation of choice	Comment
Neonatal respiratory distress	CXR	
Pulmonary infection	CXR	
Cystic fibrosis	CXR	
Abdominal mass	US for initial assessment CT/MRI for further characterization and staging	
Urinary tract infection	US	MAG3 scintigraphy for suspected obstruction MCU ± DMSA in selected cases
Hydronephrosis	US MAG3 scintigraphy	
Neonatal gut obstruction/bile-stained vomiting	AXR	Contrast studies in selected cases, e.g. suspected malrotation or Hirschsprung disease
Oesophageal atresia and tracheo-oesophageal fistula	CXR and AXR	
Hypertrophic pyloric stenosis	US	
Intussusception	AXR and US	Imaging-guided reduction unless contraindicated
Non-accidental injury	Radiography (skeletal survey)	
Developmental dysplasia of the hip	US	Radiography in older children (>6–9 months)
Osteomyelitis	MRI	Radiography at time of presentation often negative
Acutely painful hip (suspected septic arthritis or transient synovitis)	US	
Perthes disease	Radiography	Bone scintigraphy or MRI if radiography negative
Slipped capital femoral epiphysis	Radiography	
Langerhans cell histiocytosis	Radiography	CT/MRI in complex areas, e.g. temporal bone

MCU, micturating cystourethrogram.

14 Imaging in oncology

Imaging of patients with cancer is a highly complex field that includes virtually all subspecialties and imaging modalities. Many of the imaging techniques relevant to oncology have been outlined in other chapters. This chapter provides a summary and overview of imaging in oncology. Roles of imaging in oncology include:

- Establishing the primary diagnosis of cancer as a cause of presenting symptoms
- Screening for cancer in asymptomatic individuals, e.g. screening mammography
- Screening for cancer in patients with known cancer predisposition syndromes (e.g. von Hippel–Lindau or Beckwith–Weidemann syndrome), genetic mutations (e.g. *BRCA1/2* gene mutations) or exposure to known risk factors (e.g. asbestos, tobacco)
- Staging of known malignancy
- Assessment of response to therapy
- Diagnosis of complications of therapy
- Guidance of interventional procedures: interventional oncology.

Investigation of clinical symptoms and screening for cancer have been covered in other chapters. This chapter will outline the basic principles behind staging of malignancy, assessment of response to therapy, diagnosis of complications of therapy and interventional oncology.

14.1 STAGING OF KNOWN MALIGNANCY

Tumours are classified according to organ of origin and histological type. Cancer staging describes a process whereby patients with a specific type of tumour are categorized, depending on tumour extent, into groups. Patients are generally categorized into four stages, although for many tumours some stages have subcategories. With continuing improvements in treatment regimes in oncology, accurate staging of cancer is increasingly important. Purposes of cancer staging include:

- Definition of the anatomical extent of tumour
- Selection of appropriate therapy
- Estimation of prognosis
- Provision of a pretreatment baseline to allow monitoring of effects of therapy.

CT is the most commonly used modality for tumour staging (Figs 14.1 and 14.2). MRI has an increasing role, especially in children. FDG-PET has improved the accuracy of staging in certain tumours. Other modalities may be used for specific instances, e.g. MRI for rectal cancer, radionuclide bone scan for suspected skeletal metastases, US-

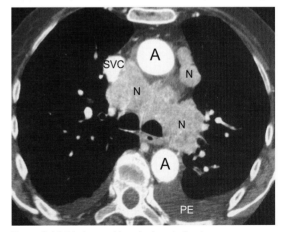

Figure 14.1 Mediastinal lymphadenopathy due to bronchogenic carcinoma: CT. Note enlarged mediastinal lymph nodes (N), superior vena cava (SVC), aorta (A), pleural effusions (PE).

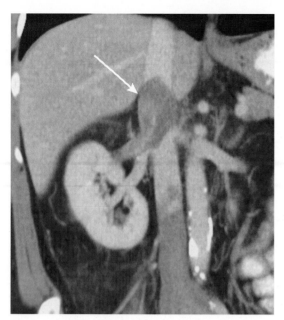

Figure 14.2 Renal cell carcinoma with invasion of the inferior vena cava (IVC): CT. Renal cell carcinoma upper pole right kidney (not shown). Coronal CT shows abnormal soft tissue extending superiorly in the IVC (arrow).

guided FNA for suspected lymph node metastases from head and neck cancer.

Cancer staging is an increasingly complex process, based on numerous factors including anatomical extent of tumour and other prognostic factors.

Various prognostic factors are described for individual tumours. Prognostic factors include:

- Tumour marker serum levels, e.g. prostate-specific antigen (PSA) in prostate cancer
- Histological grade, e.g. Gleason score in prostate cancer
- Specific locoregional features, e.g. extramural venous invasion in colorectal cancer
- Other clinical features, e.g. ascites in hepatocellular carcinoma
- Genetic factors, e.g. vascular endothelial growth factor (VEGF) expression in colorectal cancer.

For some tumours, especially lymphomas, histological classification and prognostic factors are more important than anatomical extent in planning therapy. With the exception of lymphomas and brain tumours, anatomical extent of most solid tumours is categorized according to the TNM system. The TNM system is published and updated by the American Joint Committee on Cancer (AJCC) and the International Union Against Cancer (UICC). Under the TNM classification system, features of local tumour growth plus pattern of tumour metastasis are categorized as follows:

- 'T' = primary tumour and local extent
- 'N' = regional lymph nodes
- 'M' = distant metastases.

The TNM staging system is individualized for each type of tumour. Different types of tumour will have varying prognostic factors, such as mode of growth within organ of origin, tendency to invade adjacent structures, and pattern of metastatic spread. The TNM system should reflect these prognostic factors and therefore assist in directing treatment decisions. As an example of how cancer staging incorporates the TNM system let us consider adenocarcinoma of the prostate.

14.1.1 Staging of adenocarcinoma of the prostate

Most prostate cancers are adenocarcinomas. Tumours grow initially within the prostate. With continued growth tumour may invade through the prostate capsule into surrounding fat planes. Tumour may then invade local structures including seminal vesicles and bladder base. All of these factors are expressed in the 'T' component of TNM staging for prostate cancer. The 'N' component categorizes spread to regional lymph nodes in the pelvis, including the internal iliac and obturator groups. Metastatic spread to distant sites including skeleton and non-regional lymph nodes, and less commonly to liver or lungs is expressed in the 'M' component. The TNM staging system for prostate cancer therefore reflects the typical behaviour of the tumour and is summarized in Table 14.1.

Based on anatomical extent as described by the TNM system plus other relevant prognostic factors, patients with prostate cancer are grouped into staging categories as shown in Table 14.2.

Based on these groupings treatment options may be summarized as follows:

- Stage I or II: offered curative therapy with surgery (radical prostatectomy) or radiotherapy
- Stage III: radiotherapy
- Stage IV: hormonal therapy.

Table 14.1 TNM staging of prostate cancer.

Category	Subcategory	Clinical feature
TX		Primary tumour cannot be assessed
T0		No evidence of primary tumour
T1		Tumour not clinically apparent or visible on imaging
	T1a	Incidental histological finding in <5% tissue
	T1b	Incidental histological finding in >5% tissue
	T1c	Tumour found on needle biopsy, e.g. prostate-specific antigen elevation
T2		Tumour confined within prostate
	T2a	Involves 50% of one lobe or less
	T2b	Involves more than 50% of one lobe
	T2c	Involves both lobes
T3		Extension through prostate capsule
	T3a	Extracapsular extension
	T3b	Seminal vesicle invasion
T4		Fixed tumour or invasion of other structures, e.g. rectum, bladder
NX		Regional lymph nodes not assessed
N0		No regional lymph node metastsis
N1		Metastasis in regional lymph node(s)
M0		No distant metastasis
M1		Distant metastasis
	M1a	Non-regional lymph node(s)
	M1b	Bone(s)
	M1c	Other sites(s) ± bone

It can be seen from the above that in the absence of lymph node involvement or distant metastasis, the absence or presence of prostate capsule invasion is a major determinant as to whether the patient is offered curative or non-curative therapy.

CT is unable to visualize stage T1 and T2 carcinomas. CT is not sensitive enough to diagnose subtle extracapsular extension, i.e. CT cannot differentiate T1–2 from T3a. More obvious locally invasive disease (T3b) is usually seen with CT including invasion of seminal vesicles and other structures. CT is also accurate for the diagnosis of pelvic and abdominal lymphadenopathy. MRI is the imaging investigation of choice for local staging of prostate carcinoma. Extracapsular

extension of tumour is shown accurately with MRI (Fig. 14.3).

The commonest approach to staging of prostate carcinoma is to first perform a scintigraphic bone scan to exclude bone metastases, plus CT of the abdomen and pelvis. If no bony or lymph node metastases are diagnosed, and if the CT shows no evidence of obvious locally invasive disease, MRI may be performed to exclude focal extracapsular extension.

The above principles can be applied to other tumours. Imaging regimes are tailored to demonstrate features relevant to the TNM staging of individual tumours. These regimes are summarized in the relevant chapters throughout this book.

Table 14.2 Prognostic grouping of prostate cancer.

Group	T	N	M	PSA	Gleason
I	T1a–c	N0	M0	<10	≤6
	T2a	N0	M0	<10	≤6
	T1-2a	N0	M0	X	X
IIA	T1a–c	N0	M0	<20	7
	T1a–c	N0	M0	≥10<20	≤6
	T2a	N0	M0	≥10<20	≤6
	T2a	N0	M0	<20	7
	T2b	N0	M0	<20	≤7
	T2b	N0	M0	X	X
IIB	T2c	N0	M0	Any	Any
	T1–2	N0	M0	≥20	Any
	T1–2	N0	M0	Any	≥8
III	T3a–b	N0	N0	Any	Any
IV	T4	N0	M0	Any	Any
	Any	N1	M0	Any	Any
	Any	Any N	M1	Any	Any

PSA, prostate-specific antigen.

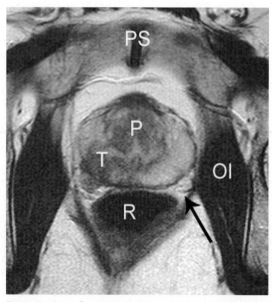

Figure 14.3 Locally invasive prostate carcinoma: MRI. Transverse T2-weighted MRI shows a prostatic carcinoma as a low signal tumour (T) in the posterior right peripheral zone of the prostate (P). Tumour tissue is extending through the prostate capsule and invading the right neurovascular bundle. By comparison, the normal left neurovascular bundle is well seen (arrow). Note also the pubic symphysis (PS) and obturator internus muscle (OI).

14.2 ASSESSMENT OF RESPONSE TO THERAPY

Assessment of response to therapy is an essential part of patient management in oncology. Depending on response, therapy may be continued, discontinued or modified. Two assessment guidelines have been used to evaluate tumour response to therapy: WHO (World Health Organization) and RECIST (Response Evaluation Criteria in Solid Tumours).

The modified RECIST criteria (RECIST 1.1) are widely accepted in clinical practice, and used in clinical trials. RECIST criteria use cross-sectional measurements of up to five target lesions, such as liver metastases or enlarged lymph nodes. Measurements may be obtained by CT or MRI. Response according to RECIST criteria may be classified as follows:

- Complete response (CR): disappearance of all lesions; remaining lymph nodes <10 mm short axis
- Partial response (PR): at least 30 per cent reduction in summated diameters of target lesions

- Progressive disease (PD): at least 20 per cent increase in summated diameters or any new lesion
- Stable disease: neither PR nor PD.

The major limitation of the RECIST criteria is that only anatomical size response is measured. Response criteria not measured by RECIST include:
- Tumour necrosis, which may occur without change in tumour size
- Metabolic activity.

FDG-PET may be used to assess metabolic response in certain malignancies (Fig. 14.4). Positron emission tomography–CT (PET–CT) combines functional and anatomical information. PET–CT is now the standard investigation for staging and response measurement in many malignancies including the lymphomas. Reduced tracer uptake on serial PET–CT scans correlates with reduced tumour activity and tumour cell death. In some malignancies, PET–CT may be used after the first or second cycle of therapy, allowing earlier modification of therapy as required.

As research progresses, other types of functional imaging, such as diffusion-weighted MR will be accepted for clinical use in certain instances, and may be incorporated into future RECIST criteria modifications.

14.3 DIAGNOSIS OF COMPLICATIONS OF THERAPY

Therapies used in oncology include surgery, chemotherapy, radiotherapy and haematopoietic stem cell transplant (HSCT). Newer therapies include monoclonal antibodies and tyrosine kinase inhibitors. Each of these therapies is associated with acute and chronic complications.

Examples of particular problems associated with oncology therapies include:
- Immunosuppression causing increased susceptibility to infection, including opportunistic infections (Fig. 14.5)

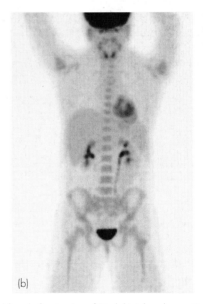

(a)   (b)

Figure 14.4 Hodgkin's lymphoma: FDG-PET. (a) FDG-PET in a 15-year-old female for staging of Hodgkin's lymphoma. Scan shows multiple areas of abnormal activity in the chest and neck indicating neoplastic lymphadenopathy. Note normal uptake related to the brain (B), heart (H), kidneys (K) and urinary bladder (U). (b) Follow-up FDG-PET after chemotherapy shows resolution of abnormal activity indicating complete metabolic response. Note normal uptake related to brain, salivary and thyroid glands, and urinary tract.

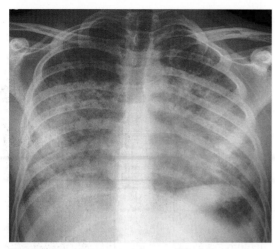

Figure 14.5 Pneumocystis pneumonia: CXR. Dry cough and shortness of breath in an immunosuppressed 15-year-old female following bone marrow transplant. Note extensive bilateral alveolar opacification.

- Fungal, e.g. aspergillosis
- TB
- *Pneumocystis jiroveci* pneumonia (PCP)
- Long-term intravenous lines may be complicated by infection or thrombosis
- Acute and chronic graft-versus-host disease (GVHD) following HSCT
  - Immune-mediated disease in which transplanted cells attack host cells with particular involvement of skin, liver, intestine and lung
- Neutropenic enterocolitis
- Radiotherapy effects
  - Radiation pneumonitis
  - Cerebral white matter disease
- Cardiac toxicity
  - Some forms of chemotherapy may cause reduced left ventricular function.

Imaging is often required to diagnose complications of therapy and to differentiate these from tumour progression or recurrence.

Examples include:
- Differentiation of radiotherapy change in the brain from progressive tumour
- Differentiation of opportunistic fungal infection of the lungs from pulmonary metastases.

Choice of imaging modality is dictated by the presenting symptom, for example:
- CXR and chest CT for respiratory symptoms
- AXR and abdomen CT for gastrointestinal symptoms
- MRI of the brain for central nervous system symptoms.

14.4 INTERVENTIONAL ONCOLOGY

Interventional radiology is used in oncology in a wide variety of roles including:
- Biopsy guidance for primary diagnosis
- Drainage of malignant ascites and pleural effusion
- Drainage and stent deployment for malignant obstruction of various structures, for example
  - Percutaneous nephrostomy and antegrade ureteric stent for malignant obstruction of the urinary tract
  - Percutaneous transhepatic cholangiogram and biliary stent for malignant biliary stricture (Fig. 14.6)
  - Superior vena cava stent for obstruction due to mediastinal tumour
  - Tracheobronchial stent for malignant airway obstruction
- Insertion of gastrostomy or gastrojejunostomy for nutritional support
- Central venous access for delivery of chemotherapy or parenteral nutrition, and repeated aspiration of blood samples
  - Peripherally inserted central catheter ('PICC line')
  - Central venous port
  - Tunnelled central venous catheter
- Arterial embolization
  - Bronchial artery embolization for massive haemoptysis due to bronchogenic carcinoma
  - Renal artery embolization for palliation of pain or haemoptysis due to inoperable renal cell carcinoma
  - Reduce bleeding risk of hypervascular tumours prior to surgical removal, e.g. renal cell carcinoma, melanoma
- Non-surgical treatments that use interventional radiology, examples of which are summarized below.

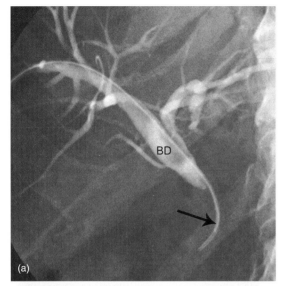

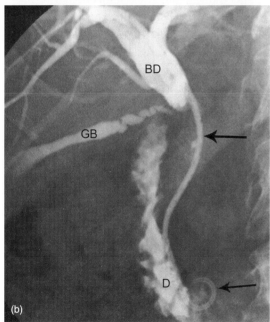

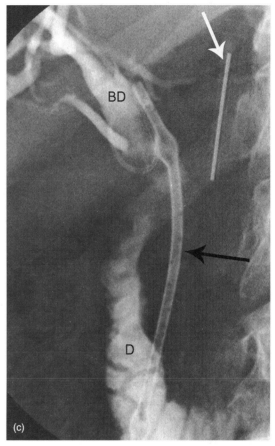

Figure 14.6 Biliary stent insertion. (a) Percutaneous transhepatic cholangiography shows obstruction of proximal bile ducts (BD) due to cholangiocarcinoma. A wire (arrow) is being passed through the obstruction. (b) A drainage catheter (arrows) has been passed over the wire into the duodenum (D). Note also the gallbladder (GB) now outlined by contrast material. (c) A biliary stent (black arrow) is placed with its ends on either side of the biliary tumour. A radiographic marker (white arrow) assists with precise positioning of the stent.

14.4.1 Percutaneous tumour ablation

Percutaneous tumour ablation may be used to treat tumours of the liver, kidney, breast, bone or lung. US, CT or MRI may be used for procedure guidance. A variety of ablation techniques is available under three broad categories:

- Injection of substances that cause cell death, such as ethanol or heated saline
- Heating
  - Radiofrequency ablation
  - Interstitial laser therapy
  - Microwave coagulation
  - High intensity focused ultrasound (HIFU)
- Freezing: cryotherapy.

Choice of technique is usually based on a number of factors including:

- Tumour type
- Anatomy of tumour, e.g. organ involved, depth from skin, proximity to adjacent structures
- Local expertise and availability of equipment.

14.4.2 Transarterial chemoembolization

Transarterial chemoembolization (TACE) is used for treatment of inoperable hepatocellular carcinoma (HCC). TACE involves the following:

- Catheter angiography of the liver to outline arterial anatomy and tumour blood supply
- Selective placement of arterial catheters into hepatic artery branches feeding the tumour
- Injection of a chemotherapeutic agent in an emulsion with iodized oil
- Injection of an arterial embolizing agent.

A modification of TACE uses drug eluting beads (DEB-TACE). Drug-eluting beads are microspheres of polyvinyl alcohol and a hydrophilic monomer loaded with doxorubicin, a chemotherapeutic agent. The microspheres lodge in the tumour and gradually release the doxorubicin.

Regardless of precise technique, TACE induces tumour necrosis through a combination of blockage of blood supply and localized delivery of a chemotherapeutic agent.

14.4.3 Selective internal radiation therapy

Selective internal radiation therapy (SIRT) is used for treatment of inoperable HCC and hepatic metastases from colorectal carcinoma. SIRT involves the following:

- High quality catheter angiography of the liver to outline arterial anatomy and tumour blood supply
- Superselective microcatheter placement into hepatic artery branches supplying tumour
- Injection of resin (or glass) microspheres loaded with a radioisotope, ^{90}yttrium
- ^{90}yttrium emits beta particle radiation
- SIRT induces tumour necrosis through a combination of blockage of blood supply and local delivery of radiotherapy (brachytherapy).

Index

Note: page numbers in **bold** refer to figures, page numbers in italics refer to information contained in tables.